Advances in
PARASITOLOGY

VOLUME 50

Advances in PARASITOLOGY

Edited by

J.R. BAKER

Royal Society of Tropical Medicine and Hygiene, London, England

R. MULLER

London School of Hygiene and Tropical Medicine, London, England

and

D. ROLLINSON

The Natural History Museum, London, England

VOLUME 50

ACADEMIC PRESS

A Division of Harcourt, Inc.

San Diego San Francisco New York
Boston London Sydney Tokyo

This book is printed on acid-free paper.

Academic Press
A division of Harcourt Inc.
Harcourt Place, 32 Jamestown Road, London NW1 7BY, UK
http://www.academicpress.com

Academic Press
A division of Harcourt Inc.
525 B Street, Suite 1900, San Diego, California 92101-4495, USA
http://www.academicpress.com

ISBN 0-12-031750-8
doi:10.1006/apar.v050

A catalogue record for this book is available from the British Library

Typeset by Charon Tec Pvt. Ltd, Chennai, India
Printed in Great Britain by MPG Books Ltd, Bodmin, Cornwall

01 02 03 04 05 06 MP 9 8 7 6 5 4 3 2 1

CONTRIBUTORS TO VOLUME 50

S.W. Attwood, *Wolfson Wellcome Biomedical Laboratories, Department of Zoology, The Natural History Museum, London, SW7 5BD, UK*

P.R. Boag, *Victorian Institute of Animal Science, Attwood, Victoria 3049; Department of Veterinary Science, The University of Melbourne, Werribee, Victoria 3030, Australia*

B.M. Cooke, *Department of Microbiology, P.O. Box 53, Monash University, Victoria 3800, Australia*

R.L. Coppel, *Department of Microbiology, P.O. Box 53, Monash University, Victoria 3800, Australia*

R.B. Gasser, *Department of Veterinary Science, The University of Melbourne, Werribee, Victoria 3030, Australia*

N. Mohandas, *Division of Life Sciences, Lawrence Berkeley Laboratories, Berkeley, California, USA*

S.E. Newton, *Victorian Institute of Animal Science, Attwood, Victoria 3049, Australia*

S. Tagboto, *Tropical Parasitic Diseases Unit, Northwick Park Institute for Medical Research, Harrow, Middlesex, HA1 3UJ, UK*

S. Townson, *Tropical Parasitic Diseases Unit, Northwick Park Institute for Medical Research, Harrow, Middlesex, HA1 3UJ, UK*

PREFACE

This, the 50th volume in the series, opens with an account by Brian Cooke, Narla Mohandas and Ross Coppel, from Monash University in Australia and the Lawrence Berkeley Laboratories in California, USA, of the molecular changes occurring in red blood cells that are infected with malaria parasites (*Plasmodium falciparum*). The infected cells develop new intracytoplasmic structures, and new proteins, derived from the parasites, appear on the red blood cell surface. These events increase the rigidity and adhesiveness of the cell membrane, and result in changes in the red blood cell's morphology and in its rheological properties. These changes, in turn, are of profound pathological significance since they are involved in the well-known phenomena of capillary blockage, cytoadherence and rosetting. The authors point out that study of these changes has not only led to increased understanding of the relationship between structure and function in the normal red blood cell but may also lead to a novel chemotherapeutic approach aimed at reducing parasite virulence.

Stephen Attwood from the Natural History Museum in London, UK, provides an authoritative account of progress made in the study of schistosomiasis in the Mekong region. The review provides a valuable update of activities following the comprehensive volume *The Mekong Schistosome* by Bruce *et al.*, 1980. Major emphasis is given to research relating to the origin and subsequent dispersal of *Schistosoma mekongi* and related taxa and a thorough account is given of the role and relationships of the intermediate snail hosts. The current status of schistosomiasis control in Laos and Cambodia is reviewed and consideration is given to the most effective approaches for future control. Zoogeography of the Southeast Asian region continues to be a perplexing issue. In this article, past ideas concerning the phylogeography of *Schistosoma* are examined and a new phylogeographic model is proposed. It is clear that the application of new molecular techniques and analytical methods are providing new insights into the past and present relationships of Asian schistosomes and their snail hosts and it seems likely that new discoveries will be forthcoming.

Studies on parasite reproduction and sexual development are recognized as being of importance and they may identify possible targets for control. For example, in the case of schistosomiasis it is well recognised that the eggs of the parasite as opposed to the adult worms are primarily responsible for pathology and related disease symptoms, and vaccines that reduce egg production are being investigated. Peter Boag, Susan Newton and Robin Gasser from the Victorian Institute of Animal Science and the University of Melbourne in Victoria, Australia provide a fascinating account of recent studies concerning the molecular aspects of sexual development in nematodes and schistosomes. Taking as their starting point relevant information on the well-studied free-living nematode *Caenorhabditis elegans* they go on to examine studies of gender-specific gene expression in free-living and parasitic nematodes and review the remarkable situation with the dioecious schistosomes. New techniques for investigating molecular reproductive processes and analysing gender-specific genes are described, including expression profiling, RNA-mediated interference and gene transformation. Rapid progress is likely in the years to come and this will surely be a most rewarding area for future research.

Finally, Senyo Tagboto and Simon Townson, at the Northwick Park Institute for Medical Research, UK, have undertaken the daunting task of reviewing, evaluating and tabulating the extensive but diffused literature on the therapeutic activity of plant extracts and other natural products against all the protozoans and helminths of medical and veterinary importance. They have gone to a great deal of trouble to verify the species of plants involved. Two recent notable advances in the use of natural products as antiparasitic agents include artemisin derivatives (from *Artemisia*) for malaria, and ivermectin (from *Streptomyces*) for onchocerciasis, and there is a new initiative led by the World Health Organization to investigate more such products, since there is now the opportunity of scientifically testing some traditional remedies in validated antiparasitic and toxicity screens. The authors outline the possibilities and difficulties involved in testing extracts of natural origin.

J. Baker
R. Muller
D. Rollinson

CONTENTS

Molecular Aspects of Sexual Development and Reproduction in Nematodes and Schistosomes

P.R. Boag, S.E. Newton and R.B. Gasser

Antiparasitic Properties of Medicinal Plants and Other Naturally Occurring Products

S. Tagboto and S. Townson

The Malaria-Infected Red Blood Cell: Structural and Functional Changes

Brian M. Cooke[1], Narla Mohandas[2] and Ross L. Coppel[1]

[1]*Department of Microbiology, P.O. Box 53, Monash University, Victoria 3800, Australia;*
[2]*Division of Life Sciences, Lawrence Berkeley Laboratories, Berkeley, California, USA*

ABSTRACT

The asexual stage of malaria parasites of the genus *Plasmodium* invade red blood cells of various species including humans. After parasite invasion, red blood cells progressively acquire a new set of properties and are converted into more typical, although still simpler, eukaryotic cells by the appearance of new structures in the red blood cell cytoplasm, and new proteins at the red blood cell membrane skeleton. The red blood cell undergoes striking morphological

ADVANCES IN PARASITOLOGY VOL 50
0065–308X $30.00

alterations and its rheological properties are considerably altered, manifesting as red blood cells with increased membrane rigidity, reduced deformability and increased adhesiveness for a number of other cells including the vascular endothelium. Elucidation of the structural changes in the red blood cell induced by parasite invasion and maturation and an understanding of the accompanying functional alterations have the ability to considerably extend our knowledge of structure–function relationships in the normal red blood cell. Furthermore, interference with these interactions may lead to previously unsuspected means of reducing parasite virulence and may lead to the development of novel antimalarial therapeutics.

ABBREVIATIONS

AARP	asparagine- and aspartate-rich protein
Ag332	antigen 332
ATP	adenosine triphosphate
ATS	acidic terminal segment
BgpA	blood group A antigen
BiP	binding protein
bp	base pairs
bporf	break point open reading frame
C32 Melanoma	C32 amelanotic melanoma cell line
CD	cluster determinant
CIDR	cysteine-rich interdomain region
CLAG	cytoadherence-linked asexual gene
CR1	complement receptor 1
CRA	circumsporozoite protein-related antigen
CRM	cysteine-rich motif
CSA	chondroitin sulphate A
CSP	circumsporozoite protein
DBL	Duffy binding ligand
DNA	deoxyribonucleic acid
ER	endoplasmic reticulum
Exp-1	exported protein-1
FEST	falciparum exported serine–threonine kinase
FIRA	falciparum interspersed repeat antigen
GAG	glycosaminoglycan
GARP	glutamic acid-rich protein
GBP	glycophorin-binding protein
Glu	glutamic acid
GPC	glycophorin C
GTP	guanosine triphosphate
HA	hyaluronic acid
HbA	haemoglobin A
HbAA	haemoglobin AA
HbAS	haemoglobin AS
HbS	haemoglobin S

HbSS	haemoglobin SS
HLA	human leucocyte antigen
HRP	histidine-rich protein
HS	heparan sulphate
HS-like GAG	heparan sulphate-like glycosaminoglycan
HUVEC	human umbilical vein endothelial cells
IC_{50}	50% inhibitory concentration
ICAM-1	intercellular adhesion molecule 1
IFN-γ	interferon gamma
IgM	immunoglobulin M
IOV	inside-out vesicle
IP	iodinatable protein
KAHRP	knob-associated histidine-rich protein
kb	kilobase-pairs
K_d	dissociation constant
kDa	kilodalton
KP	knob protein
MDa	megadalton
MESA	mature-parasite-infected erythrocyte surface antigen
mRNA	messenger ribonucleic acid
MSP	merozoite surface protein
MW	molecular weight (mass)
orf	open reading frame
PCR	polymerase chain reaction
PECAM-1	platelet–endothelial cell adhesion molecule 1
PfAARP1	*Plasmodium falciparum* asparagine- and aspartate-rich protein-1
PfEMP	*Plasmodium falciparum* erythrocyte membrane protein
PfERC	*Plasmodium falciparum* endoplasmic reticulum-located calcium-binding protein
PfHRP	*Plasmodium falciparum* histidine-rich protein
Pfsbp1	*Plasmodium falciparum* skeleton binding protein 1
PRBC	parasitized red blood cell
RAP-1	rhoptry-associated protein-1
RESA	ring-infected erythrocyte surface antigen
rif	repetitive interspersed family
RSP	ring surface protein
SDS	sodium dodecyl sulphate
SHARP	small histidine- and alanine-rich protein
SSRBC	homozygous sickle red blood cell
stevor	sub-telomeric variable open reading frame
TM	thrombomodulin
TD	transmembrane domain
TR	transferrin receptor
TRAP	thrombospondin-related anonymous protein
TSP	thrombospondin
var	variant
VARC and VAR_{CD}	equivalent terms for the cytoplasmic domain of PfEMP1
VCAM-1	vascular cell adhesion molecule 1
ves	variant erythrocyte surface
VESA	variant erythrocyte surface antigen

1. INTRODUCTION

Malaria caused by protozoa of the genus *Plasmodium*, particularly *P. falciparum*, is the most serious and widespread parasitic disease of humans. Each year, several hundred million people become infected with malaria parasites and 2–3 million (predominantly young children) die as a result of the infection. The signs and symptoms of malaria are manifested during the part of the infection in which the asexual stage parasites invade red blood cells. This process is still not well understood but involves an ordered multi-step process, which ends with the parasite residing inside the red blood cell within a membrane-lined vacuole in the red blood cell cytoplasm, called the parasitophorous vacuole. The parasites mature and undergo nuclear division, over a period of time varying between 24 and 72 hours, depending on the species of parasite. The earliest intracellular form is called the ring stage because of its signet ring-like appearance when viewed on Giemsa-stained blood films. Subsequently, the parasite matures into the pigmented trophozoite stage and then to a multinucleate form known as a schizont (or meront or segmenter), which divides to produce a number of merozoites. Finally, at the time of red blood cell rupture, the merozoites are released and, in turn, can reinvade other red blood cells to continue the cycle.

The red blood cell has traditionally been viewed as a passive container that shields the parasite from host effector mechanisms such as antibody. We now recognize that, during the maturation of the intracellular parasite, a series of dramatic and extensive changes occurs in the structural and functional properties of the infected red blood cells. These changes have been most intensively studied in *P. falciparum* and include alteration of red blood cell morphology and changes in the membrane mechanical properties of the cell and the state of phosphorylation of membrane skeletal proteins. Strikingly, the infected cells become adhesive for a number of other cells, including other parasitized red blood cells, vascular endothelial cells, normal red blood cells, dendritic cells and platelets. These changes are crucial to the survival of the parasite and, in their absence, either the parasite dies or parasitized red blood cells are rapidly eliminated from the circulation. For example, it has been suggested that the ability of red blood cells infected with mature forms of *P. falciparum* to accumulate in the microvasculature of a variety of organs (MacPherson *et al.*, 1985; Pongponratn *et al.*, 1991; Silamut *et al.*, 1999) prevents parasitized red blood cells from destruction by the reticuloendothelial system and allows the microaerophilic parasite to mature in a relatively hypoxic environment in the deep vasculature. This in turn may be linked to the enhanced virulence shown by this species of parasite, although other factors such as induction of inflammatory cytokines undoubtedly play a part (Clark *et al.*, 1994, 1997; Udomsangpetch *et al.*, 1997).

It is likely that the various structural, morphological and functional changes occurring in the red blood cell are the result of export of parasite proteins into the red blood cell cytoplasm, where they interact with the cytoplasmic, membrane skeletal and membrane components of the red blood cell. A number of reviews have examined various aspects of this issue over the years (Sherman, 1985; Tanabe, 1990a,b; Haynes, 1993; Ginsburg, 1994a,b; Cooke and Coppel, 1995; Foley and Tilley, 1995; Deitsch and Wellems, 1996; Oh *et al.*, 1997; Coppel *et al.*, 1998a,b). Several, such as that by Sherman (1985), still warrant careful reading. Recently there have been considerable advances in identifying the molecular players in phenomena such as red blood cell remodelling and cytoadherence, although knowledge of exact functional roles for many of these molecules is still missing. This review will consider a number of the key parasite molecules in turn, describe what is known of their interactions with other proteins, and indicate how these contribute to altered cellular function and the pathogenesis of malaria.

Before considering these parasite proteins, we will briefly review the structure of the normal red blood cell membrane skeleton. The red blood cell has become one of the pre-eminent systems for the analysis of structure–function relationships of biological membrane systems. It is probably the best understood eukaryotic cell in terms of the physical nature of the membrane skeleton and its relationship to the mechanical properties of the cell (Evans and Hochmuth, 1977; Mohandas *et al.*, 1984, 1992; Chasis and Mohandas, 1986; Mohandas, 1992; Mohandas and Chasis, 1993; Mohandas and Evans, 1994). The ordered arrangement of spectrin tetramers, their interconnection at the ternary complex with actin and protein 4.1, and the bonds to the overlying cell membrane via band 3 and glycophorin C (Figure 1A) provide the basis for the cell's ability to deform during repeated passage through the microcirculation during its 120 days' lifetime (Bennett, V., 1983; Gardner, K. and Bennett, 1989; Mohandas and Evans, 1994). The stability of the spectrin network is not only influenced by the primary sequence of the component proteins but can also be modulated by the levels of protein phosphorylation (Ling *et al.*, 1988; Manno *et al.*, 1995). This understanding of the relationship of the protein network to properties of the whole cell has been advanced by the study of pathological states such as inherited disorders of red blood cells including sickle cell disease, the thalassaemias and hereditary spherocytoses and ovalocytosis (Mohandas and Chasis, 1993; Mohandas and Evans, 1994). In these conditions, changes in haemoglobin structure, such as those in haemoglobin S for example, have led to altered cellular properties including changes in cell deformability and increased adhesiveness (Barabino *et al.*, 1987; Francis, 1991; Francis and Johnson, 1991; Morris *et al.*, 1993).

2. PARASITE PROTEINS EXPOSED TO THE RED BLOOD CELL MEMBRANE SKELETON

It is generally believed that almost all of the altered properties of parasitized red blood cells can be traced to the actions of a group of proteins of parasite

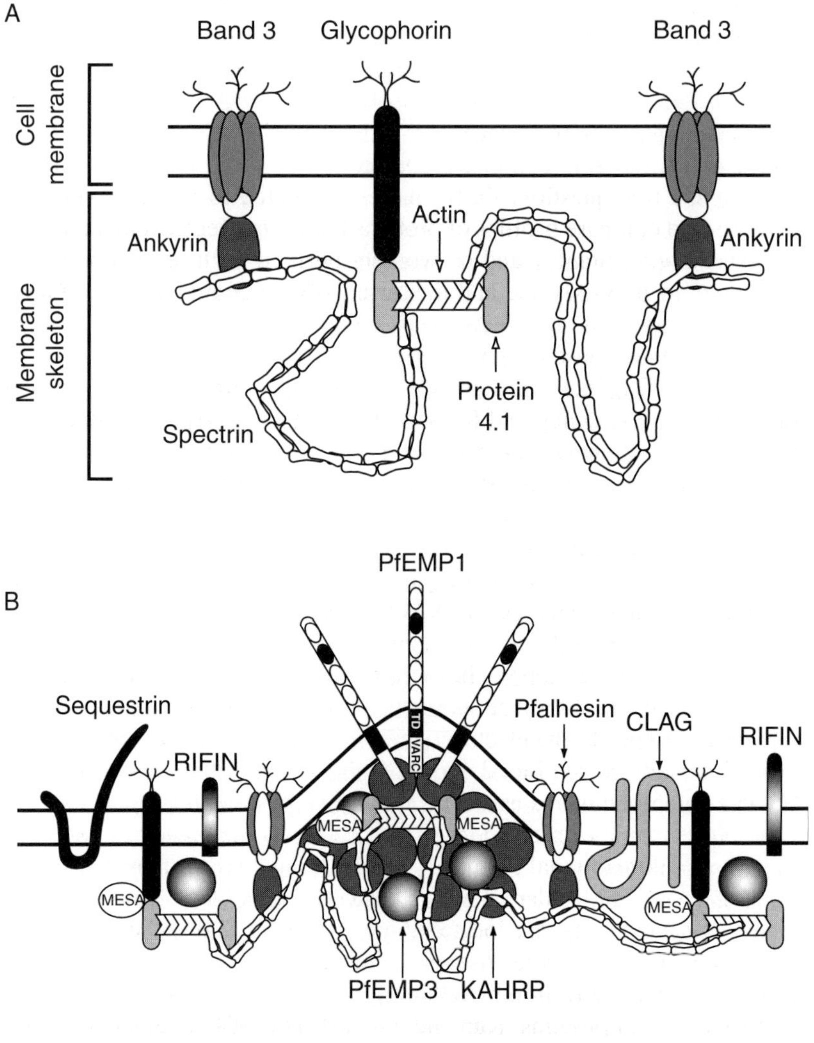

Figure 1 Schematic representation of the membrane skeleton of a red blood cell before (A) and after (B) invasion by *P. falciparum*, to indicate the changes that occur to the red blood cell as a result of infection. B depicts the typical knob structure at the infected red blood cell membrane formed by the interaction of parasite-encoded proteins such as KAHRP, PfEMP3 and MESA with the red blood cell membrane skeleton and the clustering of the major cytoadhesion ligand, PfEMP1, over the knob through interaction of its cytoplasmic tail (VARC) with KAHRP. Abbreviations are expanded on pp. 2–3.

origin that become associated with the red blood cell cytoplasm and the red blood cell membrane skeleton, either by deposition on the inner aspect of the membrane or by transient or more permanent insertion into the membrane and exposure on the red blood cell surface (Figure 1B). At present, our understanding of the number and character of the proteins that are exported to the red blood cell is far from complete. Both molecular and biochemical studies have addressed this question. Early studies attempted to isolate erythrocyte membranes and compare profiles of proteins between infected and uninfected cells. For example, Stanley and co-workers purified surface membranes by binding them to poly-L-lysine and then used silver staining and labelling to identify novel proteins in infected cells (Stanley and Reese, 1986). These studies identified at least six parasite-derived polypeptides (>240, 150, 55, 45, 35 and 20 kDa) that were associated with the infected red blood cell plasma membrane (Stanley and Reese, 1986). Interestingly, the authors suggested that four of these polypeptides (55, 45, 35 and 20 kDa) might be exposed on the surface of the infected red blood cell. Although not much was made of this observation at the time, intriguingly these protein sizes are very similar to those of the recently described products of the *rif* multi-gene family. Clearly, sensitivity of the labelling techniques or levels of expression must have been problematic, since we now know that there are more proteins associated with the red blood cell membrane than were described in this study. Alternative biochemical approaches to the identification of parasite proteins have used selective solubilization with a variety of detergents to examine membranes or to purify the electron-dense knob structures that appear on the surface of parasitized red blood cells (Chishti *et al.*, 1992; Rabilloud *et al.*, 1999). Parasite proteins that associate with the red blood cell membrane skeleton become insoluble in the non-ionic detergent Triton X-100, and this is often used as an operational definition of cytoskeletal association.

The advent of molecular cloning studies has enabled identification of a number of proteins that are located in the infected red blood cell (Tables 1 and 2). Typically such studies used antisera raised against recombinant proteins and immunolocalization by either light or electron microscopy, or both, to identify exported proteins. Kun and co-workers (1991) attempted to focus on this group of proteins by screening expression libraries with antisera made against membrane fractions. A number of proteins were identified including known exported proteins such as MESA,* but also novel sequences, some of which remain incompletely characterized at the time of writing this review. One of the novel sequences identified in this study proved to encode the exported serine–threonine kinase FEST (Kun *et al.*, 1997), so it may well be that the other sequences are also fragments encoding more, as yet unknown, exported proteins.

*Abbreviations used in the text, Tables and Figures are expanded on pp. 2–3.

Table 1 *P. falciparum* proteins associated with the red blood cell membrane skeleton and exposed on the surface of parasitized red blood cells.

Name[a]	Synonyms[a]	Molecular mass (kDa)	Comments[a]	References
PfEMP1	IP	265–285	Product of the *var* multi-gene family; mediates cytoadherence; often trypsin sensitive; clusters at knobs; antigenically variable; different forms can bind to different receptors; selection for cytoadherence selects for higher molecular mass PfEMP-1; not essential for growth *in vitro*	Leech *et al.*, 1984b; Howard, R.J., 1988; Howard, R.J. *et al.*, 1988; Magowan *et al.*, 1988; Baruch *et al.*, 1995; Smith *et al.*, 1995; Su *et al.*, 1995; Cheng *et al.*, 1998; Newbold *et al.*, 1999
Rifins	Rosettins	35–45	Product of the *rif* multi-gene family; highly polymorphic; implicated in rosetting and antigenic variation	Cheng *et al.*, 1998; Fernandez *et al.*, 1999; Kyes *et al.*, 1999
Stevor		*c.* 30	Product of the *stevor* multi-gene family; highly polymorphic; believed to be a subfamily of the *rif* genes	Cheng *et al.*, 1998; Kyes *et al.*, 1999
Clag9		–	Member of the *clag* multi-gene family; complicated multi-exon structure; believed to be exposed on the red blood cell surface; apparently necessary for cytoadherence to the receptor CD36; not required for growth *in vitro*	Holt *et al.*, 1999; Gardiner *et al.*, 2000; Trenholme *et al.*, 2000
Sequestrin		–	–	Ockenhouse *et al.*, 1991b
TR		105	Putative receptor for transferrin	Haldar *et al.*, 1986; Rodriguez and Jungery, 1986

[a] Abbreviations are expanded on pp. 2–3.

Table 2 *P. falciparum* proteins associated with the red blood cell cytosol or membrane skeleton but not exposed on the surface of parasitized red blood cells.

Name[a]	Synonyms[a]	Molecular mass (kDa)	Comments[a]	References
KAHRP	HRPI, KP	80–109	Present at knobs; isolates lacking this protein do not have knob structures detectable by electron microscopy and do not cytoadhere under flow conditions; binds to spectrin, ankyrin, actin and the cytoplasmic tail of PfEMP1; not required for growth *in vitro*	Kilejian, 1979; Hadley *et al.*, 1983; Leech *et al.*, 1984a; Culvenor *et al.*, 1987; Sharma and Kilejian, 1987; Triglia *et al.*, 1987; Kilejian *et al.*, 1991; Crabb *et al.*, 1997a; Waller, K.L. *et al.*, 1999; Oh *et al.*, 2000
MESA	PfEMP2	250–300	Phosphoprotein; binds to protein 4.1; located at knobs; extensive repetitive regions; not required for growth *in vitro*	Coppel *et al.*, 1986, 1988; Howard, R.J. *et al.*, 1987, 1988; Lustigman *et al.*, 1990; Coppel, 1992
PfEMP3	Antigen 12A	315	Located both at knobs and elsewhere at the membrane; bound to the membrane skeleton; not essential for cytoadherence, extensive repetitive regions; not required for growth *in vitro*	Handunnetti *et al.*, 1992a; Pasloske *et al.*, 1993, 1994; Van Schravendijk *et al.*, 1993; Waterkeyn *et al.*, 2000
PfHRPII	SHARP		Controversial whether this protein is secreted from the intact red blood cell	Stahl *et al.*, 1985b; Howard, R.J. *et al.*, 1986; Wellems and Howard, 1986; Wellems *et al.*, 1987
Ag332		*c.* 2500	Giant protein; present in mature parasite stages; associated with the red blood cell membrane skeleton and at knobs; some evidence of exposure on the infected red blood cell surface; function or requirement for survival remains unknown	Mattei and Scherf, 1992; Mattei *et al.*, 1992; Hinterberg *et al.*, 1994b
41-2		29	Present in schizonts, possibly localized in the schizont membrane; associated with membranous structures in the red blood cell cytoplasm and with the red blood cell's membrane skeleton	Knapp *et al.*, 1991

Table 2 *continued*

Name[a]	Synonyms[a]	Molecular mass (kDa)	Comments[a]	References
RESA	Pf155	155	Phosphoprotein; present in ring-stage parasites; minor variability; binds to spectrin; increases thermal stability of the red blood cell	Coppel *et al.*, 1984b; Perlmann *et al.*, 1984; Favaloro *et al.*, 1986; Anders *et al.*, 1987b; Foley *et al.*, 1990, 1991, 1994; Culvenor *et al.*, 1991;
FEST	Pf255	210	Serine–threonine kinase associated with the membrane skeleton; suggested to be responsible for phosphorylation of MESA and RESA	Kun *et al.*, 1991, 1997
FIRA		300	Highly antigenic during infection, present in both immature ring and mature parasite stages	Stahl *et al.*, 1987
GBP	96tr	96–130	First described as located on the merozoite surface; now generally accepted that this was artefactual and it is in fact located in the cytoplasm of the infected red blood cell	Coppel *et al.*, 1984a; Ravetch *et al.*, 1985; Kochan *et al.*, 1986; Van Schravendijk *et al.*, 1987
46 kDa cleft protein		46	Poorly characterized; localized to Maurer's clefts in the infected red blood cell cytoplasm; may be the same as the recently described Pfsbp1	Hui and Siddiqui, 1988; Etzion and Perkins, 1989; Das *et al.*, 1994; Blisnick *et al.*, 2000
Rab		23	Present in all asexual blood stages of the parasite; marker for transport studies; localization of Rab6 suggests that the early and late Golgi apparatus are separate structures in *P. falciparum*	Decastro *et al.*, 1996; Van Wye *et al.*, 1996
Exp1	CRA	23	Integral membrane protein; localized to the periphery of the parasite	Coppel *et al.*, 1985; Hope *et al.*, 1985; Simmons *et al.*, 1987; Bianco *et al.*, 1988; Günther *et al.*, 1991
PfSar1p		23	GTP-binding protein involved in protein trafficking; localized at the periphery of the parasite and in discrete vesicles and in vesicles within the red blood cell cytoplasm	Albano *et al.*, 1999a

[a] Abbreviations are expanded on pp. 2–3.

We shall discuss a number of exported proteins in detail, but first we will make a few general points. Many of the exported proteins are large, ranging in size from 100 kDa to more than 2·5 MDa. These large proteins all contain extensive regions of low complexity sequence, often occurring in the form of tandemly repeated oligopeptides (Figure 2). The repeats are characteristically present in distinct regions, with each region composed of repeats of a particular sequence. Thus KAHRP has three repeat regions and MESA has six, whereas RESA has only two repeat regions. The repeats often contain charged residues, either positive or negative, so that the repeat regions are highly charged. A common motif is a dipeptide of glutamic acid, and antibodies raised to peptides containing Glu-Glu motifs have frequently been highly cross-reactive, reacting with a number of proteins including RESA, D260, Ag332 and Pf11.1 (Mattei *et al.*, 1989; Wåhlin *et al.*, 1992; Barnes *et al.*, 1995). These charged regions of low complexity sequence are associated with non-uniform binding of sodium dodecyl sulphate (SDS) and consequent anomalous migration in SDS–polyacrylamide gels. Typically, such proteins appear to be much larger than their predicted molecular mass (Coppel *et al.*, 1994). The repeat regions are typically predicted to be either alpha-helical, random coil or coiled coil.

Many other malaria proteins contain regions of repeated sequence, including a number of proteins of the merozoite surface (Anders *et al.*, 1987a, 1993; Anders and Smythe, 1989; Coppel *et al.*, 1994). Examples include integral membrane and peripheral membrane proteins such as MSP1, MSP2 and MSP3 and the S-antigens. It should be noted that, in the case of the merozoite proteins, the repeats are typically highly variable, differing in repeat length and sequence in different isolates (Anders *et al.*, 1993; Coppel *et al.*, 1994). In MSP2, there are estimated to be several hundred distinct alleles differing in repeat sequence from each other (Eisen *et al.*, 1998). In contrast, the exported proteins that are found inside the red blood cell generally show conservation of sequence, including the repeat regions, when sequences from different isolates are compared (Stahl *et al.*, 1987; Kun *et al.*, 1999). There are exceptions, for example, in the case of the 3′ repeats of KAHRP (Kant and Sharma, 1996; Hirawake *et al.*, 1997), but in general repeat conservation is very high. The only documented differences relate to numbers of repeat units, which may vary by one to several copies. Otherwise these regions are strikingly conserved. This suggests that the repeats may in fact have some sort of functional importance and in at least one case a definite protein-binding specificity has been documented (Waller, K.L. *et al.*, 1999). This contrasts with the group of exported proteins that are found on the exterior of the red blood cell, which are highly variable, suggesting that immunological pressure is driving the alteration in sequence (Hughes and Hughes, 1995; Newbold *et al.*, 1997a, 1999; Cheng *et al.*, 1998; Fernandez *et al.*, 1999; Newbold, 1999).

Many of the exported proteins are encoded by genes containing two exons. Examples include KAHRP, RESA, MESA, FIRA, GBP and PfEMP3. The

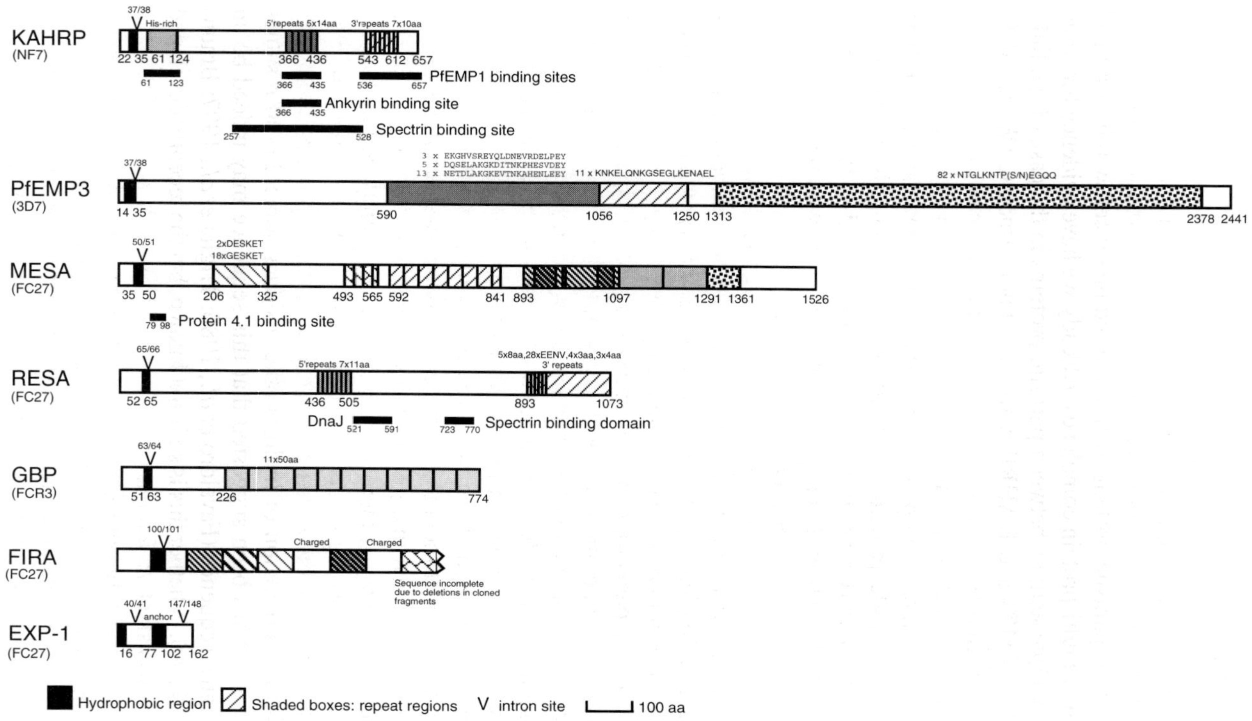

Figure 2 Schematic diagram of a number of *P. falciparum* proteins associated with the red blood cell cytoplasm and membrane skeleton. Hydrophobic and repeat regions are indicated. Abbreviations: aa, amino acids; other abbreviations are expanded on pp. 2–3.

first exon is typically short, in the range of 100–250 bp, and the second exon, which also contains the region of tandem repeats, is much larger, typically in the range of 2–6 kb (Figure 2). If one searches the malaria genome for genes with these properties, there are in fact a large number of two-exon genes containing low complexity or repeat sequences. It is likely that at least some of these are additional examples of exported proteins. This in turn suggests that it is likely that the parasite proteins within the red blood cell will be arranged in some form of multi-protein complexes. Already we have evidence for some protein–protein interactions between parasite proteins in the case of the linkages between PfEMP1 and KAHRP within the knob structure (Waller, K.L. *et al.*, 1999). Evidence from purification studies of the knob suggests that there are multiple components (Chishti *et al.*, 1992), although direct interactions between several of these components have not been demonstrated. Further, the absence of a single protein, KAHRP, is enough for this characteristic structure to disappear (Crabb *et al.*, 1997a). However, already a number of exported proteins have been found outside the knob and, with more to be discovered, it is possible that some quite complex structures will be found.

A feature noted early was that many of the exported proteins, such as MESA, RESA, KAHRP, FIRA and GBP, all lacked N-terminal hydrophobic signal sequences. Typical signal sequences of 13–15 hydrophobic residues located at the N-terminus had been found in proteins exported to the merozoite surface, in the parasitophorous vacuole and in the rhoptries, but not in these proteins exported to the red blood cell compartment. The red blood cell compartment is one that does not have an exact parallel in a typical eukaryotic cell, and it seems reasonable to suppose that the parasite requires additional trafficking machinery, perhaps a novel transport system, to place these proteins in their final cellular location. Exported proteins might then require some sort of tag to direct them to this novel export pathway or, alternatively, lack some retention signal that prevents their passage to the exterior along a default secretory pathway. If there are specific tags for transport, then there is no requirement that this tag be at the N-terminus, but it is intriguing to note that the N-terminus of these red blood cell-associated proteins is usually charged, with a short region of hydrophobic residues some 20–50 residues into the protein. It has been suggested that this sequence may indeed be an alternative signal sequence (Favaloro *et al.*, 1986; Triglia *et al.*, 1987; Braun-Breton *et al.*, 1990). Whether this is so is not known, but the recently developed techniques to transfect *P. falciparum* parasites (Van Dijk *et al.*, 1995; Wu *et al.*, 1995, 1996; Crabb and Cowman, 1996; Crabb *et al.*, 1997b) should now permit this question to be critically addressed. Once arrived within the red blood cell cytoplasm, these proteins assemble into multi-component complexes such as the knob structure. Presumably such assembly is driven by the presence of high-affinity binding domains specific for partner proteins (Table 3). The binding coefficients of such interactions described to date are

Table 3 Defined protein–protein interactions at the red blood cell membrane skeleton.

Protein partners[a]	Binding constants[b] (μM)	References
Spectrin and protein 4.1	0·1	Tyler *et al.*, 1980; Podgorski and Elbaum, 1985
Spectrin and ankyrin	0·1	Tyler *et al.*, 1980
Ankyrin and band 3	0·01	Bennett, V. and Stenbuck, 1980; Thevenin and Low, 1990
Protein 4.1 and p55	0·1	Nunomura *et al.*, 2000
Protein 4.1 and GPC	0·09	Nunomura *et al.*, 2000
p55 and GPC	1·6	Nunomura *et al.*, 2000
Protein 4.2 and ankyrin	0·1–0·4	Korsgren and Cohen, 1988
Protein 4.2 and band 3	0·2–0·8	Korsgren and Cohen, 1988
MESA and protein 4.1	0·63	Bennett, B.J. *et al.*, 1997
KAHRP and ankyrin	1·3–8·3	Magowan *et al.*, 2000
VAR_{CD} and F-actin	0·04	Oh *et al.*, 2000
VAR_{CD} and KAHRP	0·01	Oh *et al.*, 2000
VARC and KAHRP (K1A)	0·1	Waller, K.L. *et al.*, 1999
VARC and KAHRP (K2A)	3·3	Waller, K.L. *et al.*, 1999
VARC and KAHRP (K3)	13·0	Waller, K.L. *et al.*, 1999

[a] Abbreviations are expanded on pp. 2–3.
[b] Binding constants are dissociation constants (K_d) except for the MESA–protein 4.1 interaction, where the value is the IC_{50}.

generally of the order of 10^{-5} to 10^{-7} M, an affinity typical of interactions of host cell proteins of the normal red blood cell skeleton. We will now move on to discuss some of these parasite-encoded proteins in more detail.

2.1. Proteins Exposed on the Surface of Infected Red Blood Cells

2.1.1. *PfEMP1 (*Plasmodium falciparum *Erythrocyte Membrane Protein 1)*

From the mid 1960s, evidence accumulated describing the appearance of new antigens on the surface of parasitized red blood cells (e.g., Brown and Brown, 1965; Langreth and Reese, 1979; Gruenberg and Sherman, 1983; Hommel *et al.*, 1983); however, whether these molecules were parasite derived or simply altered host proteins was not known. By metabolic labelling and lactoperoxidase-catalysed radio-iodination of monkey red blood cells parasitized by *P. knowlesi*, R.J. Howard and colleagues (1983) provided the first direct evidence that a molecule of parasite origin was exposed on the surface of the parasitized cell. Using a similar biochemical approach, Leech and coworkers (1984b) later confirmed these findings using monkey red blood cells infected with *P. falciparum*. This high molecular weight (250–350 kDa) protein, now called PfEMP1, varies in size between different parasite lines and is antigenically highly variable. It is insoluble in Triton X-100 detergent, demonstrating a link to the red blood cell membrane skeleton, and frequently highly sensitive to proteases. The original definition of this molecule included the property of exquisite sensitivity to trypsin digestion (0·1 μg/mL), but PfEMP1 molecules that are resistant to trypsin have now been described (Chaiyaroj *et al.*, 1994a; Gardner, J.P. *et al.*, 1996; Smith *et al.*, 2000).

Although PfEMP1 had been associated with the phenomenon of cytoadherence for several years, defining more precisely its role in the process was hampered by the inability to identify the gene encoding this variant surface antigen. This situation changed spectacularly in 1995 when several groups simultaneously published papers describing a highly polymorphic family of genes, the *var* genes (Baruch *et al.*, 1995; Smith *et al.*, 1995; Su *et al.*, 1995), that encode PfEMP1. Initial estimates of the number of *var* genes per parasite were between 50 and 150 (Baruch *et al.*, 1995; Su *et al.*, 1995), but later studies suggest that the complement is generally 40–50 per haploid genome (Rubio *et al.*, 1996; Thompson *et al.*, 1997). The multiple copies of *var* are scattered throughout the genome and may be found on any chromosome and in either orientation (Rubio *et al.*, 1996; Fischer, K. *et al.*, 1997). They frequently occur in clusters and may be found centrally or in a subtelomeric location (Rubio *et al.*, 1996; Fischer, K. *et al.*, 1997; Hernandez-Rivas *et al.*, 1997), although their precise location in the genome varies between different parasite isolates. Although it is clear that *var* genes can be expressed irrespective of their position, it has been suggested that those in a subtelomeric position are more commonly expressed than those located centrally (Fischer, K. *et al.*, 1997). One interesting suggestion is that the subtelomeric location is prone to great variability and a high frequency of recombination, which may be part of the reason for the extreme variability of *var* genes (Rubio *et al.*, 1996; Fischer, K. *et al.*, 1997). The observation that there is quite a close relationship between some *var* genes in subtelomeric locations of different chromosomes supports this suggestion. These different genes vary in sequence, which results in antigenic heterogeneity and variability in binding specificity. It should be emphasized that different parasite isolates contain not only different numbers of *var* genes located in varying genomic locations but also different repertoires of sequences. Thus the total number of *var* gene sequences is of the order of thousands, perhaps as many as 10 000.

The primary structure of a number of *var* genes and their encoded proteins have now been determined. All the genes appear to have a similar general structure (Figure 3), comprising a long 5′ exon and a shorter 3′ exon. The 3′ exon is well conserved between different *var* genes (Bonnefoy *et al.*, 1997) and

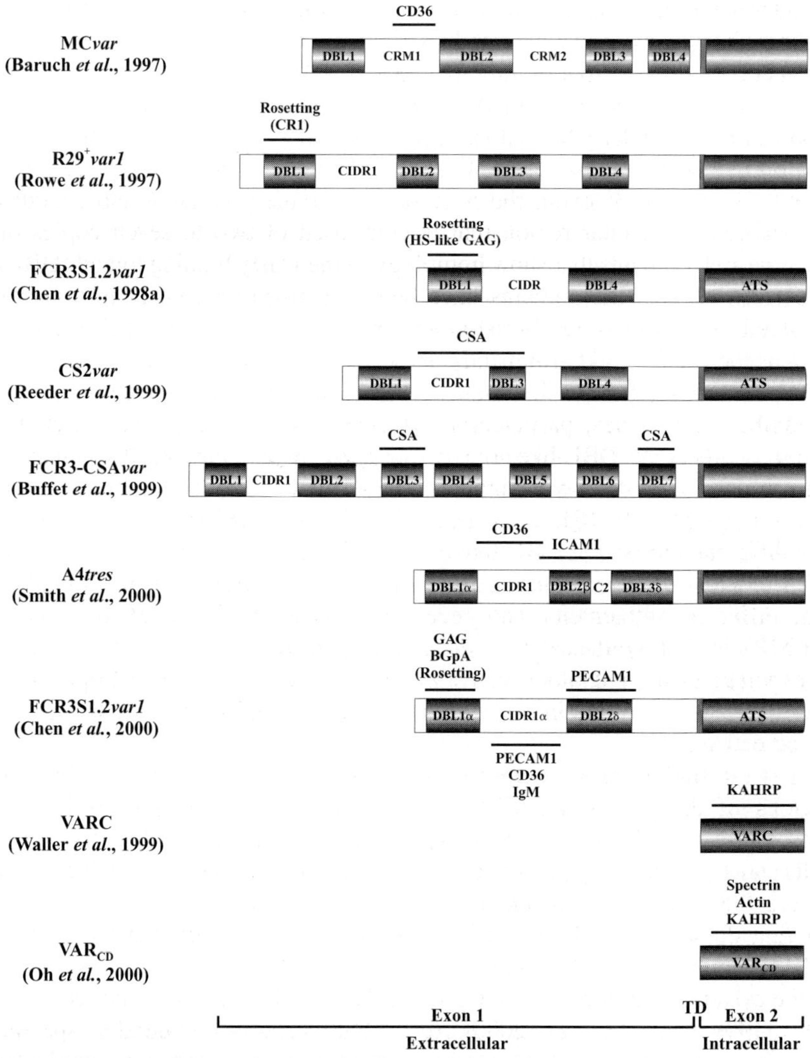

Figure 3 Structure of various cloned *var* genes from *P. falciparum* and defined functional domains in the PfEMP1 protein involved in cytoadhesion or rosetting. Specific domains of the molecule that interact with a number of endothelial cell-expressed adhesion molecules or components of the red blood cell membrane skeleton are shown where these have been determined. The terminology used to name the various structural domains of the molecule are those used by the original authors and the inconsistency demonstrates the confusing nomenclature that has developed. For example, CRM1, CIDR1 and CIDR1α are equivalent terms for the same cysteine-rich region of the molecule. Furthemore, the sequence of the DBL1 region between different *var* genes may not be identical. Abbreviations are expanded on pp. 2–3.

encodes the intracellular domain of the protein, which is rich in acidic residues. It shares homology with elements in the sequence of *Pf60*, a multi-gene family encoding quite disparate proteins (Bischoff *et al.*, 2000). This region is responsible for anchoring PfEMP1 to the membrane skeleton in infected red blood cells, particularly but not exclusively via the knob-associated histidine-rich protein, KAHRP (Waller, K.L. *et al.*, 1999; Oh *et al.*, 2000; Voigt *et al.*, 2000). Unlike the 3′ exon, the 5′ exon is extremely variable and encodes a variable extracellular region that is composed of two to seven copies of cysteine-rich domains that show homology to the Duffy binding ligand (DBL) of *P. vivax*. The DBL domains have been described previously in proteins involved in red blood cell invasion and bind to host red blood cell proteins such as the Duffy blood group antigen and glycophorin A (Adams, J.H. *et al.*, 1992; Sim *et al.*, 1994). The domains can be recognized by conservation of a number of residues, particularly cysteine, which occur in characteristic patterns. Otherwise, DBL-like domains vary greatly in sequence, although there are sub-patterns that allow recognition of DBL-1 domains from different parasites compared with DBL-4, for example. Different PfEMP1 sequences contain different numbers of DBL-like domains (Figure 3), but the significance of this is unclear. Different *var* gene sequences encode variant forms of PfEMP1 that differ in antigenicity and receptor specificity (Smith *et al.*, 1995). PfEMP1 is first synthesized by the late ring/early trophozoite stage and is transported to the red blood cell membrane where, by the late trophozoite stage, PfEMP1 is found in association with knobs and is exposed on the red blood cell surface.

Several studies have attempted to relate binding specificity to specific regions of the protein PfEMP1. Typical experimental approaches involve the expression of domains of the molecule either on the surface of COS or CHO cells and addition of receptors or cells in some form. Although such approaches ignore the potential co-operative effect of several domains, several specific binding domains have been localized (Figure 3). It appears that most or all PfEMP1 molecules contain a binding site for CD36 and this appears to reside in the cysteine-rich interdomain region (CIDR) of the molecule (Baruch *et al.*, 1997, 1999; Chen, Q. *et al.*, 2000). Additional receptors are bound by specific sequences present elsewhere in the protein and are limited to particular PfEMP1 sequences (Figure 3). Thus, the ability to bind to chondroitin sulphate A (CSA), for example, is manifested by only some isolates. Two PfEMP1 sequences from CSA-binding isolates have been reported to have this property (Buffet *et al.*, 1999; Reeder *et al.*, 1999). In one case the *PfEMP1* gene contained seven DBL-like domains (Buffet *et al.*, 1999), and in another case, only three (Reeder *et al.*, 1999) (see Figure 3). In the case of the larger protein, two isolated domains, DBL-3 and DBL-7, were capable of binding CSA, but only DBL-3 had the same spectrum of binding specificities as the parent parasite line. Accordingly it was concluded that DBL-3 was the CSA-binding region

(Buffet *et al.*, 1999). It is not yet known if the other PfEMP1 also uses DBL-3 for binding, and how similar the two binding domains may be. Human antibodies that develop after numerous pregnancies against CSA-binding variants of PfEMP1 cross-react with isolates from various locations around the world, suggesting a reasonable degree of sequence conservation (Fried *et al.*, 1998).

One of the great unknowns is the method by which *var* gene expression, and hence antigenic variation, is controlled. It has been suggested that only a single *var* gene is expressed per cell but that, within a population, several or many genes are switched on. It has been shown unequivocally that a single infected cell can bind to at least two endothelial cell-expressed receptors (Chaiyaroj *et al.*, 1994b), but this has been explained by the suggestion that a single PfEMP1 protein may have binding sites for two or more receptors (Gardner, J.P. *et al.*, 1996; Chen, Q. *et al.*, 2000). Currently, we view this question as unresolved but it has major implications for any model proposed for control of *var* gene expression. Clonal lines of parasites can change expression of PfEMP1 by some form of transcriptional control. The frequency by which cells can switch is estimated to be of the order of 2% per generation for one particular laboratory-adapted parasite line, although this is likely to be an unusually plastic clone (Roberts, D.J. *et al.*, 1992). Most cytoadherent parasites cultured *in vitro* are marked by the stability of the dominantly expressed PfEMP1 ligand. The total number of PfEMP1 molecules on the red blood cell surface is unknown but it is not believed to be an abundant molecule and the total may lie in the thousands. Finally, there is evidence that PfEMP1 transcription may be somewhat promiscuous with leaky transcription of many different *PfEMP1* genes early in the ring stage, followed by switching off transcription of all but the expressed *PfEMP1* gene as the parasite matures (Chen, Q. *et al.*, 1998b).

2.1.2. *Rifins*

In addition to the *var* gene products (PfEMP1), a second group of at least 12 radio-iodinatable proteins ranging from approximately 20 to 170 kDa can also be detected on the surface of parasitized red blood cells. Like PfEMP1, their expression is parasite stage-specific and they appear on the red blood cell surface about 14–16 hours after invasion, as the parasites develop into mature, pigmented trophozoites (Stanley and Reese, 1986; Helmby *et al.*, 1993; Fernandez *et al.*, 1999). Their precise role in adhesion is contentious, perhaps with the exception of adhesion to PECAM1 (CD31), which, in at least one parasite line, appears to be associated with the presence of one of these 35 kDa polypeptides (Fernandez *et al.*, 1999). Analysis of more than 20 different parasite lines, including both clinical isolates and laboratory-adapted cytoadherent lines and clones, has revealed that the most common and prominent of these proteins occur in the 30–45 kDa size range. Other novel radio-iodinatable bands clearly distinct from *var* gene products can be detected in some lines, but these occur much less frequently and, with the exception of a strong 170 kDa band, are relatively weak in intensity. Further, this 170 kDa polypeptide is not recognized by immune sera that immunoprecipitate multiple bands in the 30–45 kDa cluster in the same parasite line, nor is it recognized by antisera raised against the highly conserved cytoplasmic tail of PfEMP1 by Western blotting (Fernandez *et al.*, 1999).

Until recently, this family of 30–45 kDa proteins had been collectively referred to as rosettins, since they were first identified in parasite lines that showed a high and stable propensity to form rosettes of red blood cells (Helmby *et al.*, 1993). They appear to be resistant to trypsin cleavage at concentrations sufficient to remove PfEMP1 from the red blood cell surface, a distinction that was exploited to demonstrate that these molecules were involved in rosetting. It is now clear that they are not exclusively linked to this phenotype since they are frequently present in non-rosetting lines. Furthermore, they have been detected in all clinical isolates that have been examined to date, suggesting that these antigens have some other, as yet unknown, primary function, which probably plays a much more critical role in parasite survival than rosetting (Fernandez *et al.*, 1999).

Weber (1988) described a repetitive gene sequence, *rif-1* (repetitive interspersed family), in *P. falciparum*, which he claimed was expressed. Although ignored at this time, the availability of the *P. falciparum* genome revealed that *rif*-like sequences were found near *var* genes in the subtelomeric regions of chromosomes (Cheng *et al.*, 1998; Gardner, M.J. *et al.*, 1998; Bowman *et al.*, 1999). These genes, now called rifins, were shown to encode the previously described rosettins, as antisera raised against the deduced amino acid sequences from multiple *rif* genes immunoprecipitated what is apparently the same set of radio-iodinatable proteins (Fernandez *et al.*, 1999; Kyes *et al.*, 1999). It has been suggested that there may be 200–500 *rif* genes per haploid genome (Fernandez *et al.*, 1999), which would in fact make it the largest gene family described to date in *Plasmodium*. The location of the protein and large size of this gene family, together with the observation that closely related clones of *P. falciparum* express different rifins on their surface, suggest that these are clonally variant polypeptides that may play an important role in antigenic variation and evasion of immune responses (Fernandez *et al.*, 1999; Kyes *et al.*, 1999).

A further multi-gene family that has recently been defined is the *stevor* family. Details of the *stevor* gene product are still scanty, but it has been suggested, based on sequence analysis, that *stevor* genes are in fact a subfamily of the *rif* genes (Cheng *et al.*, 1998). Opinion is still divided on this point, but it should be noted that *stevor* genes are found in the subtelomeric arrangement of polymorphic genes noted in several *P. falciparum* chromosomes (Gardner, M.J. *et al.*, 1998; Bowman *et al.*, 1999).

2.1.3. *Clag9*

The involvement in cytoadherence of a gene product encoded on *P. falciparum* chromosome 9 was first suggested by observations that loss of adherence of some clinical isolates and clones during culture *in vitro* was accompanied by overgrowth of parasites possessing a smaller form of this chromosome (Day *et al.*, 1993). Loss of cytoadherence was attributed to the apparent absence of PfEMP1 on the surface of the parasitized red blood cells. The story was, however, to become increasingly more complicated.

Deletions in chromosome 9 occur frequently and typically involve loss of up to 500 kb. Deletions occur subtelomerically at both ends of the chromosome, although the majority of the loss occurs from the right arm (Foote and Kemp, 1989; Shirley *et al.*, 1990). Analysis of a number of parasite lines allowed the cytoadherence-associated locus to be precisely mapped to an open reading frame on the right arm of the chromosome (Barnes *et al.*, 1994). Interestingly, examination of a number of non-cytoadherent clones revealed that the breakpoints for deletions from the right arm of chromosome 9 always occurred within a novel open reading frame (orf), which was called the breakpoint orf (bporf) (Bourke *et al.*, 1996). Some parasite clones have been maintained in culture for many years and, despite the acquisition of a shortened right arm on chromosome 9, have retained a stable adherence phenotype. Genetic analysis has revealed that in fact the bporf has been completely removed by an internal 15 kb deletion, while 55 kb of downstream sequence, which had been lost from a non-cytoadherent sibling clone C10, was retained. This observation indicated that this 55 kb region must encode a novel gene involved in cytoadherence that was distinct from PfEMP1 since no *var* gene was contained within this region of the genome (Bourke *et al.*, 1996). Partial sequencing of the entire 55 kb region led to the identification of a candidate gene located just downstream of bporf, which was dubbed the cytoadherence-linked asexual gene (*clag9*) (Holt *et al.*, 1999; Trenholme *et al.*, 2000).

The *clag* gene is approximately 7 kb and is a complex structure comprising at least nine exons. It is transcribed in mature-stage parasites and translated into a 220 kDa protein that is distinct from PfEMP1 and can be detected in parasitized cells by Western blotting. Its precise cellular localization remains to be determined; however, prediction of the structure of the protein *in silico* (i.e., predicted by computer modelling) from its hydrophobicity profile reveals four putative transmembrane domains, suggesting that it is membrane-associated and presumably could be exposed on the surface of the parasitized cell (Trenholme *et al.*, 2000). Preliminary immunofluorescence data support this hypothesis; however, at this stage its presence on the surface of the infected red blood cell must remain speculative. Nevertheless, recent evidence that adhesion of red blood cells parasitized by the parasite line 3D7, which exhibits a stable cytoadherence phenotype, was ablated when the *clag9* gene was knocked out by transfection is compelling and confirms the essential role of *clag9* in cytoadherence, at least to CD36 (Trenholme *et al.*, 2000). Further, this same group have now confirmed their findings using an anti-sense approach (Gardiner *et al.*, 2000). Clearly, further work is required in order to determine the precise role in cytoadhesion of the clag9 protein to elucidate whether it is itself a cytoadherence ligand or whether it plays an indirect role in the adhesive process, perhaps by preventing surface expression of other adherence ligands such as PfEMP1. Further, the full range of receptors with which such gene products may interact on the surface of vascular endothelial cells remains to be determined. Recent data derived from the malaria genome sequencing project have revealed that the *clag9* gene is in fact part of a multi-gene family of homologous sequences found on a number of other chromosomes, although the nature and function of the gene products of these paralogues remain to be determined.

2.1.4. *Sequestrin*

Using anti-idiotype antibodies raised against the binding site of the anti-CD36 monoclonal antibody OKM8, Ockenhouse *et al.* (1991b) identified a novel trypsin-sensitive protein of *c.* 270 kDa in parasitized cells, which they termed sequestrin. Furthermore, the antibodies reacted with the surface of knobby parasitized cells and inhibited their ability to adhere to CD36 but did not bind to the surface of non-parasitized cells or to red blood cells infected with a knobless, non-cytoadherent parasite clone. No further characterization of this protein or the gene encoding it has ever been published and it is now widely argued that sequestrin is in fact PfEMP1. Interestingly, one recent paper describing the targeted knockout of the *clag9* gene (Trenholme *et al.*, 2000) referred to unpublished observations that these authors had knocked out the gene encoding sequestrin with no consequent reduction in the ability of the parasitized cells to adhere to CD36. Details of this protein and its function remain sketchy and we await further information.

2.2. Proteins Found in the Red Blood Cell Cytoplasm or on the Membrane Skeleton of Infected Red Blood Cells

2.2.1. *KAHRP (Knob-associated Histidine-rich Protein)*

Considerable information has been accumulated about this protein and it is now recognized to be of central importance in the changes occurring to the infected red blood cell, particularly with respect to the formation of the knob structure and its essential role in cytoadhesion. Although knobs had been described as early as 1966 (Trager *et al.*, 1966), little was known about the biochemical composition of these structures until the work of Kilejian (Kilejian, 1979; Kilejian and Olson, 1979), who compared the stage-specific proteins of 'knobby' and 'knobless' lines of the parasite isolate FCR3. Parasites were biosynthetically labelled and the proteins separated by SDS–polyacrylamide chromatography. A labelled protein of *c.* 80 kDa was found in the knobby line but not in the knobless line. Fractions of infected cells enriched for red blood cell membranes were coincidentally enriched for the presence of this protein. In a later study, Kilejian (1979) demonstrated that this protein was strongly labelled when tritiated histidine was incorporated into the culture medium. Further, an antiserum to a histidine-rich protein found in *P. lophurae* appeared by immunoelectron microscopy to label knobs. We consider the protein identified in knobby parasites by these studies to be that now referred to as KAHRP.

This work was confirmed and extended by Hadley, Leech and others in a series of papers in the early to mid 1980s (Hadley *et al.*, 1983; Gritzmacher and Reese, 1984; Leech *et al.*, 1984a; Vernot-Hernandez and Heidrich, 1984, 1985). There was general agreement that knobby parasites produced a protein that, depending on the investigator and the parasite line examined, varied in molecular mass from 80 to 108 kDa. Leech *et al.* (1984a) used a method of differential detergent extraction to show that this protein was found in the Triton X-100 insoluble fraction, and this fraction was found by thin section electron microscopy to contain knobs. Extraction with 1% SDS led to the disappearance of this protein and the consequent disappearance of the knobs. The novel protein was synthesized from about the mid-ring stage and accumulated in infected red blood cell membranes during trophozoite and schizont stages (Vernot-Hernandez and Heidrich, 1984). Although Vernot-Hernandez and Heidrich (1985) also identified a novel protein of 92 kDa that was specific to knobby parasites, they concluded that it may not be the knob-forming material. This was based on trypsin and chymotrypsin digestion of purified red blood cell membranes, which led to the disappearance of this protein, while the knob structures were still discernible by electron microscopy. More puzzling were the results from their study of intact parasitized red blood cells treated with trypsin 10 hours after invasion, before the appearance of KAHRP and of knobs. In the subsequent development of these red blood cells, knobs formed normally, but no KAHRP could be detected. Vernot-Hernandez and Heidrich (1985) postulated that enzymatic treatment might destroy the locus of insertion or anchor point of KAHRP. There has been no reported attempt to replicate these results and they remain tantalizingly enigmatic. The size of KAHRP varies in different parasite lines; it was reported to be 92 kDa in Malayan Camp and 108 kDa in the St Lucia strain (Leech *et al.*, 1984a).

The molecular cloning of the gene encoding KAHRP set the stage for a revolution in our understanding of this protein and its role in the altered properties of the infected red blood cell (Kilejian *et al.*, 1986; Ardeshir *et al.*,

1987; Pologe *et al.*, 1987; Triglia *et al.*, 1987). The gene encoding KAHRP comprises two exons of the general structure outlined earlier. The extreme N-terminal sequence of the KAHRP protein is composed of predominantly basic residues with a hydrophobic core of 11 residues found at residue 22. The protein is highly charged and contains about 8% histidine, a histidine content considerably lower than that of HRPII and HRPIII, which is closer to 70% (Stahl *et al.*, 1985b; Wellems and Howard, 1986). There are three regions of repeat sequence in the protein. The first repeat region, called the 'histidine-rich region', occurs 24 residues into the beginning of the second exon and is composed of strings of polyhistidine varying in length from 6 to 11 residues. A tetrapeptide motif HQAP is repeated three times. The next repeat region, the so-called 5′ repeats, are composed of five copies of a 13–16 residue sequence based on a canonical sequence of SKKHKDNEDAESVK. The repeats are highly charged and, overall, basic. The 3′ repeats contain seven inexact copies of a 10-mer based on the canonical sequence SKEATKEAST. Human antibodies affinity-purified on recombinant protein, or experimental sera raised to the recombinant, recognized a protein of 80–100 kDa in knobby but not knobless parasites and localized the expressed protein to knobs (Ardeshir *et al.*, 1987; Culvenor *et al.*, 1987; Pologe *et al.*, 1987; Triglia *et al.*, 1987). The protein was present at the electron-dense knobs and was confined to the inside of the red blood cell membrane. It confirmed that knobless parasites did not synthesize any of this protein, a finding now explicable as being secondary to a chromosome breakage and gene deletion event (Pologe and Ravetch, 1986).

Comparative sequencing studies suggest that the gene encoding this region is relatively highly conserved. Many of the early reports of sequence differences appear to be the result of sequencing errors caused by the presence of areas very rich in AT. The one area of clear polymorphism is found in the 3′ repeats that vary in number and sequence (Triglia *et al.*, 1987; Kant and Sharma, 1996; Hirawake *et al.*, 1997). The number of repeats varies from three to seven copies and there are variations in repeat length as well. These variations are widespread and have been reported in isolates from India, Ghana and Honduras. Although the differences are not large, the highly charged nature of these sequences accounts for the close to 20 kDa differences between some isolates. The other repeat regions are much more strongly conserved. The reason for this may relate to the observation that the repeat regions partake in the interaction that anchors PfEMP1 at the knob (Waller *et al.*, 1999). Of the three repeats, the 3′ repeat interaction is of the lowest affinity (Table 3) and thus perturbation in the repeat number of this region would be least likely to affect the overall interaction.

The function of the KAHRP protein has been studied extensively. It takes part in a number of intermolecular interactions with host cell proteins including spectrin, actin and ankyrin, and with the parasite protein PfEMP1

(Kilejian *et al.*, 1991; Waller *et al.*, 1999; Magowan *et al.*, 2000; Oh *et al.*, 2000). The consequences of these interactions are to anchor PfEMP1 securely to the membrane skeleton and provide a stable structure that allows flowing parasitized red blood cells to cytoadhere and to resist subsequent detachment by the shear forces experienced in the dynamic environment of the circulation *in vivo*. KAHRP also appears to be essential for knob formation. These latter conclusions are based on an elegant set of experiments using parasites that had lost the capacity to express KAHRP by virtue of specific targeted disruption of the *KAHRP* gene (Crabb *et al.*, 1997a). In these studies, parasites of the 3D7 line were transfected with a vector in which the *KAHRP* gene was interrupted by insertion of a gene encoding a drug resistance marker. Repeated rounds of drug treatment selected transfected parasites that had undergone integration of the marker gene. The resulting parasites were cloned by limiting dilution and a number of cloned lines examined. These lines were shown to contain a *KAHRP* gene that had been disrupted and thus did not express the KAHRP protein. Electron microscopic studies showed that these parasites lacked knob structures, strongly suggesting that KAHRP expression is necessary for knob formation (Crabb *et al.*, 1997a). The technical limitations of the malaria transfection system prevented complementation studies being performed, so it remains a formal possibility that some other secondary change led to loss of knobs. With the development of additional selectable markers, it should become possible to perform complementation and prove the requirement for KAHRP in knob formation. When the knobless transgenic parasites were examined for their capacity to cytoadhere under static conditions, they showed complete retention of the ability to bind to CD36. However, when the parasites were exposed to shear flow in a flow chamber, the capacity of the *KAHRP* knockout lines to adhere to CD36 or to platelets was markedly diminished. This was manifested as both a decrease in the number of parasitized cells able to adhere from flow, and a higher level of detachment of previously adhering parasites at any particular shear stress (Crabb *et al.*, 1997a). As the shear stresses examined were selected as those likely to be encountered in post-capillary venules, where parasitized cells preferentially sequester *in vivo* (Chen, S., 1969), it was concluded that KAHRP had a role in enabling parasitized cells to cytoadhere in the dynamic flow environment of the vasculature *in vivo*. The localization of PfEMP1 in wild-type and *KAHRP* knockouts was examined. Although PfEMP1 was able to reach the surface of mutant parasites, it appeared to be present in more localized aggregations, manifested as a punctate pattern compared with the more uniform surface location of the parent line (Crabb *et al.*, 1997a). Whether these differences were secondary to the absence of knobs or whether KAHRP is involved in the trafficking of PfEMP1 to the red blood cell surface remains to be determined. KAHRP is generally considered to be an internal protein, not exposed on the surface of the cell. However, there is at least one report of antibodies to KAHRP exerting an effect on intact parasitized cells (Carlson *et al.*, 1990b). In this study, a mononclonal antibody to KAHRP was observed to disrupt the formation of rosettes. Whether this was due to reactivity to KAHRP or cross-reactivity to some other protein is unknown, but it is certainly possible that rifins, for example, may contain sequences cross-reactive to KAHRP, which would explain these observations.

The observation that the absence of KAHRP led to a change in localization of PfEMP1 and a loss in efficiency of cytoadherence suggested some form of direct interaction between the two proteins. Previous mapping studies had identified an association between KAHRP and spectrin and actin, via a 271 residues region in the central region of KAHRP (Kilejian *et al.*, 1991). Thus the net effect of the interaction between KAHRP and PfEMP1 would be to anchor PfEMP1 indirectly to the red blood cell membrane skeleton. However the fact that PfEMP1 could still be detected on the surface of knobless parasitized cells and that cytoadherence still occurred, although to a lesser extent, suggested additional linkages to either other parasite proteins or host proteins, or both. Oh *et al.* (2000) recently identified an interaction between PfEMP1 and the spectrin–actin junction, particularly F-actin. They also noted a tendency for KAHRP to self-associate in structures that resembled knobs. In the case of the interaction of PfEMP1 with KAHRP, however, three distinct binding domains were identified and two of these have been mapped to repetitive regions of KAHRP, the histidine-rich region and the 5′ repeat region (Waller *et al.*, 1999). These two regions contain 63 and 70 residues, respectively. Such relatively short sequences make it likely that the binding motifs have a linear nature. Determination of the dissociation constants for the histidine-rich and 5′ repeats to the cytoplasmic domain of PfEMP1 gave values indicative of moderate affinity interactions (0·1 μM and 3·3 μM, respectively) (see Table 3). The third binding domain in the carboxyl terminal region of KAHRP that includes the 3′ repeats is of lower affinity (K_d = 13 μM) and the necessary experiments to map it to the repeat region have not been reported. The identification of multiple regions in KAHRP which bind to the cytoplasmic region of PfEMP1, termed VARC, contrasts with other studies focused on interactions between parasite proteins and host proteins of the red blood cell membrane skeleton. Both MESA and RESA have single binding regions for their cognate partners (Foley *et al.*, 1994; Bennett, B.J. *et al.*, 1997), as does MSP1 which is reported to bind to spectrin (Herrera *et al.*, 1993).

The histidine-rich repeats and the 5′ repeats contribute individually to the interaction between KAHRP and VARC at affinities comparable to the single binding domains identified in spectrin/protein 4.1, spectrin/ankyrin and MESA/protein 4.1 (see Table 3). Considering the data obtained for all the binding domains, its seems reasonable that the three regions may act co-operatively to result in an interaction of very high affinity. One caveat is that, in the absence of known three-dimensional structure for KAHRP, it is not certain whether it is possible for all three regions of KAHRP to interact with a single PfEMP1 molecule. Studies involving nearly full-length KAHRP do indeed show an increased affinity with PfEMP1, with dissociation constants of 10 nM reported (Oh *et al.*, 2000). However, it is also possible that one or several of the binding regions could react with separate VARC molecules providing a cross-linking effect that would serve to anchor a number of PfEMP1 molecules in a compact space. This would provide a high density of PfEMP1 ectodomains at the knob and improve binding affinity for endothelial cells. Perhaps it is the loss of clustering of PfEMP1 in the absence of knobs that explains the loss of adherence of knobless infected red blood cells under flow conditions while their binding ability appears to be maintained in the absence of flow-induced haemodynamic stress. Alternatively, the weakened adhesive properties may be due to PfEMP1 being 'pulled out' of the membrane of infected red blood cells, owing to inadequate anchoring, when subjected to the physiological shear stresses that occur in the circulation *in vivo.*

As discussed earlier, a prominent feature of many malarial proteins is the presence of extensive regions of tandemly repeated sequence (Anders *et al.*, 1987a). It has been difficult to assign functional roles to these repeat regions. They are often the target of antibody-induced immunity in individuals living in endemic areas, and it has been suggested that they act as a form of immunological 'smoke screen', diverting the immune system to low affinity non-protective antibody responses (Anders, 1986; Coppel *et al.*, 1994). Occasionally, additional roles have been suggested. For example, the repeats of the circumsporozoite protein (CSP) have been proposed to play some role in the interaction of the sporozoite with hepatocytes (Aley *et al.*, 1986). However, more recently the binding site has been mapped to a non-repetitive sequence elsewhere in the CSP (Cerami *et al.*, 1992). Similarly, the binding site of a second sporozoite protein, TRAP, for hepatocytes has also been mapped to a region of non-repetitive sequence (Muller *et al.*, 1993). The binding domains of RESA, MESA and MSP1 mentioned above are all found in a non-repetitive sequence (Herrera *et al.*, 1993; Foley *et al.*, 1994; Bennett, B.J. *et al.*, 1997). Although the 271 residues spectrin/actin-binding region of KAHRP does in fact contain the 5′ repeats (Kilejian *et al.*, 1991), the interacting domain has not been mapped to a defined peptide sequence within this region. In contrast, both high affinity KAHRP binding domains for VARC identified in this study are mapped to defined repeat regions. The interaction of KAHRP with VARC is likely to have an electrostatic component since, at the pH of the infected red blood cell (Yayon *et al.*, 1984), the overall charges on the histidine-rich and 5′ repeats are positive (+7 and +11, respectively), whereas the overall charge on VARC is negative (–28). The importance of electrostatic forces has now been confirmed by the recent studies of Voigt *et al.* (2000), who have also provided some preliminary mapping of the binding sites on PfEMP1 for KAHRP.

2.2.2. *PfEMP3* (Plasmodium falciparum *Erythrocyte Membrane Protein 3)*

P. falciparum erythrocyte membrane protein 3 (PfEMP3) was first described in a series of papers by Pasloske and co-workers (Handunnetti *et al.*, 1992a; Pasloske *et al.*, 1993, 1994). These workers had characterized a rat monoclonal antibody called 12C11 that reacted with polypeptides of 44, 95, 117, 145 and 310 kDa, and localized to material in the parasite as well as antigen aggregates in the host cell cytoplasm that extended to the plasma membrane of the infected red blood cell. Screening of an expression library with this antibody identified a clone that encoded part of the PfEMP3 coding region. The complete coding region for PfEMP3 was not known until the determination of the sequence of chromosome 2 (Gardner, M.J. *et al.*, 1998). *PfEMP3* is a two-exon gene that encodes a polypeptide of 2441 residues with a predicted iso-elelectric point of 9·18 (see Figure 2). There are extensive series of repeat regions within the protein, particularly in the carboxyl-terminal half of the protein where 82 copies of a 13-mer based on the canonical repeat NTGLKNTP(S/N)EGQQ are found. There are two other extensive repeat regions, composed of units of 19 and 22 residues. There is a buried hydrophobic region of about 20 residues starting 15 residues in from the N-terminus of the protein. Antisera raised to the recombinant protein as well as the original monoclonal antibody showed that PfEMP3 is found at the erythrocyte membrane skeleton, both within and outside knob structures (Pasloske *et al.*, 1994). Its precise linkages to host proteins at the membrane skeleton and whether it is linked to PfEMP1 or KAHRP are not known. As the *PfEMP3* gene is located immediately adjacent to the *KAHRP* gene, but closer to the telomere, spontaneous deletion events that remove KAHRP will by necessity also lead to the complete deletion of PfEMP3. Thus which of these two proteins was the major contributor to the formation of the knob structure could not be ascertained until the availability of specific knockouts (Crabb *et al.*, 1997a). Targeted deletion of *PfEMP3* produced parasites that still had numbers of knobs detectable by transmission electron microscopy, although precise knob numbers and details of morphology were not determined (Waterkeyn *et al.*, 2000). Parasites that did not express PfEMP3 appeared to cytoadhere at levels similar to those found in the parental line in both static and flow-based assays, suggesting that this protein had no direct involvement in transport or anchoring of PfEMP1 (Waterkeyn *et al.*, 2000). Further phenotypic analysis will be needed to determine the role of PfEMP3 in parasite biology.

A curious phenotype was observed in a set of mutants in which integration had occurred in the 3′ end of the gene. A truncated form of PfEMP3, lacking the C-terminal 370–470 residues, was still expressed although, curiously, expression levels were considerably higher than that found in the parental line. In these over-expression mutants, cytoadherence was markedly reduced and was concomitant with there being a reduced amount of PfEMP1 on the surface of the infected red blood cell. Instead, PfEMP1 was found to be accumulating in membrane-lined vesicles under the red blood cell membrane, a compartment in which PfEMP3 could also be found (Waterkeyn *et al.*, 2000). The authors concluded that this might be a compartment that is transiently present in normal cells, but the over-expression of PfEMP3 had led to accumulation of PfEMP1 under the surface and disruption of surface transfer. It did not appear to have affected the transport of KAHRP, which apparently moves by some other mechanism or is unsusceptible to the PfEMP3-induced blockade. The truncation of PfEMP3 did not affect its transport to the erythrocyte membrane but did interfere with its distribution on the underside of the membrane. An unresolved question is what transport processes occur after these proteins have reached these vesicles. PfEMP1 is found at knobs, with most of the protein exposed extracellularly, whereas PfEMP3 is located fairly uniformly throughout the cell, attached to the underside of the red blood cell membrane skeleton. Presumably there are further steps that traffic these proteins differently once they leave their shared location.

2.2.3. *MESA (Mature-parasite-infected Erythrocyte Surface Antigen)*

The mature-parasite-infected erythrocyte surface antigen (MESA) is a 250–300 kDa phosphoprotein (Coppel *et al.*, 1988; Howard, R.F. *et al.*, 1988) produced early in the trophozoite stage and found in association with the erythrocyte membrane skeleton (Coppel *et al.*, 1986; Howard, R.J. *et al.*, 1987). MESA interacts with the internal aspect of the host erythrocyte membrane and is not exposed on the external surface, although in late schizonts it becomes accessible to external surface-labelling reagents such as lactoperoxidase (Coppel *et al.*, 1988; Howard, R.J. *et al.*, 1988). A series of immunoprecipitation studies indicated that MESA co-precipitated with an 80 kDa phosphoprotein of host origin (Coppel *et al.*, 1988). Peptide mapping experiments suggested that this was protein 4.1 (Lustigman *et al.*, 1990). Further evidence for this interaction was provided by the observation that MESA was found in different locations in red blood cells that differed in their expression of protein 4.1 (Magowan *et al.*, 1995). In normal red blood cells, MESA is found at the periphery of the cell in association with the membrane skeleton. In contrast, in elliptocytes collected from individuals who did not express protein 4.1 in erythrocytes, MESA was found to be uniformly present in the red blood cell cytoplasm with no preference for the periphery (Magowan *et al.*, 1995). This implies that transport is a two-step process in which the protein first traffics to the red blood cell cytoplasm, followed by a second binding step to the membrane skeleton via a specific protein–protein interaction. Both MESA and protein 4.1 are phosphoproteins and in fact protein 4.1 becomes more heavily phosphorylated in infected red blood cells (Coppel *et al.*, 1988; Lustigman *et al.*, 1990; Chishti *et al.*, 1994). MESA is phosphorylated at serine residues and there are several predicted sites that are good substrates for various kinases (Coppel *et al.*, 1988; Howard, R.F. *et al.*, 1988; Coppel, 1992). Neither MESA nor protein 4.1 influence phosphorylation of their partner protein as these two proteins are phosphorylated even in mutant cells that lack the cognate binding partner (Magowan *et al.*, 1998). The kinase involved in phosphorylating MESA has an inhibitor profile characteristic of casein kinases (Magowan *et al.*, 1998), and this profile is similar to that of the kinase implicated in protein 4.1 phosphorylation in cells infected with malaria (Chishti *et al.*, 1994). Curiously, in infected cells lacking KAHRP, both MESA and protein 4.1 appear to be phosphorylated by a different kinase with a different inhibitor profile (Magowan *et al.*, 1998). A further curious observation was that MESA in red blood cells deficient in protein 4.1 was found in the Triton X-100 insoluble fraction, even though by confocal microscopy it appeared to be free in the red blood cell cytosol. This suggests that either there is an association between some parts of the infected red blood cell cytosol, perhaps via the components of the novel transport system, or different populations of MESA exist in the red blood cell that are more readily detected by the differing methods.

Determination of the primary sequence of MESA revealed that it is encoded by 2 exons (Coppel, 1992). The MESA protein is heavily charged and contains 7 distinct repeat regions, which compose over 60% of the protein. The repeat regions vary in number among different isolates and in addition there are a number of scattered mutations in non-repetitive sequence (Kun *et al.*, 1999). Overall, however, the sequence is quite strongly conserved among isolates (Kun *et al.*, 1999). The predicted secondary structure suggests that MESA is a fibrillar protein and it shows similarity to a number of cytoskeletal and neurofilament proteins, including myosin, a protein that itself binds to protein 4.1. The protein 4.1 binding domain of MESA was subsequently mapped to a 19 residues sequence (DHLYSIRNYIECLRNAPYI) near the N-terminus of the molecule, a site different from the myosin homology region. This short region appears to be capable of forming an amphipathic helix, although whether this is important for binding is not currently known. Binding of MESA to the red blood cell membrane skeleton could be inhibited by addition of exogenous protein and the 50% inhibitory concentration (IC_{50}) of this interaction was 0·63 μM, indicative of a moderate affinity interaction.

A number of studies have attempted to define the function of MESA making use of a mutant parasite line that had undergone spontaneous deletion of the end of chromosome 5 that encodes the *MESA* gene (Petersen *et al.*, 1989; Magowan *et al.*, 1995). These studies indicated that MESA was not required for cytoadherence, as measured in static assays, for formation of knobs, red blood cell invasion, or for lysis. Growth rates did not differ markedly between

MESA+ and MESA− parasite lines, although this is a difficult property to measure accurately. A curious phenotype was detected, in which MESA− parasites were able to grow in red blood cells that were deficient in protein 4.1. MESA+ parasites could not grow in such cells, and it was noted that MESA had accumulated in the infected red blood cell cytoplasm in an abnormal location. Magowan *et al.* (1995) suggested that perhaps this accumulation of MESA in an abnormal location interfered with some important cellular process such as transport of either nutrients inwards or important parasite proteins outwards in these cells. Alternatively, it may be that some other protein, also deleted by the same chromosome breakage event, gives rise to this unusual phenotype. Such questions could be answered by the generation of a gene-targeted mutant for MESA.

2.2.4. *RESA (Ring-infected Erythrocyte Surface Antigen)*

RESA was one of the first well-characterized proteins found in the ring-stage parasite, where it was noted to be associated with the periphery of the infected red blood cell (Coppel *et al.*, 1984b), and exposed to the exterior after mild glutaraldehyde treatment (Perlmann *et al.*, 1984). Biosynthetic studies suggested that this protein was synthesized in mature stages of the parasite and deposited in vesicles from which it was transferred to the red blood cell at the time of invasion (Brown, G.V. *et al.*, 1985). RESA remains detectable in the red blood cell until about 18–24 hours after invasion, when it gradually disappears about the same time as MESA appears (Coppel *et al.*, 1988). At first it was suggested that RESA accumulated in micronemes (Brown, G.V. *et al.*, 1985), but subsequently it was shown that in fact RESA was present in a population of dense granules that were released once the invading merozoite had entered the red blood cell (Aikawa *et al.*, 1990; Culvenor *et al.*, 1991). RESA was then trafficked to the red blood cell membrane skeleton by a process that is still not understood. All of this was somewhat puzzling as there were numerous reports detailing the capacity of antibodies to RESA to inhibit growth of the parasite (Wåhlin *et al.*, 1984; Berzins *et al.*, 1986; Collins *et al.*, 1986; Carlson *et al.*, 1990b). At what stage were these antibodies coming into contact with their target, as RESA was apparently not exposed during the invasion process? This question remains unresolved and RESA has continued to be assessed for its capacity to induce host protective immunity, most recently in human clinical trials in Papua New Guinea (Saul *et al.*, 1999; Genton *et al.*, 2000).

RESA was shown to be encoded by a two-exon gene on chromosome 1 (Favaloro *et al.*, 1986; Corcoran *et al.*, 1987). The protein is highly charged and contains two blocks of repetitive sequence called the 5′ and 3′ repeats. The 5′ repeats are composed of degenerate 11-mers with a consensus

DDEHVEEPTVA, whereas the 3′ repeats are composed of 8-mer and 4-mer sequences EENVEHDA and EENV. There was no typical signal sequence identified, but rather a stretch of hydrophobic residues at positions 52–65 that corresponded to the end of the first exon. Sequence conservation between *RESA* genes in different isolates was remarkably high, differing at only 3 bases over a 1500 bp stretch (Cowman *et al.*, 1984; Favaloro *et al.*, 1986). Scattered single base changes occur at the 3′ end of the gene, and these mutations appear to exist in two alternative forms such that circulating strains can be divided into one or other group (Kun *et al.*, 1994). This is similar to the dimorphic families that have been reported for merozoite surface antigens such as MSP1 and MSP2 (Anders *et al.*, 1993). It was noted that the RESA protein contained a 70 residues region with a degree of homology (39%) to a domain of the *Escherichia coli* protein DnaJ (Bork *et al.*, 1992). DnaJ is a protein that acts as a molecular chaperone and the homology was to a region of DnaJ called the DnaJ motif, a region conserved among all known homologues. The degree of homology was similar to that found between bacterial and mammalian DnaJ homologues. This has led to the proposal that RESA may itself have some sort of chaperone function, perhaps while it is bound to the red blood cell membrane skeleton.

The observation that RESA binds to the internal face of the red blood cell membrane skeleton and that it is found in the Triton X-100 extract of parasitized cells supported the idea that there was a protein–protein interaction with components of the host cell. This was confirmed by experiments in which RESA found in culture supernatant was demonstrated to bind to inside-out vesicles (IOVs) derived from normal red blood cells of several species including mouse, rabbit, sheep and human (Foley *et al.*, 1991). A second parasite protein of 73 kDa was also shown to bind to IOVs, but its identity was not known. This suggested that the RESA receptor was a well-conserved molecule and protease experiments suggested that it was protein in nature (Foley *et al.*, 1991). Binding experiments with several purified red blood cell components showed that the protein bound by RESA was in fact spectrin (Foley *et al.*, 1991; Ruangjirachuporn *et al.*, 1991). Subsequent studies localized the spectrin binding domain of RESA to 48 residues of RESA located between two blocks of repeats (Foley *et al.*, 1994). The binding domain is distinct from, but near to, the DnaJ motif. It is proposed that RESA is a modular protein with the binding domain anchoring RESA at the membrane skeleton and the DnaJ motif engaged in chaperone-like activities (see below). The region of spectrin that contains the RESA binding domain has not yet been identified. Labelling studies using [γ-^{32}P]ATP showed that RESA in ring stages was phosphorylated at serine, but not in mature stages (Foley *et al.*, 1990). This was consistent with the view that RESA is phosphorylated after spectrin binding. It is not known whether the kinase responsible is of host or parasite origin and no data are available on the inhibitor profile of the kinase involved or whether it is similar to that for the serine–threonine kinase involved in phosphorylation of MESA or protein 4.1.

Experiments with parasites that did not express RESA due to a chromosomal break showed that RESA is not required for red blood cell invasion, normal cellular growth, red blood cell lysis or cytoadherence. Experiments with nearly full-length recombinant RESA showed that binding of RESA to spectrin led to a degree of protection against heat-induced denaturation of spectrin (Da Silva *et al.*, 1994). Further, red blood cells infected with parasites lacking RESA were more susceptible to heat-induced fragmentation (Da Silva *et al.*, 1994). However, neither RESA nor anti-RESA antibodies added to resealed red blood cells before invasion seemed to inhibit the efficiency of this process, suggesting the stabilization role of RESA was not related to changing the kinetics of invasion (Da Silva *et al.*, 1994). The significance of this protection against spectrin denaturation *in vivo* is uncertain as the temperature used (50°C) was very much greater than that encountered in the bloodstream. However, there may be a number of destabilizing events, including temperature changes and the influx of calcium, that are associated with invasion.

A number of genes related to RESA have been identified, some of which contain the DnaJ motif (Cappai *et al.*, 1992; Vazeux *et al.*, 1993; Hinterberg *et al.*, 1994a; Gardner, M.J. *et al.*, 1998). The function of these various RESA-related proteins is currently unknown.

2.3. Other Less Well-Characterized Proteins in the Infected Red Blood Cell

Ag332 is a very large protein, estimated to be about 2·5 MDa, that is synthesized in young trophozoites and subsequently transported to the parasitized red blood cell, where it is found in association with large, flattened, vesicle-like structures called Maurer's clefts (Hinterberg *et al.*, 1994b). This transport process can be blocked by brefeldin A, a fungal metabolite that redistributes Golgi proteins to the endoplasmic reticulum (Hinterberg *et al.*, 1994b). The complete sequence of Ag332 is not yet available but it is known to be highly charged and to contain extensive blocks of repeats including many copies of the peptide VTEEI (Ahlborg *et al.*, 1991; Mattei *et al.*, 1992; Mattei and Scherf, 1992). This peptide is the target of Mab33G2, a monoclonal antibody that reacts with the surface of infected red blood cells and inhibits both red blood cell invasion and cytoadherence (Udomsangpetch *et al.*, 1986, 1989a). However, as antibodies to other regions of Ag332 have different reactivities and the monoclonal antibody is cross-reactive, the precise significance of these observations is unclear (Udomsangpetch *et al.*, 1989b). Such cross-reactivities bedevil the analysis of a number of proteins including D260, a 260 kDa protein that is found in the Triton X-100 insoluble fraction of proteins and varies in molecular mass between different isolates (Barnes *et al.*, 1995). Antibodies to D260 can recognize a number of other proteins including RESA and it shares sequence motifs with Ag332. Although it has many of the immunochemical properties of a protein found in the infected red blood cell, indirect fluorescent antibody studies suggest that it may be found at the periphery of the parasite, although this is by no means certain (Barnes *et al.*, 1995).

P. falciparum exported serine–threonine kinase (FEST) was first identified by screening an expression library with rabbit antiserum raised against the membrane fraction of infected cells (Kun *et al.*, 1991). The gene encoding FEST is a two-exon gene and appears not to encode a typical signal sequence at the 5′ end of the first exon. Sequence analysis indicated that the encoded protein contained all the motifs that characterize serine–threonine kinases (Kun *et al.*, 1997). These motifs were more widely separated than in other kinases due to the presence of long asparagine-rich sequences. This has been found to occur quite commonly in many *P. falciparum* sequences of housekeeping proteins, and appears to occur at regions where the presence of such extraneous loops does not interfere with protein function (Bowman *et al.*, 1999). Antibodies to fragments of this gene reacted with a doublet of 210 and 220 kDa in biosynthetically labelled proteins from infected cells. Immunofluorescence studies revealed that FEST was present throughout the life cycle but most abundant during late-trophozoite and schizont stages. It was found both within the red blood cell cytoplasm and in association with the membrane skeleton, particularly at knobs. Within the cytoplasm, it was found associated with Golgi-like stacks. Consistent with this was the observation that FEST was found in both the Triton X-100 soluble and insoluble fractions. Although it is tempting to suggest that FEST may be responsible for phosphorylation of RESA, MESA, and the 46 kDa cleft protein (see below), as yet there has been no direct demonstration of kinase activity by FEST.

The glycophorin binding protein (GBP) was first identified during a random screening of expressing clones and characterized as a mature-stage protein of 120 kDa that was immunogenic during natural infection (Coppel *et al.*, 1984a). Subsequently it was also identified using an antiserum raised against two putative merozoite surface proteins with affinity for glycophorin A. The resultant gene had a two-exon structure and encoded a protein lacking a typical N-terminal hydrophobic signal sequence and composed predominantly of 50 residues repeating units (Ravetch *et al.*, 1985; Kochan *et al.*, 1986). These repeats were implicated as the binding domain for glycophorin A (Kochan *et al.*, 1986). More recent studies have questioned these initial findings and it is now generally accepted that the glycophorin binding was artefactual (Van Schravendijk *et al.*, 1987) and that the protein is not located on the merozoite surface, but rather in the cytoplasm of the infected red blood cell. The function of GBP is not known but it is used extensively as a marker for the red blood cell compartment in transport studies.

The falciparum interspersed repeat antigen (FIRA) is another large protein of *c.* 300 kDa that is present in all asexual stages (Stahl *et al.*, 1985a; Bianco *et al.*, 1988). It is located in the red blood cell cytoplasm in an irregular punctate pattern, which becomes more intense as the parasite matures until it forms a lattice around the merozoites of the schizont (Bianco *et al.*, 1988). The gene encoding FIRA is a two-exon structure with a large second exon encoding blocks of 13 degenerate hexapeptide repeats loosely based on the consensus sequence PVTTQE (Stahl *et al.*, 1987). This protein is extremely antigenic during natural infection and is recognized by a very high proportion of individuals from their earliest infections (Stahl *et al.*, 1985a). Its function is not known but it has been suggested that it may be involved in a network of cross-reacting proteins that tend to favour induction of low affinity antibodies during infection, the so-called 'smokescreen' effect (Anders, 1986; Stahl *et al.*, 1986).

P. falciparum asparagine- and aspartate-rich protein 1 (PfAARP1) is still incompletely characterized but apparently it is a large protein of more than 700 kDa encoded by an approximately 20 kb gene found on chromosome 12 (Barale *et al.*, 1997b). Structural features of this protein include nine repeat blocks rich in asparagine and aspartate residues and a PEST domain* that is found in rapidly degraded proteins. Computer analysis predicted that PfAARP1 has multiple transmembrane domains and at least five external loops. Antisera to the PfAARP1 protein reacted with the periphery of the infected red blood cell. Antibodies affinity-purified on a repeat peptide NNDDD reacted with the surface of unfixed cells (Barale *et al.*, 1997b). Although such a result may suggest that PfAARP1 is exposed on the surface, the use of antibodies to repeat regions is fraught with technical difficulties and the possibility of artefact. There is a large family of proteins rich in asparagine and it would be extremely difficult to ensure that such anti-repeat antibodies are specific to any single protein. The authors noted that there are at least two further proteins in the PfAARP family, called PfAARP2 and PfAARP3. PfAARP2 is a protein of 150 kDa that is first synthesized about 12 hours after invasion and is transported to the red blood cell cytoplasm where it is found in a vesicular pattern reminiscent of Maurer's clefts (Barale *et al.*, 1997a). The PfAARP2 protein can be solubilized by Triton X-100, suggesting that it has no direct association with the red blood cell membrane skeleton. There are no available data on the location of PfAARP3.

The protein encoded by the *41-2* gene is reported to have a mass of 29 kDa and to be localized on the schizont membrane, the internal surface of the infected red blood cell and membranous structures in the red blood cell cytoplasm (Knapp *et al.*, 1989). The gene encoding this protein differs from

*A domain of ⩾12 amino acids containing at least one proline, one glutamic acid or aspartic acid and one serine or threonine residue.

many we have been discussing in that it is a single exon and does not encode any repeat region (Knapp *et al.*, 1989). There is an internal hydrophobic stretch of 11 residues near the N-terminus of the protein but it is shorter than that found in proteins such as GBP and FIRA.

The *P. falciparum* histidine-rich protein II (PfHRPII) is one of two low molecular mass histidine-rich proteins found in asexual stages (Wellems and Howard, 1986). The gene encoding this protein is a two-exon gene with the larger second exon containing a number of repeats that encode hexapeptides of sequence AHHAAD. The smaller protein PfHRPIII is encoded by a gene of quite similar overall structure and it is likely that the two genes resulted from a gene duplication event (Wellems and Howard, 1986). PfHRPII is a protein of *c.* 72 kDa that varies in size among isolates, based on the presence of differing numbers of repeats. The gene is not essential for growth *in vitro* or invasion, as laboratory isolates lacking this protein have been reported (Stahl *et al.*, 1985b). Immunofluorescence and immunoelectron microscopy studies localized PfHRPII to several cell compartments including the parasite cytoplasm, as discrete packets in the host erythrocyte cytoplasm and at the infected red blood cell membrane (Howard, R.J. *et al.*, 1986). The authors reported recovering approximately 50% of biosynthetically labelled PfHRPII from the cell-free supernatant of synchronized cultures at 2–24 hours and interpreted this as suggesting that the protein was secreted across several membranes (Howard, R.J. *et al.*, 1986).

PfSar1p is the *P. falciparum* homologue of a GTP-binding protein involved in trafficking proteins between the endoplasmic reticulum and the Golgi apparatus. PfSar1p shows 71% similarity to Sar1p from *Saccharomyces cerevisiae* (see Albano *et al.*, 1999a). Antibodies to PfSar1p recognized a protein of 23 kDa in immunoblots that was localized to the periphery of the parasite in discrete compartments, and that appeared distinct from the parasite endoplasmic reticulum (Albano *et al.*, 1999a). Intriguingly, PfSar1p was also found in structures in the cytoplasm of the infected red blood cell. This export was inhibited by treatment with brefeldin A. Surprisingly, there was no additional 5′ coding region in the *Sar1p* gene that might encode sequences involved in trafficking to the red blood cell, and its presence there is difficult to explain. Confirmatory experiments on the location of PfSar1p are needed but, on the basis of the paper by Albano *et al.* (1999a), there is now evidence that the parasite places components of the classical vesicle-mediated trafficking machinery inside the infected red blood cell.

The 46 kDa cleft protein is a polypeptide, identified by a several groups using various monoclonal antibodies, that has been localized to Maurer's clefts in the infected red blood cell cytoplasm (Hui and Siddiqui, 1988; Etzion and Perkins, 1989; Das *et al.*, 1994). Curiously, one of the antibodies was an anti-idiotypic reagent raised against a monoclonal antibody that reacted with the M blood group antigen on human glycophorin. The cleft protein is synthesized in red blood cells infected with ring forms and trophozoites and transported to Maurer's clefts by a brefeldin A-sensitive process (Das *et al.*, 1994). Low temperature also blocks transport, suggesting that the Golgi transport process in parasites shares many features with that found in mammalian cells. A proportion of the cleft protein becomes phosphorylated and increases slightly in size (Das *et al.*, 1994). The site of phosphorylation is suggested to be in the clefts, or at least external to the parasite. The detergent solubility of this protein can vary, suggesting that some is more tightly membrane-bound (Etzion and Perkins, 1989), and there are unresolved differences in the reports on solubility in saponin or SDS (Hui and Siddiqui, 1988). Recently, Blisnick and co-workers (2000) described a novel 1·2 kb gene in *P. falciparum* located on chromosome 7, 8 or 9, which encodes a 48 kDa protein named *Plasmodium falciparum* skeleton binding protein 1 (Pfsbp1) that appears to be associated with Maurer's clefts. The protein product, encoded by a two-exon gene, appears to bind to a 35 kDa red blood cell cytoskeletal protein, whose precise identity has not yet been defined. The relationship of Pfsbp1 to the previously described 46 kDa cleft protein is not yet known, but should be readily addressable by appropriate immunoprecipitation and co-localization studies.

Exported protein 1 (exp-1), also known as the circumsporozoite-protein-related antigen, is a protein of 23 kDa that shares sequence elements with the repeat region of the circumsporozoite protein of sporozoites (Coppel *et al.*, 1985; Hope *et al.*, 1985; Simmons *et al.*, 1987). The protein is an integral membrane protein with the membrane anchor situated in the interior of the molecule (Coppel *et al.*, 1985). The protein is localized to the periphery of the parasite and in vesicles within the red blood cell cytoplasm (Coppel *et al.*, 1985; Simmons *et al.*, 1987; Bianco *et al.*, 1988). Electron microscopic studies suggested that exp-1 is associated with the parasitophorous vacuole membrane and with membranous vesicles in the red blood cell (Simmons *et al.*, 1987; Kara *et al.*, 1988, 1990). Protease studies demonstrated that the protein is inserted in the vesicle membrane in such a way that the N-terminus is within the lumen of the vesicle and the carboxy terminus protrudes into the red blood cell cytoplasm, where it is susceptible to the exogenous protease (Günther *et al.*, 1991). The authors conclude that, based on the uniform susceptibility of exp-1 to proteases throughout its transport, it must be trafficked across the various membranes by an alternating succession of membrane fusion and membrane budding events. Whether such a process applies to all exported proteins is unknown. Also unknown is whether this is an identical set of vesicles to those that contain the 46 kDa cleft protein (Hui and Siddiqui, 1988).

Finally, the glutamic acid-rich protein (GARP) appears to be a protein in search of identity. The gene encoding this protein is absolutely typical of those encoding exported proteins, being composed of two exons with the second exon considerably larger and encoding a number of repeat regions based on tri- and penta-peptides, rich in charged amino acids (Triglia *et al.*, 1988).

Overall, the protein is predicted to be composed of 26% glutamic acid. There is no predicted hydrophobic signal sequence at the extreme N-terminus of the protein. The gene is transcribed in asexual stages and GARP is commonly recognized by sera collected from individuals living in endemic areas (Triglia *et al.*, 1988). However, neither affinity-purified antibodies nor antibodies raised to recombinant proteins react with the protein by immunoblotting, immunoprecipitation, or immunofluorescence (Triglia *et al.*, 1988), perhaps because of its unusual highly charged composition.

3. TRAFFICKING OF EXPORTED PROTEINS

The functioning of the eukaryotic cell relies on newly synthesized polypeptides being transported to the appropriate location, whether it is within the cell cytoplasm or within an organelle, at the cell membrane, or in the external milieu. A complex and highly regulated process, involving many different proteins and organelles, operates to ensure this correct targeting (Pfeffer and Rothman, 1987; Rothman and Orci, 1992; Rothman, 1994; Waters and Pfeffer, 1999). Proteins destined for any of these compartments are synthesized in the cytoplasm by a single class of ribosomes. Information encoded within the polypeptide sequence or structure itself provides instructions to the targeting machinery. Proteins that are secreted or are being transported to the cell membrane move sequentially from their site of synthesis in the rough endoplasmic reticulum (ER) through the Golgi complex by direct targeting (Allan *et al.*, 2000) for post-translational processing, and then to secretory vesicles. The secretory vesicles eventually fuse with the plasma membrane upon receipt of a signal for exocytosis and the protein contents of the vesicles either stop there by virtue of specific sequences, or pass outside the cell (Pfeffer and Rothman, 1987).

The process of protein sorting commences when mRNA molecules move into the cytoplasm of the cell and contact unbound ribosomes. Once translation commences, if the protein is bound for eventual secretion or insertion in the cell membrane, the ribosome tightly attaches to the ER in such a way that the newly synthesized polypeptide chain passes into the lumen of the ER. This targeting of secretory proteins to the ER is due to the presence of a signal sequence of approximately 15–30 residues characteristically found at the amino terminus of the protein. Typically, the signal sequence consists of one or more positively charged residues followed by a continuous stretch of about 10–12 hydrophobic residues. These sequences are usually cleaved from the polypeptide chain within the lumen of the ER by a signal peptidase. The elucidation of the role of the signal sequence in targeting proteins for movement to the cell membrane or for secretion has come from recombinant DNA experiments using chimeric gene constructs. A chimeric gene made up of a signal sequence (derived from β-lactamase) attached to the N-terminus of a protein that is not normally transported (α-globin) was made, cloned into an expression vector and transfected into cultured blood cells. The resulting protein was transported to the ER lumen, where the signal sequence was cleaved, exactly as if it had been a bona fide secreted protein (Lingappa *et al.*, 1984).

Once a polypeptide has entered the ER, it will proceed to the cell surface, unless specific signals within the protein sequence dictate its retention in an earlier compartment in the transport process, or redirection to other membrane-lined organelles. This 'bulk flow' of proteins to the cell surface passes through the cis-Golgi, the Golgi stack and the trans-Golgi before entering secretory vesicles and passing to the cell surface. Polypeptides that have been fully translocated to the lumen of the ER will be secreted, whereas those proteins that have their entry into the ER interrupted by the presence of stop-transfer or anchor sequences will be sorted to the cell surface (Pfeffer and Rothman, 1987). While in the Golgi system, polypeptides may undergo post-translational modifications such as N-linked glycosylation. Phosphorylation of N-linked oligosaccharides at mannose residues acts as a targeting signal to the lysosomes, and phosphorylation occurs in response to the presence of a particular domain structure present in the protein (Pfeffer and Rothman, 1987; Rothman and Orci, 1992).

Several protein motifs have been identified that will interfere with this default pathway. Proteins that have an N-terminal sequence of KDEL or, more generally, KXXX will become resident in the ER. This seems to occur by specific retrieval of such proteins from the Golgi system and their transport back to the ER (Rothman and Orci, 1992). Again, the importance of this sequence was elucidated by chimeric gene experiments in yeast in which the ER retention signal was added to the carboxyl terminus of a normally secreted protein (preproalpha factor fusion protein). After transfection, the resultant hybrid protein was retained in the ER (Dean and Pelham, 1990), but bore glycosylation changes typically added in the Golgi system, suggesting it had passed through that compartment before being returned to the ER. Sequences required for retention in the Golgi apparatus have also been defined by the construction of hybrid genes. In one experiment, the first of the three membrane-spanning domains of the E1 protein glycoprotein of avian coronavirus, a protein normally found in the Golgi complex, was used to replace the membrane-spanning domain of two surface proteins. This resulted in their retention in the Golgi system. Mutagenesis studies suggested that the important feature of the retention sequence appeared to be the uncharged polar residues which line one face of a predicted alpha helix (Swift and Machamer, 1991). Finally, targeting in polar cells to either the apical or basal portions of the cell appears to be in response to sequences found in the membrane-spanning and cytoplasmic domains of proteins (Weisz *et al.*, 1992). This process of protein sorting occurs in all eukaryotic cells, but the model presented above appears to be insufficient to explain the protein sorting process in the malaria parasite.

The malaria parasite appears to possess protein transport machinery that must cater for a much more complicated problem in targeting than found in the typical eukaryotic cells we have just been considering. Thus, in addition to the normal targeting locations of the parasite cytoplasm, the parasite membrane and the exterior of the cell, the parasite targets proteins to a number of cellular locations outside the parasite cell membrane. These include the red blood cell cytoplasm, the red blood cell membrane skeleton, the red blood cell surface, membrane-lined vesicles within the red blood cell cytoplasm, and possibly outside the red blood cell itself. Consideration of the infected red blood cell structure suggests that the compartment corresponding to the location of secreted proteins in a typical eukaryotic cell is the parasitophorous vacuole. No direct analogue of the compartments in the infected red blood cell exists. Thus, there appears to be no available model of protein export in eukaryotic cells that could explain the sorting of proteins to these red blood cell locations outside the parasite boundaries, nor is it clear what structures or proteins, such as chaperones or transporters, might be required to accomplish this task.

The red blood cell is, of course, devoid of the machinery for the synthesis and transport of proteins, so the parasite must somehow provide the organellar system that will allow the proteins to reach locations that are external to the parasite. Electron microscopic studies suggest the presence of clefts, loops and a complex network of tubulovesicular membranes in the red blood cell cytoplasm (Elmendorf and Haldar, 1993). These membranes appear to contain enzymes and structural proteins similar to those found in the mammalian Golgi system (Elmendorf and Haldar, 1994). In addition, there appear to be components of ABC transporters associated with these membranes (Bozdech *et al.*, 1998). Additional structures reported in this location include proteinaceous packets (Howard, R.J. *et al.*, 1986) and, recently and most controversially, a duct-like structure that allows direct connection between the parasitophorous vacuole and the external milieu (Pouvelle *et al.*, 1991). The evolving consensus is that the tubulovesicular membranes may be involved in uptake of substances to the parasite, particularly lipid, but the structures involved in the outward transport of the proteins remain largely mysterious. Importantly, however, evidence exists that both the group of exported proteins and rhoptry proteins start the export pathway in a conventional manner (Haldar, 1998). For example, the fungal metabolite brefeldin A, which inhibits protein secretion in higher eukaryotes by disrupting the integrity of the Golgi apparatus, will disrupt the transport of proteins exported to the red blood cell such as GBP and the 45 kDa cleft protein, as well as transport of rhoptry proteins to the rhoptries (Howard, R.F. and Schmidt, 1995). Thus there is at least one important similarity between the transport process used in infected red blood cells and higher eukaryotes.

In the previous section we discussed some of the extensive information about the primary amino acid sequence and cellular location of a large number of malaria proteins (Coppel *et al.*, 1994). In particular, many of the exported proteins lack typical signal sequences at their amino termini. The amino-terminal sequences of these proteins are studded with charged residues and lack a preponderance of hydrophobic residues such as phenylalanine, tyrosine, valine, leucine, or isoleucine, and instead contain many polar or hydrophilic residues such as serine or asparagine. The buried hydrophobic regions noted in proteins such as GBP, KAHRP and MESA are located approximately 20–60 residues from the N-terminus, and are hypothesized to signal export beyond the parasitophorous vacuole. For proteins that bind to the red blood cell membrane skeleton, additional cytoskeletal binding sequences, such as those described in RESA (Foley *et al.*, 1994) and MESA (Bennett, B.J. *et al.*, 1997), would guide proteins already in the red blood cell cytoplasm to these sites. Similarly, PfEMP-1 found at the red blood cell surface would have a membrane binding signal in addition to the red blood cell export signal (Baruch *et al.*, 1995). The way to test such hypotheses would be to take advantage of the new transfection technology (Waller, R.F. *et al.*, 2000) and introduce into parasites various chimeric constructs in which regions of transported proteins are added to proteins that are normally present in the cytoplasm. The location of these chimeric proteins could then be determined. It is expected that results of such experiments should be forthcoming in the not too distant future.

Beyond the question of what signals for transport may be encoded within the sequence of these proteins are the questions of what transport machinery the parasite uses to traffic proteins and what machinery it may place in the red blood cell? Also, how are the proteins able to cross so many membranes and spaces to reach their final locations? We do not yet possess a detailed understanding of the transport system but there is general agreement about at least some issues. The first of these is that the parasite possesses a conventional protein transport machinery including an ER. There are several lines of evidence for this including the identification of proteins that are components of the ER such as BiP (Peterson *et al.*, 1988) and PfERC (La Greca *et al.*, 1997) and many other proteins that are involved in vesicular transport pathways (reviewed by Albano *et al.*, 1999b). Furthermore, parasites are sensitive to the action of brefeldin A, a drug that disrupts the Golgi apparatus. When this drug is applied to cultures of parasites, several proteins are blocked from transport to their final destinations, including the rhoptry protein RAP-1 (Howard, R.F. *et al.*, 1998), the merozoite surface protein MSP1 (Wiser *et al.*, 1997), and the exported proteins GBP (Benting *et al.*, 1994) and Ag332 (Hinterberg *et al.*, 1994b). Wiser and colleagues (1997), working with *P. chabaudi*, confirmed that many exported proteins are blocked from transport to the red blood cell when parasites are exposed to brefeldin A. However, they appear to accumulate in a different location from that of proteins such as MSP1. These authors suggested that there are two distinct transport compartments, one for proteins exported to the red blood cell and the other for proteins secreted to the parasitophorous vacuole, the rhoptries and the merozoite surface. These studies were performed using a confocal microscope and it is still questionable whether this instrument has sufficient resolving power to determine if these two locations are truly distinct compartments. To complicate matters further, at least one exported protein, KAHRP, is transported by a brefeldin A-insensitive pathway (Mattei *et al.*, 1999).

There are a number of different types of vesicles present in the red blood cell cytoplasm. Dye labelling studies by Pouvelle and co-workers (1994) suggested that many of these vesicles contain membrane derived from the parasitophorous vacuole. Electron microscopic studies by Trelka *et al.* (2000) revealed the presence of electron-dense vesicles, similar in appearance to mammalian secretory vesicles, in proximity to smooth tubulovesicular elements at the periphery of the parasite cytoplasm. These vesicles appeared to be coated and were found in the red blood cell, some being close to the parasitophorous vacuole membrane. The vesicles appeared to bind to, and fuse with, the red blood cell membrane, giving rise to cup-shaped electron-dense structures. An identical appearance had already been noted in studies on MESA transport (Coppel *et al.*, 1986). Treatment of mature parasites with aluminium tetrafluoride resulted in the accumulation of the vesicles with an electron-dense limiting membrane in the erythrocyte cytosol into multiple vesicle strings (Trelka *et al.*, 2000). As this reagent prevents coat shedding of vesicles, it suggests a process that is G-protein regulated. These vesicles appeared to be involved in the transport of parasite proteins PfEMP1 and PfEMP3 as they co-localized with the vesicles.

In addition to the problem of the transport of proteins to the red blood cell, there is also the issue of transport, predominantly of nutrients, in the other direction. New permeation pathways are elaborated by the parasite within the red blood cell and these have wide-ranging effects on permeability. A detailed discussion of this is beyond the scope of this review, but one may be found in the recent Novartis Foundation symposium on transport and trafficking in the malaria-infected erythrocyte (Bock and Cardew, 1999). As has been mentioned above, the tubulovesicular network has been implicated in transport of material to the interior of the parasite cell. One aspect of internal trafficking that has been completely ignored is the removal of parasite proteins from the red blood cell membrane skeleton. As mentioned, RESA is a protein found in dense granules in the merozoite that makes its way after invasion to the red blood cell membrane skeleton where it binds to spectrin. After about 18–22 hours, RESA disappears from the red blood cell membrane at about the time that MESA appears (Coppel *et al.*, 1988). How does this happen? Is it detached and trafficked back to the parasite or is it selectively digested by proteases of host or parasite origin? We simply do not know. Certainly there appear to be one or more proteases active in the infected red blood cell cytoplasm, at least as judged by the apparent loss of spectrin during parasite development (Schrével *et al.*, 1990). Several studies have reported decrease in spectrin levels and other membrane skeleton components such as glycophorin in red blood cells infected by *P. berghei*, *P. chabaudi* and *P. lophurae* (see Weidekamm *et al.*, 1973; Konigk and Mirtsch, 1977; Sherman and Jones, 1979). However, this proteolysis of RESA would need to be selective, as there is no report of other exported proteins of parasite origin being affected. It would be interesting to know whether any other parasite proteins are also removed in this fashion, as it might be part of a previously unrecognized retrograde trafficking mechanism. However, it should be pointed out that few studies have been performed in a sufficiently quantitative manner for any strong conclusion to be drawn. Studies have noted the presence of uninfected red blood cells containing RESA in the circulation and this has been used to infer the existence of splenic removal of parasites from infected red blood cells (Angus *et al.*, 1997; Chotivanich *et al.*, 2000a). This suggests that the removal of RESA from the red blood cell membrane requires the presence of the parasite and could support the concept of a continuing trafficking process.

4. ALTERATIONS TO NATIVE RED BLOOD CELL PROTEINS DURING MALARIA INFECTION

Infection leads to several changes in antigenicity and arrangement of host red blood cell membrane proteins. The overall architecture of the red blood cell membrane skeleton does not appear to change, at least as revealed by whole cell mount electron microscopy, although electron-dense aggregates do appear (Taylor *et al.*, 1987a,b). Intramembranous particles (primarily due to glycophorins and tetramers of band 3) are specifically redistributed in the region of the knob (Allred *et al.*, 1986). This clustering of band 3 at knobs is also suggested by specific knob labelling using concanavalin A, a lectin that recognizes glycosylated band 3 (Sherman and Greenan, 1986). Band 3 undergoes several modifications to give rise to forms of >240 kDa and 65 kDa, which are more reactive with anti-band 3 autoantibodies (Winograd *et al.*, 1987). It has been reported that monoclonal antibodies that recognize band 3 only in parasitized cells (termed Pfalhesin) have also been prepared (Winograd and Sherman, 1989) and these are capable of blocking cytoadherence of infected red blood cells to C32 amelanotic melanoma cells or CD36, as are synthetic peptides based on the sequence of the altered band 3 (Crandall *et al.*, 1993).

These results appear to be contradicted by recent papers from the same group, which now highlight thrombospondin as the host receptor for modified band 3 (Lucas and Sherman, 1998; Eda *et al.*, 1999). It is not known precisely what processes lead to modification of band 3 but they are probably related to structural changes in the red blood cell secondary to malaria infection, since antibodies that react with altered band 3 on the surface of parasitized cells also react with the surface of sickle red blood cells and reduce their adhesiveness to cultured endothelial cells (Thevenin *et al.*, 1997). Levels of phosphorylation of red blood cell membrane skeletal proteins are also affected by malarial infection (Yuthavong and Limpaiboon, 1987; Murray and Perkins, 1989; Lustigman *et al.*, 1990; Chishti *et al.*, 1994). In red blood cells infected with *P. berghei*, there is a marked increase in phosphorylation of a 43 kDa red blood cell membrane skeletal protein, perhaps actin, and this increase correlates directly with filterability and inversely with the osmotic fragility of the infected cells (Yuthavong and Limpaiboon, 1987). In red blood cells infected with *P. falciparum* there is a marked increase in phosphorylation of protein 4.1, sometimes as much as tenfold, depending on the infecting parasite strain (Lustigman *et al.*, 1990; Chishti *et al.*, 1994). Since phosphorylation of protein 4.1 inhibits spectrin–actin interactions mediated by the protein (Ling *et al.*, 1988), one may expect that the parasite-induced phosphorylation would reduce membrane mechanical stability. This is accompanied by a lesser, but still measurable, increase in phosphorylation of band 3 (Chishti *et al.*, 1994).

5. ALTERATIONS IN CELLULAR PROPERTIES OF INFECTED RED BLOOD CELLS

Light and electron microscopic studies of infected red blood cells have identified a number of morphological changes within the red blood cell cytoplasm associated with infection. A number of names, such as Maurer's clefts and Schuffner's dots, have been given to these structures. Some of them can be seen by electron microscopy to be novel membranous structures that resemble Golgi stacks (Haldar, 1994). Their role is still controversial, but the balance of evidence suggests that they are most probably part of new pathways for nutrient transport by the parasite. The infected red blood cell becomes spherocytic with its surface punctuated by 5000–10 000 localized, electron-dense elevations of the red blood cell membrane called knobs (Aikawa, 1977; Aikawa and Miller, 1983; Gruenberg and Sherman, 1983). The knobs are located over the junctional complexes of the red blood cell (Chishti *et al.*, 1992; Oh *et al.*, 1997) and vary in size (70–150 nm) and density (10–70/μm^2), becoming smaller and more numerous as the parasite matures (Gruenberg *et al.*, 1983). Knobs appear to be required for parasitized red blood cells to cytoadhere *in vivo* (Howard, R.J., 1988; Crabb *et al.*, 1997a) and are invariably found on infected red blood cells isolated directly from patients (Van Schravendijk *et al.*, 1991; Nakamura *et al.*, 1992). Further ultrastructural studies suggest that adhesion actually occurs between the parasite ligand PfEMP1 localized at knobs and the surface of the other cell (Van Schravendijk *et al.*, 1991; Nakamura *et al.*, 1992). Two recent papers have examined the knob structure using atomic force microscopy (Aikawa *et al.*, 1996; Nagao *et al.*, 2000). Interestingly, these studies revealed that knobs are in fact positively charged, with a membrane potential of +20 mV, when compared with the remainder of the red blood cell membrane which is negatively charged, and they are raised above the red blood cell membrane by 18–25 nm (Aikawa *et al.*, 1996). Although one study suggested that knobs were composed of two distinct subunits (Aikawa *et al.*, 1996), this was not borne out in the second study (Nagao *et al.*, 2000), which demonstrated that the two sub-units structure was in fact an artefact of the technology used. The number of knobs is linearly related to the number of parasites infecting a particular cell (Nagao *et al.*, 2000) and, using this method of measurement, knob volume does not decrease with maturation of the parasite. It has been noted that there are a number of small electron-dense patches (30–65 nm) that are distinct from knobs in whole cell mounts of infected cells; however, the nature of these patches and their constituent molecules are not known (Taylor *et al.*, 1987b). Other species of *Plasmodium* have been reported to express knobs and these have been shown to be the site of cytoadherence (Kawai *et al.*, 1995).

6. RHEOLOGICAL CHANGES IN INFECTED RED BLOOD CELLS

Red blood cells are incredibly robust with uniquely adapted mechanical properties that enable them to circulate repeatedly up to half a million times during their 120 days' lifetime under the harsh extrinsic shear forces of the circulation *in vivo*. This is possible because red blood cells are highly deformable structures, which can undergo rapid and reversible shape changes repeatedly when exposed to haemodynamic shear. Normally biconcave discs in their 'resting' state, red blood cells deform to ellipses and align linearly in large vessels during arterial flow (Fischer, T.M. *et al.*, 1978). Furthermore, red blood cells can bend and fold to produce 'slipper' and other forms (Gaehtgens *et al.*, 1980) to enable these cells, which have diameters of approximately 8 μm, to traverse capillaries in the microcirculation with luminal diameters down to 3 μm or through the intraendothelial slits and basement membrane fenestrations in the spleen. The principle of cell deformability, and the wide array of methods available for its measurement, have been well reviewed in the past (Bull *et al.*, 1984; Stuart *et al.*, 1984; Stuart, 1985; Evans, 1989).

Fundamentally, there are three major determinants of red blood cell deformability: (i) the low viscosity of the cytoplasm (essentially just a solution of haemoglobin), (ii) the high surface area to cell volume ratio, and (iii) the highly visco-elastic membrane. Additionally, red blood cells are able to freely rotate their membrane around their cytoplasm in a ‘tank-treading’ fashion, which further facilitates transluminal passage by reducing hydraulic resistance (Bagge *et al.*, 1980; Gaehtgens *et al.*, 1980; Secomb and Skalak, 1982).

Invasion of red blood cells by malaria parasites has profound effects on all of these factors and as a consequence the rheological properties of parasitized cells are dramatically altered (Cranston *et al.*, 1984; Nash *et al.*, 1989; Paulitschke and Nash, 1993; Dondorp *et al.*, 2000). Compared with normal red blood cells, parasitized cells are more rigid, less deformable and, to a greater or lesser extent, more spherocytic. As the parasite matures, the cells' ability to circulate becomes increasingly impaired, and eventually they become completely immobilized in the microvasculature. The decreased deformability of parasitized cells is likely to impede the passage of these cells through the intraendothelial fenestrations in the spleen. It has been suggested that cytoadherence may have evolved in order to minimize exposure of rigid parasitized cells in the spleen and thus minimize splenic sequestration and their consequent destruction.

It is now almost 30 years since Miller and colleagues (1971, 1972) first demonstrated reduced deformability in monkey red blood cells parasitized by *P. knowlesi* and *P. coatneyi*, using relatively simple filtration techniques in which the rate of filtration of suspensions of parasitized cells through small diameter pores in filters was quantified. Flow rates were lowest for samples containing large numbers of mature parasites. Similar decreased filterability was reported for *P. falciparum*, using clinical isolates (Lee *et al.*, 1982). This decrease in filterability, however, was largely influenced by the presence of the rigid, spherical parasite itself, which may occupy as much as 90% of the total volume of the red blood cell. Furthermore, these filtration techniques were relatively insensitive and detected measurable differences only when the parasitaemia was high. This is frequently not the case for clinical isolates and methods for enrichment of parasitized cells would therefore be required which, themselves, may influence the results. Filtration times are also dominated by the presence of leucocytes, which must be removed from clinical samples before any meaningful result can be obtained (Chien *et al.*, 1983; Chan *et al.*, 1984). Cranston and colleagues (1984) were able to observe directly the flow behaviour of culture-derived parasitized cells in a rheoscope. They measured the extent of red blood cell elongation (length to width ratio) induced by graded levels of shear stress, the prevalence of tank-treading, and the time course for recovery of cell shape in synchronous cultures of parasitized cells and non-parasitized controls. A knobby line of *P. falciparum*, Indochina 1, and a knobless clonal line, D4, were examined. Red blood cells containing young ring-stage parasites elongated less than controls and had a tendency to tumble, rather than align in the direction of flow. Moreover, the time taken to recover cell shape following cessation of applied shear stress was slower. The magnitude of these changes increased as the parasite matured, so that red blood cells infected with more mature, pigmented stages were even less deformable than ring forms and did not linearly align or tank-tread in flow. Knobless red blood cells were also relatively non-deformable, but quantitative data were not reported. This provided the first direct evidence that the extent of cellular modification was directly linked to the degree of parasite maturation. Although, in contrast to filtration, the rheoscope enabled individual cells to be observed directly, alterations in the mechanical properties of the cell membrane could not be precisely dissected from the influence of the parasite. Nash *et al.* (1989), however, addressed this problem by examining the membrane mechanical properties of individual cells using glass micropipettes. They aspirated individual red blood cells infected by both the uncharacterized cultured line WL and clinical isolates into micropipettes (3 μm diameter) and measured the time and pressure required for complete aspiration of the cell. They also demonstrated a loss of deformability that was greater for red blood cells infected with mature stages of parasites. Further, by measuring the increase in the length of a 'tongue' of red blood cell membrane aspirated into micropipettes with a much smaller diameter (*c.* 1·5 μm) at defined increasing pressures, they were able to calculate the shear elastic modulus for the cell membrane. Then, by simple geometry, they were able to estimate the surface area and volume of infected red blood cells. This was the first time that parasite-induced changes to the mechanical properties of the red blood cell membrane itself, which were not influenced by the presence of the parasite, had been quantified. There was some loss of deformability at the ring stage of infection, which was attributed to a reduction in the surface area to volume ratio and a slight rigidification of the cell membrane. Membrane rigidity was even higher for red blood cells containing mature forms, although no distinction was made between trophozoites and schizonts. The importance of particular parasite proteins in changing red blood cell properties has been suggested by Paulitschke and Nash (1993), who examined a series of knobby and knobless parasites. Although there was considerable inter-strain variation, a trend for increased membrane rigidity in knobby red blood cells was observed. A caveat to this study, however, was that the parasite lines tested came from a wide variety of different genetic backgrounds and from diverse geographical locations. This may explain the relatively high level of inter-strain variation and, moreover, may have masked detection of any subtle change that may have existed between different parasite lines.

Many cellular changes observed in the infected red blood cell cannot yet be related to specific molecular interactions. For example, the parasite exerts considerable oxidative stress on the red blood cell, which can contribute to loss of membrane deformability, presumably by affecting a number of different proteins (Hunt and Stocker, 1990). Nor do we know what events result in the predictable lysis of the infected red blood cell about 48 hours after invasion, in the case of *P. falciparum*. It is reasonable to suppose that the reported decrease in the amount of red blood cell spectrin may be involved (Schrével *et al.*, 1990), as could alteration in the polarity and components of the red blood cell lipid bilayer.

Interestingly, some studies have shown that the deformability of non-parasitized red blood cells is also reduced during malaria infection (Lee *et al.*, 1982; Areekul and Yamarat, 1988) and appears to be related to an increase in the rigidity of the red blood cell membrane itself (Dondorp *et al.*, 2000). Furthermore, the degree of red blood cell rigidification appears to be greater in individuals with more severe disease, when measured by ektacytometry (Dondorp *et al.*, 1997). Others, however, have failed to confirm such observations by examining the rigidity of individual non-parasitized red blood cells from malaria cultures by micropipette analysis (Paulitschke and Nash, 1993). The mechanism by which the deformability of non-parasitized cells might be affected by malaria parasites is not known, but one possibility is the binding to the surface of non-parasitized red blood cells of exoantigens released by malaria parasites (Read *et al.*, 1990; Naumann *et al.*, 1991). When examined by immunofluorescence, a number of non-parasitized red blood cells from the peripheral blood of infected individuals also appeared to contain RESA in association with the red blood cell membrane skeleton (Angus *et al.*, 1997; Chotivanich *et al.*, 2000a). The presence of RESA in red blood cells that clearly did not contain parasites is difficult to explain, but could result from the selective removal of the parasite from some red blood cells in the spleen, followed by re-sealing and return of the red blood cell to the peripheral circulation. Although the deformability of such 'pitted' cells has not been quantified, it is reasonable to expect that rheological properties would be measurably altered. Clearly, more work is required to resolve this issue; however, the phenomenon could provide an explanation for the beneficial effects of exchange transfusion in individuals with severe malaria.

Changes in the rheological properties of uninfected red blood cells may also be implicated in the phenomenon of anaemia secondary to malaria infection. This is a common and severe complication of malaria, especially in young children, and is suggested to account for approximately 50% of malaria mortality in some endemic areas. The pathogenesis of this anaemia is not well understood and is almost certainly multifactorial (see Menendez *et al.*, 2000 and Wickramasinghe and Abdalla, 2000 for recent reviews). In addition to the obligatory lysis of parasitized red blood cells during schizont rupture, the greatest contributor to the reduction in haematocrit appears to be an accelerated destruction of uninfected red blood cells (Looareesuwan *et al.*, 1991; Salmon *et al.*, 1997). The mechanism by which uninfected red blood cells are destroyed has not been fully elucidated; however, reduced cell deformability (Dondorp *et al.*, 2000), inversion of the membrane lipid bilayer (Joshi *et al.*, 1986) and increased red blood cell immunoglobulin binding resulting in premature phagocytosis or complement-mediated lysis (Waitumbi *et al.*, 2000) have all been suggested to play an important role. Clearly, further studies are needed to provide a convincing explanation for the pathogenesis of the anaemia during malaria.

7. ALTERED ADHESIVE PROPERTIES OF INFECTED RED BLOOD CELLS

Essentially, we can conveniently divide the altered adhesive properties of parasitized red blood cells into four distinct cytoadhesive phenotypes. Parasitized cells can adhere directly to the vascular endothelial cells (cytoadhesion), to uninfected red blood cells (rosetting), to other infected red blood cells (autoagglutination) and, most recently described, to dendritic cells (Urban *et al.*, 1999). Undoubtedly the most extensively studied of these is the interaction of infected red blood cells with the endothelial cells that line the vascular intima. As a consequence of this, red blood cells infected by mature parasites accumulate in the microvasculature and are notably absent from the peripheral circulation, a diagnostic feature of falciparum malaria. This phenomenon, known as sequestration, protects parasitized cells from entrapment and destruction in the spleen and maintains the microaerophilic parasites in a relatively hypoxic environment. While clearly beneficial for the parasite, sequestered red blood cells can perturb or completely obstruct blood flow in small diameter vessels of the microcirculation (Raventos-Suarez *et al.*, 1985), with serious vaso-occlusive consequences. Furthermore, high levels of inflammatory cytokines that are released locally at sites of sequestration can both increase the number of parasitized cells that accumulate or increase disease severity by a more generalized systemic effect of increased levels of circulating cytokines (Udomsangpetch *et al.*, 1997). The dogma that it is only red blood cells infected with mature stages of *P. falciparum* that are capable of cytoadherence has recently been challenged (Pouvelle *et al.*, 2000). These investigators examined parasite lines that had been selected *in vitro* for their ability to bind to CSA, or clinical isolates collected from a number of sources including the placentas of pregnant women. They noted significant numbers of red blood cells containing immature ring-stage parasites, which were capable of binding to cultured vascular endothelial cells derived from monkey brain. The adherent parasitized red blood cells had not matured sufficiently to express PfEMP1, but were shown to have two as yet uncharacterized polypeptides of approximately 200 kDa and 40 kDa, designated ring surface protein-1 (RSP-1) and RSP-2 respectively, on the red blood cell surface. The receptor that these putative ligands recognized on the endothelial cell surface is also not certain but the interaction may involve heparan-like proteoglycans. Interestingly, as the parasites mature to trophozoites and PfEMP1 begins to appear on the red blood cell surface, the parasitized red blood cells switch to an exclusively CSA-binding phenotype and RSP-1 and RSP-2 disappear. Novel findings of this type undoubtedly require replication, and further studies will be needed to assess the significance of ring-stage adhesion in the pathogenesis of malaria. Again, however, this emphasizes the complexity of this ancient host–parasite relationship. The existence of rosettes and autoagglutinates in the circulation *in vivo* remains uncertain, although several studies have shown a correlation between both of these phenomena, when quantified in patients' blood *in vitro*, and the severity of clinical disease (Carlson *et al.*, 1990a; Treutiger *et al.*, 1992; Rowe *et al.*, 1995; Roberts *et al.*, 2000). Neither is their contribution to vascular obstruction well understood; however, both rosettes and autoagglutinates have been observed to form in flow-based adhesion assays that mimic the circulation *in vivo* using parasites taken directly from individuals with malaria (Cooke *et al.*, 1993). The force of interaction between uninfected and parasitized red blood cells in rosettes is at least five times higher than that between parasitized red blood cells and endothelial cells (see Table 4) when measured by single cell micromanipulation (Nash *et al.*, 1992a). Furthermore, rosettes from both laboratory-adapted parasite lines and clinical isolates can withstand disruption by physiologically relevant shear stresses applied using a rotational viscometer *in vitro* (Chotivanich *et al.*, 2000b).

7.1. Cytoadhesion

Because of the association of cytoadherence and sequestration with severe clinical syndromes such as cerebral malaria, where infected red blood cells preferentially sequester in the brain (MacPherson *et al.*, 1985; Pongponratn *et al.*, 1991; Silamut *et al.*, 1999), numerous studies have examined this phenomenon. Adhesion appears to be a critical process for maintenance of parasite virulence, as isolates that have lost the capacity to bind cause mild or inapparent infections in laboratory animals (Langreth and Peterson, 1985). Cytoadherence has been studied in a number of systems *in vitro* and infected red blood cells have been shown to be capable of adhering to at least 11 different receptors that are expressed on the surface of vascular endothelial cells or in the placenta, which differ in structure from members of the immunoglobulin super family and integrins to glycosamino- and proteoglycans (Figure 4 and Table 4). Although adhesion to some of these receptors

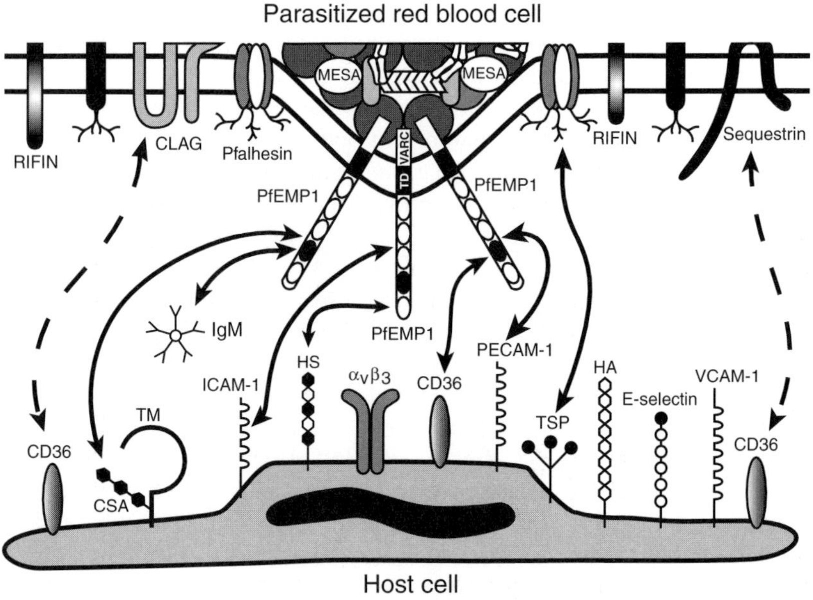

Figure 4 Schematic representation of the diverse array of molecules implicated in the adhesive interaction between red blood cells infected with *P. falciparum* and vascular endothelial cells or placental syncytiotrophoblasts (host cell). The figure shows a typical knob at the infected red blood cell membrane formed by the interaction of parasite-encoded proteins such as KAHRP, PfEMP3 and MESA with the red blood cell membrane skeleton. Solid arrows indicate interactions between specific receptors on the surface of the infected red blood cell and the host cell only where these have been unequivocally determined. Broken arrows indicate interactions for which there is currently less compelling evidence. References describing these interactions are provided in Table 3. Abbreviations: $\alpha_V\beta_3$, $\alpha_V\beta_3$ integrin; other abbreviations are expanded on pp. 2–3.

appears to be associated with particular forms of severe malaria (e.g., CSA and HA in placental malaria, or CD36 and ICAM-1 in the brain in the case of cerebral malaria), it is not, however, clear how relevant several of these interactions are *in vivo* (Cooke and Coppel, 1995). For example, the strength of binding of parasitized red blood cells to thrombospondin appears to be too low to allow formation of this interaction in normal post-capillary venules, where parasitized cells preferentially sequester (Cooke *et al.*, 1994). Similarly, adhesion of parasitized cells to hyaluronic acid (HA) appears to be critically shear-dependent (Table 5), so that high levels of adhesion occur only at shear stresses lower than those predicted to exist in post-capillary venules (Beeson *et al.*, 2000). This might indicate, however, that HA could be used only as a receptor for sequestration of parasitized cells in the placenta, where blood

Table 4 Receptor–ligand interactions implicated in cytoadherence and rosetting of red blood cells infected with *P. falciparum.*

Host receptor[a]	Parasite ligand[a]	Comments[a]	References
Cytoadherence			
CD36	PfEMP1	Most common binding phenotype of parasites; CIDR region of PfEMP1 appears to be involved; polymorphisms exist in CD36 in Africans, which appear to affect disease severity	Oquendo *et al.*, 1989; Baruch *et al.*, 1995, 1996; Chen, Q. *et al.*, 2000
ICAM-1 (CD54)	PfEMP1	Member of the immunoglobulin superfamily; rolling receptor for parasitized cells under flow; polymorphisms exist in ICAM-1 in Africans, which may influence adhesion and affect disease severity	Berendt *et al.*, 1989, 1992; Baruch *et al.*, 1996; Smith *et al.*, 2000
TSP	PfEMP1	Physiological role is in question due to low affinity of the binding under flow conditions	Roberts *et al.*, 1985; Sherwood *et al.*, 1987; Cooke *et al.*, 1994; Baruch *et al.*, 1996
TSP	Pfalhesin	Pfalhesin represents altered host red blood cell band 3, the anion transporter; previously reported to bind to CD36 but recently disputed	Crandall *et al.*, 1993, 1994; Lucas and Sherman, 1998; Eda *et al.*, 1999
Chondroitin-4-sulphate	PfEMP1	Found in association with thrombomodulin on the endothelial cell surface and on syncytiotrophoblasts of the placenta; appears to be important in malaria during pregnancy	Rogerson *et al.*, 1995; Fried and Duffy, 1996; Buffet *et al.*, 1999; Reeder *et al.*, 1999; Maubert *et al.*, 2000
HA	?	Appears to be important in malaria during pregnancy; low affinity binding under flow conditions	Beeson *et al.*, 2000
PECAM-1 (CD31)	PfEMP1	Appears to be an uncommon binding target for parasitized cells	Newbold *et al.*, 1997b; Treutiger *et al.*, 1997; Chen, Q. *et al.*, 2000
E-selectin (CD62E)	?	Appears to be an uncommon binding target for parasitized cells	Ockenhouse *et al.*, 1992

Table 4 continued

Host receptor[a]	Parasite ligand[a]	Comments[a]	References
VCAM-1 (CD106)	?	Member of the immunoglobulin superfamily; appears to be an uncommon binding receptor	Ockenhouse *et al.*, 1992; Newbold *et al.*, 1997b
CD36	Sequestrin	Obtained using an unusual approach with anti-idiotype reagents; role in cytoadhesion remains questionable	Ockenhouse *et al.*, 1991b
?	Clag9	Knockout of the *clag9* gene ablates binding of parasitized cells to CD36; precise role in adhesion remains unknown	Gardiner *et al.*, 2000; Trenholme *et al.*, 2000
$\alpha_v\beta_3$	?	First integrin receptor described for parasitized cells; remains to be independently confirmed or shown to be a receptor for clinical isolates	Siano *et al.*, 1998
Rosetting			
CR1 (CD35)	PfEMP1	CD35 polymorphisms exist in Africans, which may confer protection against detrimental effects of rosetting	Rowe, A. *et al.*, 1995
HS-like GAG	PfEMP1	Suggested to be heparan sulphate on red blood cell via GAG binding motifs on PfEMP1 DBL-1 domain; likely to be involved in heparin-sensitive rosetting	Chen, Q. *et al.*, 1998a, 2000; Barragan *et al.*, 2000a
CD36	PfEMP1	The level of CD36 present on older red blood cells is very low; the importance of this interaction is unknown	Handunnetti *et al.*, 1992b
Rosettins/rifins	?	Poorly defined, low molecular weight proteins implicated in rosetting and possibly adhesion to CD31	Helmby *et al.*, 1993; Chen, Q. *et al.*, 1998a; Cheng *et al.*, 1998; Fernandez *et al.*, 1999
ABO blood group antigens	PfEMP1	Appear to influence size rather than frequency of rosetting; blood group A appears to be particularly important	Carlson and Wählgren, 1992; Barragan *et al.*, 2000b; Chen, Q. *et al.*, 2000

[a] Abbreviations are expanded on pp. 2–3.

Table 5 Force required to detach red blood cells from other cells or purified receptors *in vitro*.

Red blood cells[a]	Cell/Receptor[a]	Force (pN)	References
RBC	HUVEC	4[b]	Nash *et al.*, 1992b; Rowland *et al.*, 1993
SSRBC	HUVEC	8[b]	Rowland *et al.*, 1993
PRBC	C32 melanoma	60[c]	Nash *et al.*, 1992b
PRBC	HUVEC	86[b,c]	Nash *et al.*, 1992b
PRBC	ICAM-1	Note d	–
PRBC	CD36	50[b]	Cooke *et al.*, 1994; Crabb *et al.*, 1997a
PRBC	CSA	42[b]	Cooke *et al.*, 1996
PRBC	TSP	Note e	–
PRBC	TM	50[b]	Rogerson *et al.*, 1997
PRBC	HA	14[b]	Beeson *et al.*, 2000
PRBC	Normal RBC	440[c]	Nash *et al.*, 1992a

[a] Abbreviations are expanded on pp. 2–3.
[b] Force calculated from the wall shear stress required to detach adherent red blood cells in a parallel-plate flow chamber.
[c] Force measured by single cell micropipette manipulation.
[d] Detachment force not quantified since PRBC continuously roll on this receptor under flow (Cooke *et al.*, 1994).
[e] PRBC do not adhere to TSP under flow conditions (Cooke *et al.*, 1994).

flow is slower than elsewhere in the body (Ramsey and Donner, 1980). The significance of the interaction with PECAM-1 (CD31) is also hard to gauge, as CD31 appears to be confined to areas of cell–cell contact between endothelial cells and to be absent from the luminal face to which parasitized cells adhere (Treutiger *et al.*, 1997). Although CD31 may redistribute to the luminal face under IFN-γ stimulation, both the timing and extent to which this happens during malaria infection are unknown.

For endothelial adhesion, the most common interaction appears to be between PfEMP1 and CD36, with studies suggesting that most if not all parasites can adhere to this receptor (Hasler *et al.*, 1990; Ho *et al.*, 1991; Ockenhouse *et al.*, 1991a, 1992; Cooke *et al.*, 1995; Newbold *et al.*, 1997b). The binding site on PfEMP1 has been localized within the CIDR (Baruch *et al.*, 1997) and it has been demonstrated that recombinant proteins from this region are capable of blocking and even reversing adherence of several isolates expressing antigenically distinct forms of PfEMP1 (Cooke *et al.*, 1998). It has proved difficult to detect CD36 on endothelial cells of the cerebral circulation, particularly in post-mortem studies of patients who have died of cerebral malaria (Turner *et al.*, 1994). In fact these individuals appear to be preferentially infected by parasites that adhere to both CD36 and ICAM-1, a receptor readily identified in cerebral vessels. Chondroitin-4-sulphate appears to be present at high levels on the surface of syncytiotrophoblasts in the placenta (Maubert *et al.*, 2000) and isolates that recognize this receptor (but not CD36 or ICAM-1) appear to be preferentially involved in malaria during pregnancy (Rogerson *et al.*, 1995; Fried and Duffy, 1996; Maubert *et al.*, 2000). Such isolates may constitute a relatively restricted population, and development of strain-specific immunity to these may limit subsequent infection. This could explain why primigravidae are so much more susceptible to malaria than multigravidae.

One point of interest is the behaviour of parasitized red blood cells when they interact with different receptors under conditions of flow. When parasitized cells interact with CD36 they remain stationary, whereas they continuously roll over ICAM-1 (Cooke *et al.*, 1994). This is reminiscent of the interactions between activated white blood cells and the endothelium, although the receptors and their roles are clearly different. ICAM-1, for example, is an immobilizing receptor for white blood cells and a rolling receptor for parasitized red blood cells. Cytoadherence *in vivo* will most probably result from the sum of several interactions between parasitized cells and endothelial receptors, perhaps acting synergistically or in concert to determine the final pattern of adhesion (Cooke *et al.*, 1994; McCormick *et al.*, 1997; Newbold *et al.*, 1997b). Again, the complicated influence of upregulation of various endothelial-cell-expressed molecules by inflammatory cytokines released into the circulation in response to infection must also be taken into account.

7.2. Rosetting

A second form of adhesion is rosetting, the binding of two or more uninfected red blood cells around a single infected red blood cell (David *et al.*, 1988; Udomsangpetch *et al.*, 1989c). By transmission electron microscopy, the membranes of the infected red blood cell and surrounding uninfected red blood cells appear to be in close association (Udomsangpetch *et al.*, 1989c). Rosetting requires both calcium and magnesium (Carlson *et al.*, 1990a,b) and is inhibited by trypsin, heparin (Udomsangpetch *et al.*, 1991) — in some but not all strains — and, perhaps surprisingly, antibodies against KAHRP (Carlson *et al.*, 1990b). Rosetting is a property of only some strains of *P. falciparum*, and freshly collected field isolates can vary quite dramatically in the extent to which they rosette (Wahlgren *et al.*, 1994). The importance of rosetting in host–parasite relations has been under intense study. There is a good deal of controversy, but on balance it appears that rosetting parasites are responsible for more severe disease. Epidemiological studies in endemic areas have shown that severe clinical disease, such as cerebral malaria, is more common in individuals infected with strains capable of rosetting. Further, those patients with antibodies capable of disrupting rosettes are found to suffer less severe clinical forms of malaria (Carlson *et al.*, 1990a; Ringwald *et al.*, 1993; Rowe, A. *et al.*, 1995). Contradictory results have been obtained in other epidemiological settings (al-Yaman *et al.*, 1995), and it may be that the variability in rosetting ability of the parasite, added to markedly different host factors such as HLA status, degree of endemicity of malaria, and presence of other infections, can give rise to different clinical outcomes. The molecules reported to mediate rosetting are also beginning to become increasingly diverse and complex (Figure 5). Both PfEMP1 and the rifins have been implicated as the parasite-encoded ligands responsible for rosetting (Helmby *et al.*, 1993; Rowe, J.A. *et al.*, 1997; Chen, Q. *et al.*, 1998a), although recent evidence suggests that PfEMP1 is the most likely candidate (Fernandez *et al.*, 1999; Barragan *et al.*, 2000b; Chen, Q. *et al.*, 2000). A number of counter receptors on the surface of red blood cells have been described to which PfEMP1 can

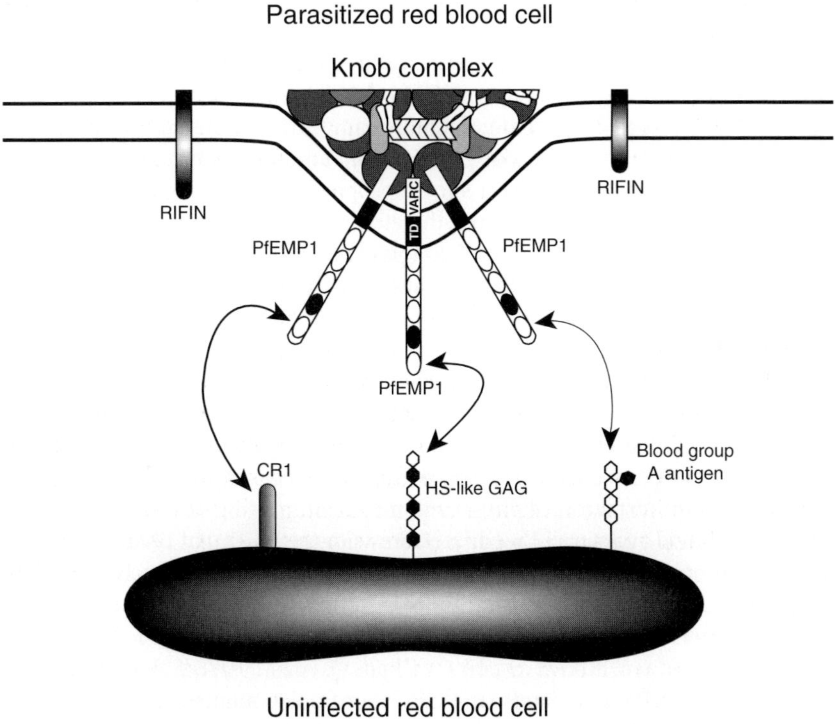

Figure 5 Schematic representation of the molecules implicated in the interaction between red blood cells infected with *P. falciparum* and non-parasitized cells (rosetting). Abbreviations are expanded on pp. 2–3.

bind, including complement receptor 1 (CR1) (Rowe, J.A. *et al.*, 1997), heparan sulphate or heparan sulphate-like glycosaminoglycans (Chen, Q. *et al.*, 1998a, 2000; Barragan *et al.*, 2000a,b), and the ABO blood group antigens, particularly blood group A (Carlson and Wählgren, 1992; Barragan *et al.*, 2000b; Chen, Q. *et al.*, 2000). The physical forces binding cells into a rosette have been measured using both dual micropipetting techniques (see Table 4) and viscometry, and, as stated above, are estimated to be at least five times higher than those involved in cytoadherence to endothelial cells (Nash *et al.*, 1992a; Chotivanich *et al.*, 2000b). Finally, there is evidence to suggest that some blood groups and thalassaemic red blood cells hinder rosette formation to the benefit of the patient (Carlson *et al.*, 1994). Rosetting has been observed in other malaria species that sequester, such as *P. chabaudi* and *P. fragile*, but it has also been described in *P. vivax* and *P. ovale*, which do not cause cerebral malaria and in general cause less serious disease (David *et al.*, 1988; Udomsangpetch *et al.*, 1991, 1995; Angus *et al.*, 1996; Lowe *et al.*, 1998). This still needs to be explained, and it may be that a better operational definition of what constitutes a rosette is required, particularly with respect to size and ability to resist forces of disruption.

If rosetting is a parasite virulence factor, the mechanism by which this occurs is still unclear. One suggestion is that the parasite, cocooned within a group of uninfected red blood cells, may rapidly and efficiently invade these cells, leading to higher levels of parasitaemia and more severe disease. There is little experimental support for such a proposition at present, and it appears that there is no difference in growth rates of parasites capable of rosetting compared with those that cannot (Clough *et al.*, 1998). A second possibility is that the rosettes interfere with circulation of the blood, leading to a greater degree of microvascular obstruction, and perhaps increased pathology. Consistent with this is the observation that in the rat *ex vivo* mesoappendix model, perfusion of rosetting parasites showed higher levels of vascular resistance than with non-rosetting parasites (Kaul *et al.*, 1991). Alternatively, the parasite in a rosette may have less exposure to serum antibodies directed to parasite antigens on the surface of the infected red blood cells, such as PfEMP1, or to surface proteins of the merozoite during invasion. The uninfected red blood cells could well interfere with the ability of phagocytic cells, such as monocytes, to destroy parasites by a process of antibody-dependent killing (Bouharoun-Tayoun *et al.*, 1990).

Two studies examined populations of parasites either enriched or depleted for rosetting (Rowe, J.A. *et al.*, 1997; Chen, Q. *et al.*, 1998a). Examination of expressed PfEMP1 sequences by PCR identified sequences greatly enriched in the rosetting population, and absent or almost entirely so from non-rosetting parasites. Expression of the DBL-1 regions of the identified genes produced proteins capable of binding to uninfected red blood cells. The two genes identified were not identical in sequence and their protein products bound to different receptors, complement receptor 1 and glycosoaminoglycans (GAG), on an as yet unidentified proteoglycan, but at present presumed to be heparan sulphate. It is suggested that the binding to GAG is mediated by a number of basic GAG-binding motifs found scattered through the particular PfEMP1 sequence (Chen, Q. *et al.*, 1998a). These findings explain why it is that only certain isolates rosette, as these must be isolates that both contain and express a PfEMP1 capable of interacting with uninfected red blood cells. The relative frequency of rosetting suggests that more PfEMP1 sequences capable of rosetting will be identified; otherwise, it would mean that one or other of these two genes is expressed at a very high frequency. These observations also help to explain why some but not all rosetting strains could have their rosettes disrupted by the addition of heparin (Rogerson *et al.*, 1994; Wahlgren *et al.*, 1994). Presumably heparin-sensitive isolates are rosetting via a PfEMP1–GAG interaction. Further, since the highly variable PfEMP1 is involved in this interaction, it is possible that additional red blood cell receptors will be identified. It should be noted that specific proteins that also bind to heparan sulphate have been described in the sporozoite stage. It is not clear why it was necessary to evolve two such markedly different genes, unless this is related to the differing cellular locations of the two genes and differing requirements for transport. The relative importance of the various ligand–receptor combinations (see Figure 4), particularly in cases of severe malaria, is yet to be determined. The observation that CR1 polymorphisms are common in Africans is consistent with this rosetting interaction being common and associated with significant clinical disease and, hence, selective pressure (Rowe, J.A. *et al.*, 1997).

8. COMPARISON BETWEEN MALARIA AND *BABESIA* INFECTION OF RED BLOOD CELLS

Babesia bovis and *B. bigemina* are closely related intraerythrocytic protozoan parasites that infect cattle and cause bovine babesiosis. The pathogenesis and clinical picture of this disease bear striking resemblances to malaria in humans (Commins *et al.*, 1988; Wright *et al.*, 1988; Allred, 1995; Schetters and Eling, 1999), particularly when *B. bovis* and *P. falciparum* infections are compared with each other. Like malaria parasites, *Babesia* spp. are also members of the phylum Apicomplexa, and thus specialized for invasion and growth inside red blood cells. During their development inside bovine red blood cells, *Babesia* parasites also make a large number of modifications to the red blood cells, which inevitably affect their function. A major difference between *Plasmodium* and *Babesia*, however, is the time taken to complete the life cycle inside the red blood cell. For *B. bovis*, the cycle time is c. 15 hours, and thus it can complete more than three life cycles during the time taken for *P. falciparum* to complete only one. The cellular modifications in bovine red blood cells infected with *Babesia*, therefore, occur much more rapidly and persist in the cell for a much shorter time than those that occur in red blood cells infected with *P. falciparum*. Although comparatively little is known at the molecular level about the precise nature or identity of the proteins that are involved in such modifications, their relative lability and the speed at which they must occur may indicate that these alterations are less complex than those that occur in malaria-infected red blood cells. *B. bovis* can also be cultured with ease *in vitro*, which, together with the relatively short doubling time, makes it an ideal model to explore parasite protein–red blood cell cytoskeleton interactions more thoroughly. Accumulation of parasitized red blood cells in microvasculature also accompanies *Babesia* infection (Hoyte, 1971), which frequently develops into severe and almost invariably fatal syndromes characterized by organ-specific sequestration, such as cerebral babesiosis (Callow and McGavin, 1963). Intimate interaction of parasitized cells with the vascular endothelium, and with each other (similar to rosetting), appears to be via 'stellate protrusions' of the infected red blood cell membrane (Wright, 1972; Aikawa *et al.*, 1985; Everitt *et al.*, 1986; O'Connor *et al.*, 1999). Although these have frequently been likened to the knobs of malaria-infected cells, they appear to be much larger projections (320 nm × 160 nm) than the knobs on *P. falciparum*-infected red blood cells (150 nm × 65 nm) and show much lower focal electron density (Aikawa *et al.*, 1985; O'Connor *et al.*, 1999).

B. bigemina, on the other hand, behaves quite differently and more resembles *P. vivax*. There is no evidence of sequestration at any stage of the infection (Callow and Johnston, 1963; Hoyte, 1971) and, in fatal cases, death usually results from anaemia. There is a marked difference between *B. bovis* and *B. bigemina* in their tendency to sequester in the brain (Callow and Johnston, 1963), which is a consistent finding that has been useful in diagnosis (Hoyte, 1971). In infected cattle, *B. bigemina* is rarely observed in brain capillaries (Callow and Johnston, 1963). Moreover, the virulence of *B. bovis*, but not that of *B. bigemina*, is reduced by repeated blood passage in splenectomized cattle and restored by passage in intact cattle or transmission by ticks. Compared with malaria, virtually nothing is known at the molecular level about the structural and functional alterations that occur in *Babesia*-infected red blood cells. The infected cells do demonstrate rheological abnormalities. For example, there is a profound reduction in whole cell deformability, as measured by rheoscope, and a reduction in the ability of the red blood cell membrane to tank-tread. The parasitized red blood cells also become abnormally adhesive for vascular endothelial cells (O'Connor *et al.*, 1999), although no specific adhesion molecule has yet been identified on the surface of the endothelial cells to mediate this process. However, a variant antigen

(VESA) appears to cluster over the knob-like protrusions on the surface of *Babesia*-infected red blood cells (O'Connor *et al.*, 1997, 1999) and is the product of the newly described *ves* multi-gene family (Allred *et al.*, 2000); this may be the cytoadherence ligand. Clearly more work is warranted on this parasite system since it offers great potential to serve as a much simpler and more amenable model, both *in vitro* and *in vivo*, for human malaria infection.

9. THE HOST–PARASITE RELATIONSHIP

The fact that *P. falciparum* manifests its mortality predominantly in young children ensures that it exerts extraordinary selective pressure on humans living in endemic areas. Thus it is no surprise to observe the presence of a number of phenotypes in humans that appear to confer resistance to malaria infection. These may manifest as individuals with more effective immune responses to malaria antigens or individuals with red blood cells that resist parasite invasion and growth by virtue of either haemoglobin or membrane protein mutations. Of those that act through changes in the red blood cell, the best known are probably the haemoglobinopathies such as sickle cell disease and the thalassaemias. The pathobiology of red blood cells in these conditions has been reviewed in detail (Evans and Hochmuth, 1977; Mohandas *et al.*, 1984, 1992; Chasis and Mohandas, 1986; Mohandas, 1992; Mohandas and Chasis, 1993; Mohandas and Evans, 1994) and description of the pathophysiology of these conditions is outside the scope of this current review. Many of these conditions induce rheological changes in the red blood cell that parallel those caused by malaria infection, and it is instructive to compare them.

Homozygous sickle cell disease is a devastating condition with protean clinical manifestations, most of which are undoubtedly the result of physical trapping of grossly mechanically impaired sickle red blood cells in the microvasculature leading to painful, vaso-occlusive crises with accumulative organ damage. In sickle cells, normal adult haemoglobin (HbA) is replaced by abnormal sickle haemoglobin (HbS), which can be inherited in either a heterozygous or homozygous state. In heterozygotes (sickle-cell trait), acquisition of only one copy of the *HbS* gene results in HbAS red blood cells that contain approximately equal proportions of HbA and HbS. Except under extreme conditions of low oxygen tension or oxidative stress, these individuals remain clinically unaffected by their condition. In fact, there is some advantage to acquisition of the trait in individuals living in areas endemic for malaria, since this condition offers relative protection against severe malaria. In these areas, malaria exerts a strong positive selective pressure on the sickle gene and is the primary reason it is maintained in the human gene pool. In contrast, homozygotes who inherit two copies of the sickle gene and whose red blood cells contain only HbS (HbSS) bear the full brunt of this condition. Unlike HbA, HbS forms long rigid rods of polymer (nematic tactoids) upon deoxygenation, which leads to profound changes in red blood cell morphology. Furthermore, during repeated cycles of deoxygenation and reoxygenation, sickle cells become progressively dehydrated, most probably as a consequence of potassium loss via the Gardos channel (McGoron *et al.*, 2000), although other membrane transport pathways, including the KCl co-transporter, may also play a role (Joiner, 1993; Brugnara, 1997). Dehydration further exacerbates the reduction in cell deformability by increasing the intracellular haemoglobin concentration, which in turn dramatically increases the red blood cells' internal viscosity. The overall loss of cell deformability is also due in part to a marked decrease in the elasticity of the red blood cell membrane itself (Chien *et al.*, 1970, 1982; Nash *et al.*, 1984, 1986; Green *et al.*, 1988). While these changes occur to a substantial degree even when the cells are fully oxygenated, the degree of impairment is much greater upon deoxygenation, when they assume their characteristic sickle shape.

Although, like malaria-infected red blood cells, sickle cells have also been shown to be abnormally adhesive, the alteration occurs to a much lesser extent than in red blood cells parasitized by *P. falciparum*. In a direct comparison of adhesion of normal (HbAA), HbAS, HbSS and *P. falciparum*-infected red blood cells with cultured vascular endothelial cells under physiologically relevant flow conditions, the relative levels of adhesion were in the ratio of 1 : 1 : 3 : 1000 (Rowland *et al.*, 1993). Thus, it seems likely that the direct physical mechanical trapping of sickle cells in the small diameter vessels of the microcirculation, consequent upon their abnormal mechanical properties, is the primary event in the genesis of the vaso-occlusive pathology seen in sickle cell anaemia. In contrast, cell adhesion is the most likely key pathogenic event in malaria infection, with abnormal mechanics playing a secondary role. It has been suggested, however, that mechanical trapping of parasitized red blood cells in the bone marrow sinuses may exacerbate anaemia by inhibiting the release of new red blood cells into the circulation (Wickramasinghe *et al.*, 1987).

Interactions between host and parasite can become extremely complex and we do not yet understand many of these. For example, it is clear that the parasite requires a normal red blood cell membrane skeleton for parasite growth. Several groups have examined the capacity of red blood cells with an abnormal membrane skeleton to support the growth of *P. falciparum* in culture *in vitro* (Schulman *et al.*, 1990; Facer, 1995; Magowan *et al.*, 1995). Schulman and co-workers (1990) demonstrated that culture over two to three cycles resulted in diminished growth rates, which were proportional to the amount of spectrin in the red blood cell membrane skeleton. The reason for this is not clear but it may be related to some requirement for cytoskeletal components in the formation of a competent invasion complex on the merozoite surface. This may explain the otherwise unexpected observation that MSP1 binds to spectrin (Herrera *et al.*, 1993). MSP1 is believed to be important for invasion and interacts with the outside of the red blood cell. Thus, the only time it comes into contact with spectrin is during red blood cell lysis before invasion. Spectrin-binding ability would be relevant only at this stage, perhaps by securing spectrin molecules to the surface of the merozoite. The most profound growth inhibition was noted in red blood cells deficient in protein 4.1, whereas red blood cells with abnormal band 3 proteins supported parasite growth as well as controls (Schulman *et al.*, 1990). The inability of parasites to grow in red blood cells deficient in protein 4.1 was confirmed by Magowan and co-workers (1995), who suggested that this growth failure was secondary to accumulation of MESA in the cytoplasm of the red blood cell because of the absence of its binding partner protein 4.1. Abnormalities of haemoglobin may have secondary effects on the integrity of the red blood cell membrane skeleton and this may also perturb the host–parasite relationship (Nagel and Roth, 1989; Yuan *et al.*, 1995). Examples include the apparent change in PfEMP1 accessibility to antibody in thalassaemic red blood cells, which appears to make parasites more susceptible to clearance by immune mechanisms (Luzzi *et al.*, 1991a,b). Transgenic mice with specific abnormalities of red blood cells have been examined for susceptibility to malaria infection (Shear, 1993; Shear *et al.*, 1993, 1998; Hood *et al.*, 1996). In general, these studies have confirmed the importance of abnormal haemoglobin in restricting parasite growth.

Another phenomenon in which the complex interplay of host and parasite factors is seen is that of cytoadherence, where it appears that modulating the level of cytoadherence can be of benefit to the host. *P. falciparum* parasites that do not cytoadhere cause milder disease than adherent strains (Langreth and Peterson, 1985). From this it could be argued that there may be a selective advantage for the host if it can decrease the level of adhesion. Accordingly, the structural genes encoding host receptors for PfEMP1 have been examined for evidence of polymorphism that may result from mutations that decrease the extent of sequestration (Fernandez-Reyes *et al.*, 1997; Adams *et al.*, 2000; Craig *et al.*, 2000; Smith *et al.*, 2000). There is a high frequency polymorphism in the human *ICAM-1* gene in a malaria-endemic population in Kilifi, Kenya. Studies *in vitro* showed that infected red blood cells bound less well to the mutant recombinant ICAM-1, termed ICAM-1^{Kilifi} (Adams *et al.*, 2000; Craig *et al.*, 2000). Paradoxically, however, individuals homozygous for this polymorphism, at least in this region of Africa, were twice as likely to develop the severe form of malaria known as cerebral malaria (Fernandez-Reyes *et al.*, 1997). The significance of this result is unclear but it challenges the contention that lowered levels of adhesion are beneficial for the host. However, these adhesion studies were performed using laboratory-adapted parasite lines, which may not accurately reflect those circulating in the field. Perhaps in this particular area of Africa, where malaria transmission is high, compensatory mutations in PfEMP1 may have arisen that bind to ICAM-1^{Kilifi} with much higher avidity. Sequence analyses of African populations showed a surprisingly high frequency of mutations in the *CD36* gene that result in loss of expression of CD36 (Aitman *et al.*, 2000). Again, one might expect this to be protective against malaria, based on the widely professed importance of CD36 in cytoadherence. Surprisingly, however, individuals deficient in CD36 were in fact more susceptible to severe malaria, particularly cerebral malaria, than individuals expressing normal levels of wild-type CD36. Clearly more needs to be learnt about the importance of quantitative differences in adhesion levels in the causation of disease.

Finally, if cytoadherence really is a virulence factor, then preventing or reversing adhesion with anti-adhesive substances should significantly ameliorate the severity of the disease. Laboratory studies have identified potential anti-adherence reagents including recombinant fragments of PfEMP1 (Cooke *et al.*, 1998), but these have not been subjected to clinical trial. Further work over the next few years will undoubtedly improve our knowledge of the interaction between the malaria parasite and the host red blood cell. This in turn may suggest further strategies that could interfere with processes critical for parasite survival.

REFERENCES

Adams, J.H., Sim, B.K., Dolan, S.A., Fang, X., Kaslow, D.C. and Miller, L.H. (1992). A family of erythrocyte binding proteins of malaria parasites. *Proceedings of the National Academy of Sciences of the USA* **89**, 7085–7089.

Adams, S., Turner, G.D., Nash, G.B., Micklem, K., Newbold, C.I. and Craig, A.G. (2000). Differential binding of clonal variants of *Plasmodium falciparum* to allelic forms of intracellular adhesion molecule 1 determined by flow adhesion assay. *Infection and Immunity* **68**, 264–269.

Ahlborg, N., Berzins, K. and Perlmann, P. (1991). Definition of the epitope recognized by the *Plasmodium falciparum*-reactive human monoclonal antibody 33G2. *Molecular and Biochemical Parasitology* **46**, 89–96.

Aikawa, M. (1977). Variations in structure and function during the life cycle of malarial parasites. *Bulletin of the World Health Organization* **55**, 139–156.

Aikawa, M. and Miller, L.H. (1983). Structural alteration of the erythrocyte membrane during malarial parasite invasion and intraerythrocytic development. *Ciba Foundation Symposium* **94**, 45–63.

Aikawa, M. Rabbege, J., Uni, S., Ristic, M. and Miller, L.H. (1985). Structural alteration of the membrane of erythrocytes infected with *Babesia bovis*. *American Journal of Tropical Medicine and Hygiene* **34**, 45–49.

Aikawa, M., Torii, M., Sjölander, A., Berzins, K., Perlmann, P. and Miller, L.H. (1990). Pf155/resa antigen is localized in dense granules of *Plasmodium falciparum* merozoites. *Experimental Parasitology* **71**, 326–329.

Aikawa, M., Kamanura, K., Shiraishi, S., Matsumoto, Y., Arwati, H., Torii, M., Ito, Y., Takeuchi, T. and Tandler, B. (1996). Membrane knobs of unfixed *Plasmodium falciparum* infected erythrocytes — new findings as revealed by atomic force microscopy and surface potential spectroscopy. *Experimental Parasitology* **84**, 339–343.

Aitman, T.J., Cooper, L.D., Norsworthy, P.J., Wahid, F.N., Gray, J.K., Curtis, B.R., McKeigue, P.M., Kwiatkowski, D., Greenwood, B.M., Snow, R.W., Hill, A.V. and Scott, J. (2000). Malaria susceptibility and CD36 mutation. *Nature* **405**, 1015–1016.

Albano, F.R., Berman, A., La Greca, N., Hibbs, A.R., Wickham, M., Foley, M. and Tilley, L. (1999a). A homologue of Sar1p localises to a novel trafficking pathway in malaria-infected erythrocytes. *European Journal of Cell Biology* **78**, 453–462.

Albano, F.R., Foley, M. and Tilley, L. (1999b). Export of parasite proteins to the erythrocyte cytoplasm: secretory machinery and traffic signals. In: *Transport and Trafficking in the Malaria-Infected Erythrocyte* (G.R. Bock and G. Cardew, eds). Novartis Foundation Symposium Vol. 226, pp. 157–172. Chichester: John Wiley and Sons.

Aley, S.B., Bates, M.D., Tam, J.P. and Hollingdale, M.R. (1986). Synthetic peptides from the circumsporozoite proteins of *Plasmodium falciparum* and *Plasmodium knowlesi* recognize the human hepatoma cell line HepG2-A16 *in vitro*. *Journal of Experimental Medicine* **164**, 1915–1922.

Allan, B.B., Moyer, B.D. and Balch, W.E. (2000). Rab1 recruitment of p115 into a cis-snare complex: programming budding COPII vesicles for fusion. *Science* **289**, 444–448.

Allred, D.R. (1995). Immune evasion by *Babesia bovis* and *Plasmodium falciparum*: cliff-dwellers of the parasite world. *Parasitology Today* **11**, 100–105.

Allred, D.R., Gruenberg, J.E. and Sherman, I.W. (1986). Dynamic rearrangements of erythrocyte membrane internal architecture induced by infection with *Plasmodium falciparum*. *Journal of Cell Science* **81**, 1–16.

Allred, D.R., Carlton, J.M., Satcher, R.L., Long, J.A., Brown, W.C., Patterson, P.E., O'Connor, R.M. and Stroup, S.E. (2000). The *ves* multigene family of *B. bovis* encodes components of rapid antigenic variation at the infected erythrocyte surface. *Molecular Cell* **5**, 153–162.

Al-Yaman, F., Genton, B., Mokela, D., Raiko, A., Kati, S., Rogerson, S., Reeder, J. and Alpers, M. (1995). Human cerebral malaria: lack of significant association between erythrocyte rosetting and disease severity. *Transactions of the Royal Society of Tropical Medicine and Hygiene* **89**, 55–58.

Anders, R.F. (1986). Multiple cross-reactivities amongst antigens of *Plasmodium falciparum* impair the development of protective immunity against malaria. *Parasite Immunology* **8**, 529–539.

Anders, R.F. and Smythe, J.A. (1989). Polymorphic antigens in *Plasmodium falciparum*. *Blood* **74**, 1865–1875.

Anders, R.F., Barzaga, N., Shi, P.-T., Scanlon, D.B., Brown, L.E., Thomas, L.M., Brown, G.V., Stahl, H.D., Coppel, R.L. and Kemp, D.J. (1987a). Repetitive sequences in malaria antigens. In: *Molecular Strategies of Parasitic Invasion* (N. Agabian, H. Goodman and N. Noguiera, eds), pp. 333–342. New York: Alan R. Liss.

Anders, R.F., Murray, L.J., Thomas, L.M., Davern, K.M., Brown, G.V. and Kemp, D.J. (1987b). Structure and function of candidate vaccine antigens in *Plasmodium falciparum*. *Biochemical Society Symposia* **53**, 103–114.

Anders, R.F., McColl, D.J. and Coppel, R.L. (1993). Molecular variation in *Plasmodium falciparum*; polymorphic antigens of asexual erythrocytic stages. *Acta Tropica* **53**, 239–253.

Angus, B.J., Thanikkul, K., Silamut, K., White, N.J. and Udomsangpetch, R. (1996). Rosette formation in *Plasmodium* ovale infection. *American Journal of Tropical Medicine and Hygiene* **55**, 560–561.

Angus, B.J., Chotivanich, K., Udomsangpetch, R. and White, N.J. (1997). *In vivo* removal of malaria parasites from red blood cells without their destruction in acute falciparum malaria. *Blood* **90**, 2037–2040.

Ardeshir, F., Flint, J.E., Matsumoto, Y., Aikawa, M., Reese, R.T. and Stanley, H. (1987). cDNA sequence encoding a *Plasmodium falciparum* protein associated with knobs and localization of the protein to electron-dense regions in membranes of infected erythrocytes. *EMBO Journal* **6**, 1421–1427.

Areekul, S. and Yamarat, P. (1988). Alterations in the viscosity and deformability of red cells in patients with *Plasmodium falciparum. Journal of the Medical Association of Thailand* **71**, 196–202.

Bagge, U., Branemark, P.I., Karlsson, R. and Skalak, R. (1980). Three-dimensional observations of red blood cell deformation in capillaries. *Blood Cells* **6**, 231–239.

Barabino, G.A., McIntire, L.V., Eskin, S.G., Sears, D.A. and Udden, M. (1987). Endothelial cell interactions with sickle cell, sickle trait, mechanically injured, and normal erythrocytes under controlled flow. *Blood* **70**, 152–157.

Barale, J.C., Attal-Bonnefoy, G., Brahimi, K., Pereira da Silva, L. and Langsley, G. (1997a). *Plasmodium falciparum* asparagine and aspartate rich protein 2 is an evolutionarily conserved protein whose repeats identify a new family of parasite antigens. *Molecular and Biochemical Parasitology* **87**, 169–181.

Barale, J.C., Candelle, D., Attalbonnefoy, G., Dehoux, P., Bonnefoy, S., Ridley, R., Dasilva, L.P. and Langsley, G. (1997b). *Plasmodium falciparum* AARP1, a giant protein containing repeated motifs rich in asparagine and aspartate residues, is associated with the infected erythrocyte membrane. *Infection and Immunity* **65**, 3003–3010.

Barnes, D.A., Thompson, J., Triglia, T., Day, K. and Kemp, D.J. (1994). Mapping the genetic locus implicated in cytoadherence of *Plasmodium falciparum* to melanoma cells. *Molecular and Biochemical Parasitology* **66**, 21–29.

Barnes, D.A., Wollish, W., Nelson, R.G., Leech, J.H. and Petersen, C. (1995). *Plasmodium falciparum*-d260, an intraerythrocytic parasite protein, is a member of the glutamic acid dipeptide-repeat family of proteins. *Experimental Parasitology* **81**, 79–89.

Barragan, A., Fernandez, V., Chen, Q., von Euler, A., Wahlgren, M. and Spillmann, D. (2000a). The duffy-binding-like domain 1 of *Plasmodium falciparum* erythrocyte membrane protein 1 (PfEMP1) is a heparan sulfate ligand that requires 12mers for binding. *Blood* **95**, 3594–3599.

Barragan, A., Kremsner, P.G., Wahlgren, M. and Carlson, J. (2000b). Blood group A antigen is a coreceptor in *Plasmodium falciparum* rosetting. *Infection and Immunity* **68**, 2971–2975.

Baruch, D.I., Pasloske, B.L., Singh, H.B., Bi, X.H., Ma, X.C., Feldman, M., Taraschi, T.F. and Howard, R.J. (1995). Cloning the *P. falciparum* gene encoding PfEMP1, a malarial variant antigen and adherence receptor on the surface of parasitized human erythrocytes. *Cell* **82**, 77–87.

Baruch, D.I., Gormley, J.A., Ma, C., Howard, R.J. and Pasloske, B.L. (1996). *Plasmodium falciparum* erythrocyte membrane protein 1 is a parasitized erythrocyte receptor for adherence to CD36, thrombospondin, and intercellular adhesion molecule 1. *Proceedings of the National Academy of Sciences of the USA* **93**, 3497–3502.

Baruch, D., Ma, X., Singh, H., Bi, X., Pasloske, B. and Howard, R. (1997). Identification of a region of pfemp1 that mediates adherence of *Plasmodium falciparum* infected erythrocytes to cd36: conserved function with variant sequence. *Blood* **90**, 3766–3775.

Baruch, D.I., Ma, X.C., Pasloske, B., Howard, R.J. and Miller, L.H. (1999). CD36 peptides that block cytoadherence define the CD36 binding region for *Plasmodium falciparum*-infected erythrocytes. *Blood* **94**, 2121–2127.

Beeson, J.G., Rogerson, S.J., Cooke, B.M., Reeder, J.C., Chai, W., Lawson, A.M., Molyneux, M.E. and Brown, G.V. (2000). Adhesion of *Plasmodium falciparum*-infected erythrocytes to hyaluronic acid in placental malaria. *Nature Medicine* **6**, 86–90.

Bennett, B.J., Mohandas, N. and Coppel, R.L. (1997). Defining the minimal domain of the *Plasmodium falciparum* protein mesa involved in the interaction with the red blood cell membrane skeletal protein 4.1. *Journal of Biological Chemistry* **272**, 15299–15306.

Bennett, V. (1983). Proteins involved in membrane–cytoskeleton association in human erythrocytes: spectrin, ankyrin, and band 3. *Methods in Enzymology* **96**, 313–323.

Bennett, V. and Stenbuck, P.J. (1980). Association between ankyrin and the cytoplasmic domain of band 3 isolated from the human erythrocyte membrane. *Journal of Biological Chemistry* **255**, 6424–6432.

Benting, J., Mattei, D. and Lingelbach, K. (1994). Brefeldin a inhibits transport of the glycophorin-binding protein from *Plasmodium falciparum* into the host erythrocyte. *Biochemical Journal* **300**, 821–826.

Berendt, A.R., Simmons, D.L., Tansey, J., Newbold, C.I. and Marsh, K. (1989). Intracellular adhesion molecule 1 is an endothelial cell adhesion molecule for *Plasmodium falciparum*. *Nature* **341**, 57–59.

Berendt, A.R., McDowall, A., Craig, A.G., Bates, P.A., Sternberg, M.J.E., Marsh, K., Newbold, C.I. and Hogg, N. (1992). The binding site on ICAM-1 for *Plasmodium falciparum*-infected erythrocytes overlaps, but is distinct from the LFA-1 binding site. *Cell* **68**, 71–81.

Berzins, K., Perlmann, H., Wåhlin, B., Carlsson, J., Wahlgren, M., Udomsangpetch, R., Björkman, A., Patarroyo, M.E. and Perlmann, P. (1986). Rabbit and human antibodies to a repeated amino acid sequence of a *Plasmodium falciparum* antigen, Pf 155, react with the native protein and inhibit merozoite invasion. *Proceedings of the National Academy of Sciences of the USA* **83**, 1065–1069.

Bianco, A.E., Crewther, P.E., Coppel, R.L., Stahl, H.D., Kemp, D.J., Anders, R.F. and Brown, G.V. (1988). Patterns of antigen expression in asexual blood stages and gametocytes of *Plasmodium falciparum*. *American Journal of Tropical Medicine and Hygiene* **38**, 258–267.

Bischoff, E., Guillotte, M., Mercereau-Puijalon, O. and Bonnefoy, S. (2000). A member of the *Plasmodium falciparum* Pf60 multigene family codes for a nuclear protein expressed by readthrough of an internal stop codon. *Molecular Microbiology* **35**, 1005–1016.

Blisnick, T., Morales-Betoulle, M.E., Barale, J-C., Uzureau, P., Berry, L., Desroses, S., Fujioka, H., Mattei, D. and Braun-Breton, C. (2000). Pfsbp1, a Maurer's cleft *Plasmodium falciparum* protein, is associated with the erythrocyte skeleton. *Molecular and Biochemical Parasitology* **111**, 107–121.

Bock, G. and Cardew, G., eds (1999). *Transport and Trafficking in the Malaria-Infected Erythrocyte*. Novartis Foundation Symposium Vol. 226. Chichester: John Wiley and Sons.

Bonnefoy, S., Bischoff, E., Guillotte, M. and Mercereau Puijalon, O. (1997). Evidence for distinct prototype sequences within the *Plasmodium falciparum* Pf60 multigene family. *Molecular and Biochemical Parasitology* **87**, 1–11.

Bork, P., Sander, C., Valencia, A. and Bukau, B. (1992). A module of the DnaJ heat shock proteins found in malaria parasites. *Trends in Biochemical Sciences* **17**, 129.

Bouharoun-Tayoun, H., Attanath, P., Sabchareon, A., Chongsuphajaisiddhi, T. and Druilhe, P. (1990). Antibodies that protect humans against *Plasmodium falciparum* blood stages do not on their own inhibit parasite growth and invasion *in vitro*, but act in cooperation with monocytes. *Journal of Experimental Medicine* **172**, 1633–1641.

Bourke, P.F., Holt, D.C., Sutherland, C.J., Currie, B. and Kemp, D.J. (1996). Positional cloning of a sequence from the breakpoint of chromosome 9 commonly associated with the loss of cytoadherence. *Annals of Tropical Medicine and Parasitology* **90**, 353–357.

Bowman, S., Lawson, D., Basham, D., Brown, D., Chillingworth, T., Churcher, C.M., Craig, A., Davies, R.M., Devlin, K., Feltwell, T., Gentles, S., Gwilliam, R., Hamlin, N., Harris, D., Holroyd, S., Hornsby, T., Horrocks, P., Jagels, K., Jassal, B., Kyes, S., McLean, J., Moule, S., Mungall, K., Murphy, L., Oliver, K., Quail, M.A.,

Rajandream, M.-A., Rutter, S., Skelton, J., Squares, R., Squares, S., Sulston, J.E., Whitehead, S., Woodward, J.R., Newbold, C. and Barrell, B.G. (1999). The complete nucleotide sequence of chromosome 3 of *Plasmodium falciparum. Nature* **400**, 532–538.

Bozdech, Z., Van Wye, J., Haldar, K. and Schurr, E. (1998). The human malaria parasite *Plasmodium falciparum* exports the ATP-binding cassette protein PfGCN20 to membrane structures in the host red blood cell. *Molecular and Biochemical Parasitology* **97**, 81–95.

Braun-Breton, C., Langsley, G., Mattei, D. and Scherf, A. (1990). Intra- and extracellular routing in *P. falciparum. Blood Cells* **16**, 396–400.

Brown, G.V., Culvenor, J.G., Crewther, P.E., Bianco, A.E., Coppel, R.L., Saint, R.B., Stahl, H.D., Kemp, D.J. and Anders, R.F. (1985). Localization of the ring-infected erythrocyte surface antigen (RESA) of *Plasmodium falciparum* in merozoites and ring-infected erythrocytes. *Journal of Experimental Medicine* **162**, 774–779.

Brown, K.N. and Brown, I.N. (1965). Immunity to malaria: antigenic variation in chronic infections of *Plasmodium knowlesi. Nature* **208**, 1286–1288.

Brugnara, C. (1997). Erythrocyte membrane transport physiology. *Current Opinion in Hematology* **4**, 122–127.

Buffet, P.A., Gamain, B., Scheidig, C., Baruch, D., Smith, J.D., Hernandez-Rivas, R., Pouvelle, B., Oishi, S., Fujii, N., Fusai, T., Parzy, D., Miller, L.H., Gysin, J. and Scherf, A. (1999). *Plasmodium falciparum* domain mediating adhesion to chondroitin sulfate A: a receptor for human placental infection. *Proceedings of the National Academy of Sciences of the USA* **96**, 12743–12748.

Bull, B., Stuart, J. and Juhan-Vague, I. (1984). Normal and pathological determinants of erythrocyte deformability. In: *Investigative Microtechniques in Medicine and Biology* (J. Chayen, and L. Bitensky, eds), pp. 257–295. New York: Marcel Dekker.

Callow, L.L. and Johnston, L.A.Y. (1963). *Babesia* spp. in the brains of clinically normal cattle and their detection by a brain smear technique. *Australian Veterinary Journal* **39**, 25–31.

Callow, L.L. and McGavin, M.D. (1963). Cerebral babesiosis due to *Babesia argentina. Australian Veterinary Journal* **39**, 15–21.

Cappai, R., Kaslow, D.C., Peterson, M.G., Cowman, A.F., Anders, R.F. and Kemp, D.J. (1992). Cloning and analysis of the *RESA-2* gene – a DNA homologue of the ring-infected erythrocyte surface antigen gene of *Plasmodium falciparum. Molecular and Biochemical Parasitology* **54**, 213–222.

Carlson, J. and Wählgren, M. (1992). *Plasmodium falciparum* erythrocyte rosetting is mediated by promiscuous lectin-like interactions. *Journal of Experimental Medicine* **176**, 1311–1317.

Carlson, J., Helmby, H., Hill, A.V.S., Brewster, D., Greenwood, B.M. and Wählgren, M. (1990a). Human cerebral malaria: association with erythrocyte rosetting and lack of anti-rosetting antibodies. *Lancet* **336**, 1457–1460.

Carlson, J., Holmquist, G., Taylor, D.W., Perlmann, P. and Wählgren, M. (1990b). Antibodies to a histidine-rich protein (PfHRP1) disrupt spontaneously formed *Plasmodium falciparum* erythrocyte rosettes. *Proceedings of the National Academy of Sciences of the USA* **87**, 2511–2515.

Carlson, J., Nash, G.B., Gabutti, V., Alyaman, F. and Wählgren, M. (1994). Natural protection against severe *Plasmodium falciparum* malaria due to impaired rosette formation. *Blood* **84**, 3909–3914.

Cerami, C., Kwakye, B.F. and Nussenzweig, V. (1992). Binding of malarial circumsporozoite protein to sulfatides [Gal(3-SO_4)beta 1-Cer] and cholesterol-3-sulfate and its dependence on disulfide bond formation between cysteines in region II. *Molecular and Biochemical Parasitology* **54**, 1–12.

Chaiyaroj, S.C., Coppel, R.L., Magown, C. and Brown, G. (1994a). A *Plasmodium falciparum* isolate with a chromosome 9 deletion expresses a trypsin-resistant cytoadherence molecule. *Molecular and Biochemical Parasitology* **67**, 21–30.

Chaiyaroj, S.C., Coppel, R.L., Novakovic, S. and Brown, G.V. (1994b). Multiple ligands for cytoadherence can be present simultaneously on the surface of *Plasmodium falciparum*-infected erythrocytes. *Proceedings of the National Academy of Sciences of the USA* **91**, 10805–10808.

Chan, M.T., Catry, E., Weill, D., Marcel, G.A. and George, C. (1984). Assessment of erythrocyte deformability by constant flow filtration technique: analysis of factors influencing the initial pressure. *Biorheology* **1**, supplement 1, 267–270.

Chasis, J. and Mohandas, N. (1986). Erythrocyte membrane deformability and stability: two distinct membrane properties which are independently regulated by skeletal protein associations. *Journal of Cell Biology* **103**, 343–350.

Chen, Q., Barragan, A., Fernandez, V., Sundstrom, A., Schlichtherle, M., Sahlen, A., Carlson, J., Datta, S. and Wahlgren, M. (1998a). Identification of *Plasmodium falciparum* erythrocyte membrane protein 1 (PfEMP1) as the rosetting ligand of the malaria parasite *P. falciparum*. *Journal of Experimental Medicine* **187**, 15–23.

Chen, Q., Fernandez, V., Sundstrom, A., Schlichtherle, M., Datta, S., Hagblom, P. and Wahlgren, M. (1998b). Developmental selection of *var* gene expression in *Plasmodium falciparum*. *Nature* **394**, 392–395.

Chen, Q., Heddini, A., Barragan, A., Fernandez, V., Pearce, S.F.A. and Wahlgren, M. (2000). The semiconserved head structure of *Plasmodium falciparum* erythrocyte membrane protein 1 mediates binding to multiple independent host receptors. *Journal of Experimental Medicine* **192**, 1–10.

Chen, S. (1969). Blood rheology and its relation to flow resistance and transcapillary exchange with special reference to shock. *Advances in Microcirculation* **2**, 89–103.

Cheng, Q., Cloonan, N., Fischer, K., Thompson, J., Waine, G., Lanzer, M. and Saul, A. (1998). *Stevor* and *rif* are *Plasmodium falciparum* multicopy gene families which potentially encode variant antigens. *Molecular and Biochemical Parasitology* **97**, 161–176.

Chien, S., Usami, S. and Bertles, J.F. (1970). Abnormal rheology of oxygenated blood in sickle cell anemia. *Journal of Clinical Investigation* **49**, 623–634.

Chien, S., King, R.G., Kaperonis, A.A. and Usami, S. (1982). Viscoelastic properties of sickle cells and hemoglobin. *Blood Cells* **8**, 53–64.

Chien, S., Schmalzer, E.A., Lee, M.M., Impelluso, T. and Skalak, R. (1983). Role of white blood cells in filtration of blood cell suspensions. *Biorheology* **20**, 11–27.

Chishti, A.H., Andrabi, K.I., Derick, L.H., Palek, J. and Liu, S.C. (1992). Isolation of skeleton-associated knobs from human red blood cells infected with malaria parasite *Plasmodium falciparum*. *Molecular and Biochemical Parasitology* **52**, 283–288.

Chishti, A.H., Maalouf, G.J., Marfatia, S., Palek, J., Wang, W., Fisher, D. and Liu, S.C. (1994). Phosphorylation of protein 4.1 in *Plasmodium falciparum*-infected human red blood cells. *Blood* **83**, 3339–3345.

Chotivanich, K., Udomsangpetch, R., Dondorp, A., Williams, T., Angus, B., Simpson, J.A., Pukrittayakamee, S., Looareesuwan, S., Newbold, C.I. and White, N.J. (2000a). The mechanisms of parasite clearance after antimalarial treatment of *Plasmodium falciparum* malaria. *Journal of Infectious Diseases* **182**, 629–633.

Chotivanich, K.T., Dondorp, A.M., White, N.J., Peters, K., Vreeken, J., Kager, P.A. and Udomsangpetch, R. (2000b). The resistance to physiological shear stresses of the erythrocytic rosettes formed by cells infected with *Plasmodium falciparum*. *Annals of Tropical Medicine and Parasitology* **94**, 219–226.

Clark, I.A., Cowden, W.B. and Rockett, K.A. (1994). The pathogenesis of human cerebral malaria. *Parasitology Today* **10**, 417–418.

Clark, I.A., al Yaman, F.M. and Jacobson, L.S. (1997). The biological basis of malarial disease. *International Journal for Parasitology* **27**, 1237–1249.

Clough, B., Atilola, F. and Pasvol, G. (1998). The role of rosetting in the multiplication of *Plasmodium falciparum*: rosette formation neither enhances nor targets parasite invasion into uninfected red blood cells. *British Journal of Haematology* **100**, 99–104.

Collins, W.E., Anders, R.F., Pappaioanou, M., Campbell, G.H., Brown, G.V., Kemp, D.J., Coppel, R.L., Skinner, J.C., Andrysiak, P.M., Favaloro, J.M., Corcoran, L.M., Broderson, J.R., Mitchell, G.F. and Campbell, C.C. (1986). Immunization of *Aotus* monkeys with recombinant proteins of an erythrocyte surface antigen of *Plasmodium falciparum*. *Nature* **323**, 259–262.

Commins, M.A., Goodger, B.V., Waltisbuhl, D.J. and Wright, I.G. (1988). *Babesia bovis*: studies of parameters influencing microvascular stasis of infected erythrocytes. *Research in Veterinary Science* **44**, 226–228.

Cooke, B.M. and Coppel, R.L. (1995). Cytoadhesion and falciparum malaria: going with the flow. *Parasitology Today* **11**, 282–287.

Cooke, B.M., Morris-Jones, S., Greenwood, B.M. and Nash, G.B. (1993). Adhesion of parasitized red blood cells to cultured endothelial cells: a flow-based study of isolates from Gambian children with falciparum malaria. *Parasitology* **107**, 359–368.

Cooke, B.M., Berendt, A.R., Craig, A.G., MacGregor, J., Newbold, C.I. and Nash, G.B. (1994). Rolling and stationary cytoadhesion of red blood cells parasitised by *Plasmodium falciparum*: separate roles for ICAM-1, CD36 and thrombospondin. *British Journal of Haematology* **87**, 162–170.

Cooke, B.M., Morris-Jones, S., Greenwood, B.M. and Nash, G.B. (1995). Mechanisms of cytoadhesion of flowing, parasitized red blood cells from Gambian children with falciparum malaria. *American Journal of Tropical Medicine and Hygiene* **53**, 29–35.

Cooke, B.M., Rogerson, S.J., Brown, G.V. and Coppel, R.L. (1996). Adhesion of malaria-infected red blood cells to chondroitin sulfate A under flow conditions. *Blood* **88**, 4040–4044.

Cooke, B.M., Nicoll, C.L., Baruch, D.I. and Coppel, R.L. (1998). A recombinant peptide based on PfEMP-1 blocks and reverses adhesion of malaria-infected red blood cells to CD36 under flow. *Molecular Microbiology* **30**, 83–90.

Coppel, R.L. (1992). Repeat structures in a *Plasmodium falciparum* protein (MESA) that binds human erythrocyte protein 4.1. *Molecular and Biochemical Parasitology* **50**, 335–347.

Coppel, R.L., Brown, G.V., Mitchell, G.F., Anders, R.F. and Kemp, D.J. (1984a). Identification of a cDNA clone encoding a mature blood stage antigen of *Plasmodium falciparum* by immunization of mice with bacterial lysates. *EMBO Journal* **3**, 403–407.

Coppel, R.L., Cowman, A.F., Anders, R.F., Bianco, A.E., Saint, R.B., Lingelbach, K.R., Kemp, D.J. and Brown, G.V. (1984b). Immune sera recognize on erythrocytes *Plasmodium falciparum* antigen composed of repeated amino acid sequences. *Nature* **310**, 789–791.

Coppel, R.L., Favaloro, J.M., Crewther, P.E., Burkot, T.R., Bianco, A.E., Stahl, H.D., Kemp, D.J., Anders, R.F. and Brown, G.V. (1985). A blood stage antigen of *Plasmodium falciparum* shares determinants with the sporozoite coat protein. *Proceedings of the National Academy of Sciences of the USA* **82**, 5121–5125.

Coppel, R.L., Culvenor, J.G., Bianco, A.E., Crewther, P.E., Stahl, H.D., Brown, G.V., Anders, R.F. and Kemp, D.J. (1986). Variable antigen associated with the surface of erythrocytes infected with mature stages of *Plasmodium falciparum*. *Molecular and Biochemical Parasitology* **20**, 265–277.

Coppel, R.L., Lustigman, S., Murray, L. and Anders, R.F. (1988). MESA is a *Plasmodium falciparum* phosphoprotein associated with the erythrocyte membrane skeleton. *Molecular and Biochemical Parasitology* **31**, 223–231.

Coppel, R.L., Davern, K.M. and McConville, M.J. (1994). Immunochemistry of parasite antigens. In: *Immunochemistry* (C.J. van Oss and M.H.V. van Regenmortel, eds), pp. 475–532. New York: Marcel Dekker.

Coppel, R.L., Brown, G.V. and Nussenzweig, V. (1998a). Adhesive proteins of the malaria parasite. *Current Opinion in Microbiology* **1**, 472–481.

Coppel, R.L., Cooke, B.M., Magowan, C. and Mohandas, N. (1998b). Malaria and the erythrocyte. *Current Opinion in Hematology* **5**, 132–138.

Corcoran, L.M., Forsyth, K.P., Bianco, A.E., Brown, G.V. and Kemp, D.J. (1987). Chromosome size polymorphisms in *Plasmodium falciparum* can involve deletions and are frequent in natural parasite populations. *Cell* **44**, 87–95.

Cowman, A.F., Coppel, R.L., Saint, R.B., Favaloro, J., Crewther, P.E., Stahl, H.D., Bianco, A.E., Brown, G.V., Anders, R.F. and Kemp, D.J. (1984). The ring-infected erythrocyte surface antigen (RESA) polypeptide of *Plasmodium falciparum* contains two separate blocks of tandem repeats encoding antigenic epitopes that are naturally immunogenic in man. *Molecular Biology and Medicine* **2**, 207–221.

Crabb, B.S. and Cowman, A.F. (1996). Characterization of promoters and stable transfection by homologous and nonhomologous recombination in *Plasmodium falciparum. Proceedings of the National Academy of Sciences of the USA* **93**, 7289–7294.

Crabb, B., Cooke, B.M., Reeder, J.C., Waller, R.F., Caruana, S.R., Davern, K.M., Wickham, M.E., Brown, G.V., Coppel, R.L. and Cowman, A.F. (1997a). Targeted gene disruption shows that knobs enable malaria-infected red blood cells to cytoadhere under physiological shear stress. *Cell* **89**, 287–296.

Crabb, B.S., Triglia, T., Waterkeyn, J.G. and Cowman, A.F. (1997b). Stable transgene expression in *Plasmodium falciparum. Molecular and Biochemical Parasitology* **90**, 131–144.

Craig, A., Fernandez-Reyes, D., Mesri, M., McDowall, A., Altieri, D.C., Hogg, N. and Newbold, C. (2000). A functional analysis of a natural variant of intercellular adhesion molecule-1 (ICAM-1^{Kilifi}). *Human Molecular Genetics* **9**, 525–530.

Crandall, I., Collins, W.E., Gysin, J. and Sherman, I.W. (1993). Synthetic peptides based on motifs present in human band 3 protein inhibit cytoadherence/sequestration of the malaria parasite *Plasmodium falciparum. Proceedings of the National Academy of Sciences of the USA* **90**, 4703–4707.

Crandall, I., Land, K.M. and Sherman, I.W. (1994). *Plasmodium falciparum*: Pfalhesin and CD36 form an adhesin/receptor pair that is responsible for the pH dependent portion of cytoadherence/sequestration. *Experimental Parasitology* **78**, 203–209.

Cranston, H.A., Boylan, C.W., Carroll, G.L., Sutera, S.P. and Williamson, J.R. (1984). *Plasmodium falciparum* maturation abolishes physiologic red blood cell deformability. *Science* **223**, 400–403.

Culvenor, J.G., Langford, C.J., Crewther, P.E., Saint, R.B., Coppel, R.L., Kemp, D.J., Anders, R.F. and Brown, G.V. (1987). *Plasmodium falciparum*: identification and localization of a knob protein antigen expressed by a cDNA clone. *Experimental Parasitology* **63**, 58–67.

Culvenor, J.G., Day, K.P. and Anders, R.F. (1991). *Plasmodium falciparum* ring-infected erythrocyte surface antigen is released from merozoite dense granules after erythrocyte invasion. *Infection and Immunity* **59**, 1183–1187.

Das, A., Elmendorf, H.G., Li, W.I. and Haldar, K. (1994). Biosynthesis, export and processing of a 45 kDa protein detected in membrane clefts of erythrocytes infected with *Plasmodium falciparum. Biochemical Journal* **302**, 487–496.

Da Silva, E., Foley, M., Dluzewski, A.R., Murray, L.J., Anders, R.F. and Tilley, L. (1994). The *Plasmodium falciparum* protein RESA interacts with the erythrocyte cytoskeleton and modifies erythrocyte thermal stability. *Molecular and Biochemical Parasitology* **66**, 59–69.

David, P.H., Handunnetti, S.M., Leech, J.H., Gamage, P. and Mendis, K.N. (1988). Rosetting: a new cytoadherence property of malaria-infected erythrocytes. *American Journal of Tropical Medicine and Hygiene* **38**, 289–297.

Day, K.P., Karamalis, F., Thompson, J., Barnes, D.A., Peterson, C., Brown, H., Brown, G.V. and Kemp, D.J. (1993). Genes necessary for expression of a virulence determinant and for transmission of *Plasmodium falciparum* are located on a 0·3-megabase region of chromosome 9. *Proceedings of the National Academy of Sciences of the USA* **90**, 8292–8296.

Dean, N. and Pelham, H. (1990). Recycling of proteins from the Golgi compartment to the ER in yeast. *Journal of Cell Biology* **111**, 369–377.

Decastro, F.A., Ward, G.E., Jambou, R., Attal, G., Mayau, V., Jaureguiberry, G., Braunbreton, C., Chakrabarti, D. and Langsley, G. (1996). Identification of a family of RAB G-proteins in *Plasmodium falciparum* and a detailed characterisation of PfRab6. *Molecular and Biochemical Parasitology* **80**, 77–88.

Deitsch, K.W. and Wellems, T.E. (1996). Membrane modifications in erythrocytes parasitized by *Plasmodium falciparum. Molecular and Biochemical Parasitology* **76**, 1–10.

Dondorp, A.M., Angus, B.J., Hardeman, M.R., Chotivanich, K.T., Silamut, K., Ruangveerayuth, R., Kager, P.A., White, N.J. and Vreeken, J. (1997). Prognostic significance of reduced red blood cell deformability in severe falciparum malaria. *American Journal of Tropical Medicine and Hygiene* **57**, 507–511.

Dondorp, A.M., Kager, P.A., Vreeken, J. and White, N.J. (2000). Abnormal blood flow and red blood cell deformability in severe malaria. *Parasitology Today* **16**, 228–232.

Eda, S., Lawler, J. and Sherman, I.W. (1999). *Plasmodium falciparum*-infected erythrocyte adhesion to the type 3 repeat domain of thrombospondin-1 is mediated by a modified band 3 protein. *Molecular and Biochemical Parasitology* **100**, 195–205.

Eisen, D., Billman-Jacobe, H., Marshall, V.F., Fryauff, D. and Coppel, R.L. (1998). Temporal variation of the merozoite surface protein-2 gene of *Plasmodium falciparum. Infection and Immunity* **66**, 239–246.

Elmendorf, H.G. and Haldar, K. (1993). Secretory transport in *Plasmodium. Parasitology Today* **9**, 98–102.

Elmendorf, H.G. and Haldar, K. (1994). *Plasmodium falciparum* exports the Golgi marker sphingomyelin synthase into a tubovesicular network in the cytoplasm of mature erythrocytes. *Journal of Cell Biology* **124**, 449–462.

Etzion, Z. and Perkins, M.E. (1989). Localization of a parasite encoded protein to erythrocyte cytoplasmic vesicles of *Plasmodium falciparum*-infected cells. *European Journal of Cell Biology* **48**, 174–179.

Evans, E. (1989). Structure and deformation properties of red blood cells: concepts and quantitative methods. *Methods in Enzymology* **173**, 3–35.

Evans, E. and Hochmuth, R. (1977). A solid–liquid composite model of the red blood cell membrane. *Journal of Membrane Biology* **30**, 351–362.

Everitt, J.I., Shadduck, J.A., Steinkamp, C. and Clabaugh, W. (1986). Experimental *Babesia bovis* infection in Holstein calves. *Veterinary Pathology* **23**, 556–562.

Facer, C.A. (1995). Erythrocytes carrying mutations in spectrin and protein 4.1 show differing sensitivities to invasion by *Plasmodium falciparum. Parasitology Research* **81**, 52–57.

Favaloro, J.M., Coppel, R.L., Corcoran, L.M., Foote, S.J., Brown, G.V., Anders, R.F. and Kemp, D.J. (1986). Structure of the *RESA* gene of *Plasmodium falciparum. Nucleic Acids Research* **14**, 8265–8277.

Fernandez, V., Hommel, M., Chen, Q., Hagblom, P. and Wahlgren, M. (1999). Small, clonally variant antigens expressed on the surface of the *Plasmodium falciparum*-infected erythrocyte are encoded by the *rif* gene family and are the target of human immune responses. *Journal of Experimental Medicine* **190**, 1393–1404.

Fernandez-Reyes, D., Craig, A.G., Kyes, S.A., Peshu, N., Snow, R.W., Berendt, A.R., Marsh, K. and Newbold, C.I. (1997). A high frequency African coding polymorphism in the N-terminal domain of ICAM-1 predisposing to cerebral malaria in Kenya. *Human Molecular Genetics* **6**, 1357–1360.

Fischer, K., Horrocks, P., Preuss, M., Wiesner, J., Wunsch, S., Camargo, A.A. and Lanzer, M. (1997). Expression of *var* genes located within polymorphic subtelomeric domains of *Plasmodium falciparum* chromosomes. *Molecular and Cellular Biology* **17**, 3679–3686.

Fischer, T.M., Stohr-Lissen, M. and Schmid-Schonbein, H. (1978). The red blood cell as a fluid droplet: tank tread-like motion of the human erythrocyte membrane in shear flow. *Science* **202**, 894–896.

Foley, M. and Tilley, L. (1995). Home improvements: malaria and the red blood cell. *Parasitology Today* **11**, 436–439.

Foley, M., Murray, L.J. and Anders, R.F. (1990). The ring-infected erythrocyte surface antigen protein of *Plasmodium falciparum* is phosphorylated upon association with the host cell membrane. *Molecular and Biochemical Parasitology* **38**, 69–76.

Foley, M., Tilley, L., Sawyer, W.H. and Anders, R.F. (1991). The ring-infected erythrocyte surface antigen of *Plasmodium falciparum* associates with spectrin in the erythrocyte membrane. *Molecular and Biochemical Parasitology* **46**, 137–148.

Foley, M., Corcoran, L., Tilley, L. and Anders, R. (1994). *Plasmodium falciparum*: mapping the membrane-binding domain in the ring-infected erythrocyte surface antigen. *Experimental Parasitology* **79**, 340–350.

Foote, S.J. and Kemp, D.J. (1989). Chromosomes of malarial parasites. *Trends in Genetics* **5**, 337–342.

Francis, R.B. (1991). Large-vessel occlusion in sickle cell disease: pathogenesis, clinical consequences, and therapeutic implications. *Medical Hypotheses* **35**, 88–95.

Francis, R.B., jr, and Johnson, C.S. (1991). Vascular occlusion in sickle cell disease: current concepts and unanswered questions. *Blood* **77**, 1405–1414.

Fried, M. and Duffy, P.E. (1996). Adherence of *Plasmodium falciparum* to chondroitin sulfate A in the human placenta. *Science* **272**, 1502–1504.

Fried, M., Nosten, F., Brockman, A., Brabin, B.J. and Duffy, P.E. (1998). Maternal antibodies block malaria. *Nature* **395**, 851–852.

Gaehtgens, P., Duhrssen, C. and Albrecht, K.H. (1980). Motion, deformation, and interaction of blood cells and plasma during flow through narrow capillary tubes. *Blood Cells* **6**, 799–817.

Gardiner, D.L., Holt, D.C., Thomas, E.A., Kemp, D.J. and Trenholme, K.R. (2000). Inhibition of *Plasmodium falciparum clag9* gene function by antisense RNA. *Molecular and Biochemical Parasitology* **110**, 33–41.

Gardner, J.P., Pinches, R.A., Roberts, D.J. and Newbold, C.I. (1996). Variant antigens and endothelial receptor adhesion in *Plasmodium falciparum*. *Proceedings of the National Academy of Sciences of the USA* **93**, 3503–3508.

Gardner, K. and Bennett, G.V. (1989). Recently identified erythrocyte membrane-skeletal proteins and interactions. Implications for structure and function. In: *Red Blood Cell Membranes: Structure, Function, Clinical Implications* (P. Agre and J.C. Parker, eds), pp. 1–29. New York: Marcel Dekker.

Gardner, M.J., Tettelin, H., Carucci, D.J., Cummings, L.M., Aravind, L., Koonin, E.V., Shallom, S., Mason, T., Yu, K., Fujii, C., Pederson, J., Shen, K., Jing, J., Aston, C., Lai, Z., Schwartz, D.C., Pertea, M., Salzberg, S., Zhou, L., Sutton, G.G., Clayton, R., White, O., Smith, H.O., Fraser, C.M., Adams, M.D., Venter, J.C. and Hoffman, S.L. (1998). Chromosome 2 sequence of the human malaria parasite *Plasmodium falciparum*. *Science* **282**, 1126–1132.

Genton, B., Al-Yaman, F., Anders, R., Saul, A., Brown, G., Pye, D., Irving, D.O., Briggs, W.R., Mai, A., Ginny, M., Adiguma, T., Rare, L., Giddy, A., Reber-Liske, R., Stuerchler, D. and Alpers, M.P. (2000). Safety and immunogenicity of a three-component blood-stage malaria vaccine in adults living in an endemic area of Papua New Guinea. *Vaccine* **18**, 2504–2511.

Ginsburg, H. (1994a). How *Plasmodium* secures nutrients: new targets for drugs. *Parasitology Today* **10**, 102–103.

Ginsburg, H. (1994b). Transport pathways in the malaria-infected erythrocyte — characterization and their use as potential targets for chemotherapy. *Memórias do Instituto Oswaldo Cruz* **89**, 99–109.

Green, M.A., Noguchi, C.T., Keidan, A.J., Marwah, S.S. and Stuart, J. (1988). Polymerization of sickle cell hemoglobin at arterial oxygen saturation impairs erythrocyte deformability. *Journal of Clinical Investigation* **81**, 1669–1674.

Gritzmacher, C.A. and Reese, R.T. (1984). Reversal of knob formation on *Plasmodium falciparum*-infected erythrocytes. *Science* **226**, 65–67.

Gruenberg, J. and Sherman, I.W. (1983). Isolation and characterization of the plasma membrane of human erythrocytes infected with the malarial parasite *Plasmodium falciparum. Proceedings of the National Academy of Sciences of the USA* **80**, 1087–1091.

Gruenberg, J., Allred, D. and Sherman, I. (1983). Scanning electron microscope-analysis of the protrusions (knobs) present on the surface of *Plasmodium falciparum*-infected erythrocytes. *Journal of Cell Biology* **97**, 795–802.

Günther, K., Tummler, M., Arnold, H.H., Ridley, R., Goman, M., Scaife, J.G. and Lingelbach, K. (1991). An exported protein of *Plasmodium falciparum* is synthesized as an integral membrane protein. *Molecular and Biochemical Parasitology* **46**, 149–157.

Hadley, T.J., Leech, J.H., Green, T.J., Daniel, W.A., Wahlgren, M., Miller, L.H. and Howard, R.J. (1983). A comparison of knobby (k+) and knobless (k–) parasites from two strains of *Plasmodium falciparum. Molecular and Biochemical Parasitology* **9**, 271–278.

Haldar, K. (1994). Ducts, channels and transporters in *Plasmodium*-infected erythrocytes. *Parasitology Today* **10**, 393–395.

Haldar, K. (1998). Intracellular trafficking in *Plasmodium*-infected erythrocytes. *Current Opinion in Microbiology* **1**, 466–471.

Haldar, K., Henderson, C.L. and Cross, G.A. (1986). Identification of the parasite transferrin receptor of *Plasmodium falciparum*-infected erythrocytes and its acylation via 1,2-diacyl-sn-glycerol. *Proceedings of the National Academy of Sciences of the USA* **83**, 8565–8569.

Handunnetti, S.M., Pasloske, B.L., van Schravendijk, M.R., Aguiar, J.C., Taraschi, T.F., Gormley, J.A. and Howard, R.J. (1992a). The characterization of two monoclonal antibodies which react with high molecular weight antigens of asexual *Plasmodium falciparum. Molecular and Biochemical Parasitology* **54**, 231–246.

Handunnetti, S.M., van Schravendijk, M.R., Hasler, T., Barnwell, J.W., Greenwalt, D.E. and Howard, R.J. (1992b). Involvement of CD36 on erythrocytes as a rosetting receptor for *Plasmodium falciparum*-infected erythrocytes. *Blood* **80**, 2097–2104.

Hasler, T., Handunnetti, S.M., Aguiar, J.C., Van, S.M., Greenwood, B.M., Lallinger, G., Cegielski, P. and Howard, R.J. (1990). *In vitro* rosetting, cytoadherence, and microagglutination properties of *Plasmodium falciparum*-infected erythrocytes from Gambian and Tanzanian patients. *Blood* **76**, 1845–1852.

Haynes, J. (1993). Erythrocytes and malaria. *Current Opinion in Hematology* **1**, 79–89.

Helmby, H., Cavelier, L., Pettersson, U. and Wahlgren, M. (1993). Rosetting *Plasmodium falciparum*-infected erythrocytes express unique strain-specific antigens on their surface. *Infection and Immunity* **61**, 284–288.

Hernandez-Rivas, R., Mattei, D., Sterkers, Y., Peterson, D.S., Wellems, T.E. and Scherf, A. (1997). Expressed *var* genes are found in *Plasmodium falciparum* subtelomeric regions. *Molecular and Cellular Biology* **17**, 604–611.

Herrera, S., Rudin, W., Herrera, M., Clavijo, P., Mancilla, L., De, P.C., Matile, H. and Certa, U. (1993). A conserved region of the MSP-1 surface protein of *Plasmodium falciparum* contains a recognition sequence for erythrocyte spectrin. *EMBO Journal* **12**, 1607–1614.

Hinterberg, K., Mattei, D., Wellems, T.E. and Scherf, A. (1994a). Interchromosomal exchange of a large subtelomeric segment in a *Plasmodium falciparum* cross. *EMBO Journal* **13**, 4174–4180.

Hinterberg, K., Scherf, A., Gysin, J., Toyoshima, T., Aikawa, M., Mazie, J.C., Dasilva, L.P. and Mattei, D. (1994b). *Plasmodium falciparum*: the Pf332 antigen is secreted from the parasite by a brefeldin A-dependent pathway and is translocated to the erythrocyte membrane via the Maurer's clefts. *Experimental Parasitology* **79**, 279–291.

Hirawake, H., Kita, K. and Sharma, Y.D. (1997). Variations in the C-terminal repeats of the knob-associated histidine-rich protein of *Plasmodium falciparum. Biochimica et Biophysica Acta* **1360**, 105–108.

Ho, M., Singh, B., Looareesuwan, S., Davis, T., Bunnag, D. and White, N.J. (1991). Clinical correlates of *in vitro Plasmodium falciparum* cytoadherence. *Infection and Immunity* **59**, 873–878.

Holt, D.C., Gardiner, D.L., Thomas, E.A., Mayo, M., Bourke, P.F., Sutherland, C.J., Carter, R., Myers, G., Kemp, D.J. and Trenholme, K.R. (1999). The cytoadherence linked asexual gene family of *Plasmodium falciparum*: are there roles other than cytoadherence? *International Journal for Parasitology* **29**, 939–944.

Hommel, M., David, P.H. and Oligino, L.D. (1983). Surface alterations of erythrocytes in *Plasmodium falciparum* malaria. *Journal of Experimental Medicine* **157**, 1137–1148.

Hood, A.T., Fabry, M.E., Costantini, F., Nagel, R.L. and Shear, H.L. (1996). Protection from lethal malaria in transgenic mice expressing sickle hemoglobin. *Blood* **87**, 1600–1603.

Hope, I.A., Mackay, M., Hyde, J.E., Goman, M. and Scaife, J. (1985). The gene for an exported antigen of the malaria parasite *Plasmodium falciparum* cloned and expressed in *Escherichia coli. Nucleic Acids Research* **13**, 369–379.

Howard, R.F. and Schmidt, C.M. (1995). The secretory pathway of *Plasmodium falciparum* regulates transport of P82/RAP-1 to the rhoptries. *Molecular and Biochemical Parasitology* **74**, 43–54.

Howard, R.F., Stanley, H.A. and Reese, R.T. (1988). Characterization of a high-molecular-weight phosphoprotein synthesized by the human malarial parasite *Plasmodium falciparum. Gene* **64**, 65–75.

Howard, R.F., Narum, D.L., Blackman, M. and Thurman, J. (1998). Analysis of the processing of *Plasmodium falciparum* rhoptry-associated protein 1 and localization of Pr86 to schizont rhoptries and p67 to free merozoites. *Molecular and Biochemical Parasitology* **92**, 111–122.

Howard, R.J. (1988). Malarial proteins at the membrane of *Plasmodium falciparum*-infected erythrocytes and their involvement in cytoadherence to endothelial cells. *Progress in Allergy* **41**, 98–147.

Howard, R.J., Barnwell, J.W. and Kao, V. (1983). Antigenic variation of *Plasmodium knowlesi* malaria: identification of the variant antigen on infected erythrocytes. *Proceedings of the National Academy of Sciences of the USA* **80**, 4129–4133.

Howard, R.J., Uni, S., Aikawa, M., Aley, S.B., Leech, J.H., Lew, A.M., Wellems, T.E., Rener, J. and Taylor, D.W. (1986). Secretion of a malarial histidine-rich protein (PfHRPII) from *Plasmodium falciparum*-infected erythrocytes. *Journal of Cell Biology* **103**, 1269–1277.

Howard, R.J., Lyon, J.A., Uni, S., Saul, A.J., Aley, S.B., Klotz, F., Panton, L.J., Sherwood, J.A., Marsh, K., Aikawa, M. and Rock, E.P. (1987). Transport of an M_r approximately 300,000 *Plasmodium falciparum* protein (PfEMP2) from the intraerythrocytic asexual parasite to the cytoplasmic face of the host cell membrane. *Journal of Cell Biology* **104**, 1269–1280.

Howard, R.J., Barnwell, J.W., Rock, E.P., Neequaye, J., Ofori, A.D., Maloy, W.L., Lyon, J.A. and Saul, A. (1988). Two approximately 300 kilodalton *Plasmodium falciparum* proteins at the surface membrane of infected erythrocytes. *Molecular and Biochemical Parasitology* **27**, 207–224.

Hoyte, H.M.D. (1971). Differential diagnosis of *Babesia argentina* and *Babesia bigemina* infections in cattle using thin blood smears and brain smears. *Australian Veterinary Journal* **47**, 248–250.

Hughes, M.K. and Hughes, A.L. (1995). Natural selection on *Plasmodium* surface proteins. *Molecular and Biochemical Parasitology* **71**, 99–113.

Hui, G.S. and Siddiqui, W.A. (1988). Characterization of a *Plasmodium falciparum* polypeptide associated with membrane vesicles in the infected erythrocytes. *Molecular and Biochemical Parasitology* **29**, 283–293.

Hunt, N.H. and Stocker, R. (1990). Oxidative stress and the redox status of malaria-infected erythrocytes. *Blood Cells* **16**, 499–526.

Joiner, C.H. (1993). Cation transport and volume regulation in sickle red blood cells. *American Journal of Physiology* **264**, C251–C270.

Joshi, P., Alam, A., Chandra, R., Puri, S.K. and Gupta, C.M. (1986). Possible basis for membrane changes in nonparasitized erythrocytes of malaria-infected animals. *Biochimica et Biophysica Acta* **862**, 220–222.

Kant, R. and Sharma, Y. (1996). Allelic forms of the knob associated histidine-rich protein gene of *Plasmodium falciparum*. *FEBS Letters* **380**, 147–151.

Kara, U.A., Stenzel, D.J., Ingram, L.T. and Kidson, C. (1988). The parasitophorous vacuole membrane of *Plasmodium falciparum*: demonstration of vesicle formation using an immunoprobe. *European Journal of Cell Biology* **46**, 9–17.

Kara, U., Murray, B., Pam, C., Lahnstein, J., Gould, H., Kidson, C. and Saul, A. (1990). Chemical characterization of the parasitophorous vacuole membrane antigen QF116 from *Plasmodium falciparum*. *Molecular and Biochemical Parasitology* **38**, 19–23.

Kaul, D.K., Roth, E.J., Nagel, R.L., Howard, R.J. and Handunnetti, S.M. (1991). Rosetting of *Plasmodium falciparum*-infected red blood cells with uninfected red blood cells enhances microvascular obstruction under flow conditions. *Blood* **78**, 812–819.

Kawai, S., Kano, S. and Suzuki, M. (1995). Rosette formation by *Plasmodium coatneyi*-infected erythrocytes of the Japanese macaque (*Macaca fuscata*). *American Journal of Tropical Medicine and Hygiene* **53**, 295–299.

Kilejian, A. (1979). Characterization of a protein correlated with the production of knob-like protrusions on membranes of erythrocytes infected with *Plasmodium falciparum*. *Proceedings of the National Academy of Sciences of the USA* **76**, 4650–4653.

Kilejian, A. and Olson, J. (1979). Proteins and glycoproteins from human erythrocytes infected with *Plasmodium falciparum*. *Bulletin of the World Health Organization* **57**, 101–107.

Kilejian, A., Sharma, Y.D., Karoui, H. and Naslund, L. (1986). Histidine-rich domain of the knob protein of the human malaria parasite *Plasmodium falciparum*. *Proceedings of the National Academy of Sciences of the USA* **83**, 7938–7941.

Kilejian, A., Rashid, M.A., Aikawa, M., Aji, T. and Yang, Y.F. (1991). Selective association of a fragment of the knob protein with spectrin, actin and the red blood cell membrane. *Molecular and Biochemical Parasitology* **44**, 175–182.

Knapp, B., Hundt, E. and Kupper, H.A. (1989). A new blood stage antigen of *Plasmodium falciparum* transported to the erythrocyte surface. *Molecular and Biochemical Parasitology* **37**, 47–56.

Knapp, B., Nau, U., Hundt, E. and Küpper, H.A. (1991). A new blood stage antigen of *Plasmodium falciparum* highly homologous to the serine-stretch protein SERP. *Molecular and Biochemical Parasitology* **44**, 1–14.

Kochan, J., Perkins, M. and Ravetch, J.V. (1986). A tandemly repeated sequence determines the binding domain for an erythrocyte receptor binding protein of *P. falciparum*. *Cell* **44**, 689–696.

Konigk, E. and Mirtsch, S. (1977). *Plasmodium chabaudi*-infection of mice: specific activities of erythrocyte membrane-associated enzymes and patterns of proteins and glycoproteins of erythrocyte membrane preparations. *Tropenmedizin und Parasitologie* **28**, 17–22.

Korsgren, C. and Cohen, C.M. (1988). Associations of human erythrocyte band 4.2. Binding to ankyrin and to the cytoplasmic domain of band 3. *Journal of Biological Chemistry* **263**, 10212–10218.

Kun, J., Hesselbach, J., Schreiber, M., Scherf, A., Gysin, J., Mattei, D., Pereira da Silva, L. and Muller-Hill, B. (1991). Cloning and expression of genomic DNA sequences coding for putative erythrocyte membrane-associated antigens of *Plasmodium falciparum*. *Research in Immunology* **142**, 199–210.

Kun, J.F.J., Leet, M., Anthony, R.L., Kun, J.E. and Anders, R.F. (1994). *Plasmodium falciparum*: a region of polymorphism in the 3′ end of the gene for the ring-infected erythrocyte surface antigen. *Experimental Parasitology* **78**, 418–421.

Kun, J.F.J., Hibbs, A.R., Saul, A., McColl, D.J., Coppel, R.L. and Anders, R.F. (1997). A putative *Plasmodium falciparum* exported serine/threonine protein kinase. *Molecular and Biochemical Parasitology* **85**, 41–51.

Kun, J.F.J., Waller, K. and Coppel, R.L. (1999). *Plasmodium falciparum*: structural and functional domains of the mature-parasite-infected erythrocyte surface antigen. *Experimental Parasitology* **91**, 258–267.

Kyes, S.A., Rowe, J.A., Kriek, N. and Newbold, C.I. (1999). Rifins: a second family of clonally variant proteins expressed on the surface of red blood cells infected with *Plasmodium falciparum*. *Proceedings of the National Academy of Sciences of the USA* **96**, 9333–9338.

La Greca, N., Hibbs, A.R., Riffkin, C., Foley, M. and Tilley, L. (1997). Identification of an endoplasmic reticulum-resident calcium-binding protein with multiple EF-hand motifs in asexual stages of *Plasmodium falciparum*. *Molecular and Biochemical Parasitology* **89**, 283–293.

Langreth, S.G. and Peterson, E. (1985). Pathogenicity, stability, and immunogenicity of a knobless clone of *Plasmodium falciparum* in Colombian owl monkeys. *Infection and Immunity* **47**, 760–766.

Langreth, S.G. and Reese, R.T. (1979). Antigenicity of the infected-erythrocyte and merozoite surfaces in falciparum malaria. *Journal of Experimental Medicine* **150**, 1241–1254.

Lee, M.V., Ambrus, J.L., DeSouza, J.M. and Lee, R.V. (1982). Diminished red blood cell deformability in uncomplicated human malaria. A preliminary report. *Journal of Medicine* **13**, 479–485.

Leech, J.H., Barnwell, J.W., Aikawa, M., Miller, L.H. and Howard, R.J. (1984a). *Plasmodium falciparum* malaria: association of knobs on the surface of infected erythrocytes with a histidine-rich protein and the erythrocyte skeleton. *Journal of Cell Biology* **98**, 1256–1264.

Leech, J.H., Barnwell, J.W., Miller, L.H. and Howard, R.J. (1984b). Identification of a strain-specific malarial antigen exposed on the surface of *Plasmodium falciparum*-infected erythrocytes. *Journal of Experimental Medicine* **159**, 1567–1575.

Ling, E., Danilov, Y.N. and Cohen, C.M. (1988). Modulation of red blood cell band 4.1 function by cAMP-dependent kinase and protein kinase C phosphorylation. *Journal of Biological Chemistry* **263**, 2209–2216.

Lingappa, V., Chaidez, J., Yost, C. and Hedgpeth, J. (1984). Determinants for protein localization: beta-lactamase signal sequence directs globin across microsomal membranes. *Proceedings of the National Academy of Sciences of the USA* **81**, 456–460.

Looareesuwan, S., Davis, T., Pukrittayakamee, S., Supanaranond, W., Desakorn, V., Silamut, K., Krishna, S., Boonamrung, S. and White, N.J. (1991). Erythrocyte survival in severe falciparum malaria. *Acta Tropica* **48**, 372–373.

Lowe, B.S., Mosobo, M. and Bull, P.C. (1998). All four species of human malaria parasites form rosettes. *Transactions of the Royal Society of Tropical Medicine and Hygiene* **92**, 526.

Lucas, J.Z. and Sherman, I.W. (1998). *Plasmodium falciparum*: thrombospondin mediates parasitized erythrocyte band 3-related adhesin binding. *Experimental Parasitology* **89**, 78–85.

Lustigman, S., Anders, R.F., Brown, G.V. and Coppel, R.L. (1990). The mature-parasite-infected erythrocyte surface antigen (MESA) of *Plasmodium falciparum* associates with the erythrocyte membrane skeletal protein, band 4.1. *Molecular and Biochemical Parasitology* **38**, 261–270.

Luzzi, G., Merry, A., Newbold, C., Marsh, K., Pasvol, G. and Weatherall, D. (1991a). Surface antigen expression on *Plasmodium falciparum*-infected erythrocytes is modified in alpha- and beta-thalassemia. *Journal of Experimental Medicine* **173**, 785–791.

Luzzi, G.A., Merry, A.H., Newbold, C.I., Marsh, K. and Pasvol, G. (1991b). Protection by alpha-thalassaemia against *Plasmodium falciparum* malaria: modified surface antigen expression rather than impaired growth or cytoadherence. *Immunology Letters* **30**, 233–240.

MacPherson, G.G., Warrell, M.J., White, N.J., Looareesuwan, S. and Warrell, D.A. (1985). Human cerebral malaria. A quantitative ultrastructural analysis of parasitized erythrocyte sequestration. *American Journal of Pathology* **119**, 385–401.

Magowan, C., Wollish, W., Anderson, L. and Leech, J. (1988). Cytoadherence by *Plasmodium falciparum*-infected erythrocytes is correlated with the expression of a family of variable proteins on infected erythrocytes. *Journal of Experimental Medicine* **168**, 1307–1320.

Magowan, C., Coppel, R.L., Lau, A., Moronne, M.M., Tchernia, G. and Mohandas, N. (1995). Role of the *Plasmodium falciparum* mature-parasite infected erythrocyte surface antigen (MESA/PfEMP-2) in malarial infection of erythrocytes. *Blood* **86**, 3196–3204.

Magowan, C., Liang, J., Yeung, J., Takakuwa, Y., Coppel, R.L. and Mohandas, N. (1998). *Plasmodium falciparum*: influence of malarial and host erythrocyte skeletal protein interactions on phosphorylation in infected erythrocytes. *Experimental Parasitology* **89**, 40–49.

Magowan, C., Nunomora, W., Waller, K.L., Yeung, J., Liang, J., Van Dort, H., Low, P.S., Coppel, R.L. and Mohandas, N. (2000). *Plasmodium falciparum* histidine-rich protein 1 associates with the band 3 binding domain of ankyrin in the infected red blood cell membrane. *Biochimica et Biophysica Acta* **1502**, 461–470.

Manno, S., Takakuwa, Y., Nagao, K. and Mohandas, N. (1995). Modulation of erythrocyte membrane mechanical function by beta-spectrin phosphorylation and dephosphorylation. *Journal of Biological Chemistry* **270**, 5659–5665.

Mattei, D. and Scherf, A. (1992). The Pf332 gene of *Plasmodium falciparum* codes for a giant protein that is translocated from the parasite to the membrane of infected erythrocytes. *Gene* **110**, 71–79.

Mattei, D., Berzins, K., Wahlgren, M., Udomsangpetch, R., Perlmann, P., Griesser, H.W., Scherf, A., Muller-Hill, B., Bonnefoy, S., Guillotte, M., Langsley, G., Pereira Da Silva, L.

and Mercereau-Puijalon, O. (1989). Cross-reactive antigenic determinants present on different *Plasmodium falciparum* blood-stage antigens. *Parasite Immunology* **11**, 15–29.

Mattei, D., Hinterberg, K. and Scherf, A. (1992). Pf11-1 and Pf332: two giant proteins synthesized in erythrocytes infected with *Plasmodium falciparum. Parasitology Today* **8**, 426–428.

Mattei, D., Berry, L., Couffin, S. and Richard, O. (1999). The transport of the histidine-rich protein I from *Plasmodium falciparum* is insensitive to brefeldin A. In: *Transport and Trafficking in the Malaria-Infected Erythrocyte* (G.R. Bock and G. Cardew, eds). Novartis Foundation Symposium Vol. 226, pp. 215–226. Chichester: John Wiley and Sons.

Maubert, B., Fievet, N., Tami, G., Boudin, C. and Deloron, P. (2000). Cytoadherence of *Plasmodium falciparum*-infected erythrocytes in the human placenta. *Parasite Immunology* **22**, 191–199.

McCormick, C., Craig, A., Roberts, D., Newbold, C. and Berendt, A. (1997). Intercellular adhesion molecule-1 and CD36 synergise to mediate adherence of *Plasmodium falciparum*-infected erythrocytes to human microvascular endothelial cells. *Journal of Clinical Investigation* **100**, 2521–2529.

McGoron, A.J., Joiner, C.H., Palascak, M.B., Claussen, W.J. and Franco, R.S. (2000). Dehydration of mature and immature sickle red blood cells during fast oxygenation/deoxygenation cycles: role of KCl cotransport and extracellular calcium. *Blood* **95**, 2164–2168.

Menendez, C., Fleming, A.F. and Alonso, P.L. (2000). Malaria-related anaemia. *Parasitology Today* **16**, 469–476.

Miller, L.H., Usami, S. and Chien, S. (1971). Alteration in the rheologic properties of *Plasmodium knowlesi*-infected red blood cells. A possible mechanism for capillary obstruction. *Journal of Clinical Investigation* **50**, 1451–1455.

Miller, L.H., Chien, S. and Usami, S. (1972). Decreased deformability of *Plasmodium coatneyi*-infected red blood cells and its possible relation to cerebral malaria. *American Journal of Tropical Medicine and Hygiene* **21**, 133–136.

Mohandas, N. (1992). Molecular basis for red blood cell membrane viscoelastic properties. *Biochemical Society Transactions* **20**, 776–782.

Mohandas, N. and Chasis, J.A. (1993). Red blood cell deformability, membrane material properties and shape: regulation by transmembrane, skeletal and cytosolic proteins and lipids. *Seminars in Hematology* **30**, 171–192.

Mohandas, N. and Evans, E. (1994). Mechanical properties of the red blood cell membrane in relation to molecular structure and genetic defects. *Annual Review of Biophysics and Biomolecular Structure* **23**, 787–818.

Mohandas, N., Lie-Injo, L.E., Friedman, M. and Mak, J.W. (1984). Rigid membranes of Malayan ovalocytes: a likely genetic barrier against malaria. *Blood* **63**, 1385–1392.

Mohandas, N., Winardi, R., Knowles, D., Leung, A., Parra, M., George, E., Conboy, J. and Chasis, J. (1992). Molecular basis for membrane rigidity of hereditary ovalocytosis. A novel mechanism involving the cytoplasmic domain of band 3. *Journal of Clinical Investigation* **89**, 686–692.

Morris, C.L., Rucknagel, D.L. and Joiner, C.H. (1993). Deoxygenation-induced changes in sickle cell–sickle cell adhesion. *Blood* **81**, 3138–3145.

Muller, H.M., Reckman, I., Hollingdale, M.R., Bujard, H., Robson, K.J. and Crisanti, A. (1993). Thrombospondin related anonymous protein (TRAP) of *Plasmodium falciparum* binds specifically to sulfated glycoconjugates and to HepG2 hepatoma cells suggesting a role for this molecule in sporozoite invasion of hepatocytes. *EMBO Journal* **12**, 2881–2889.

Murray, M.C. and Perkins, M.E. (1989). Phosphorylation of erythrocyte membrane and cytoskeleton proteins in cells infected with *Plasmodium falciparum. Molecular and Biochemical Parasitology* **34**, 229–236.

Nagao, E., Kaneko, O. and Dvorak, J.A. (2000). *Plasmodium falciparum*-infected erythrocytes: qualitative and quantitative analyses of parasite-induced knobs by atomic force microscopy. *Journal of Structural Biology* **130**, 34–44.

Nagel, R.L. and Roth, E.F., jr (1989). Malaria and red blood cell genetic defects. *Blood* **74**, 1213–1221.

Nakamura, K., Hasler, T., Morehead, K., Howard, R.J. and Aikawa, M. (1992). *Plasmodium falciparum*-infected erythrocyte receptor(s) for CD36 and thrombospondin are restricted to knobs on the erythrocyte surface. *Journal of Histochemistry and Cytochemistry* **40**, 1419–1422.

Nash, G.B., Johnson, C.S. and Meiselman, H.J. (1984). Mechanical properties of oxygenated red blood cells in sickle cell (HbSS) disease. *Blood* **63**, 73–82.

Nash, G.B., Johnson, C.S. and Meiselman, H.J. (1986). Influence of oxygen tension on the viscoelastic behavior of red blood cells in sickle cell disease. *Blood* **67**, 110–118.

Nash, G.B., O'Brien, E., Gordon, S.E. and Dormandy, J.A. (1989). Abnormalities in the mechanical properties of red blood cells caused by *Plasmodium falciparum*. *Blood* **74**, 855–861.

Nash, G.B., Cooke, B.M., Carlson, J. and Wahlgren, M. (1992a). Rheological properties of rosettes formed by red blood cells parasitized by *Plasmodium falciparum*. *British Journal of Haematology* **82**, 757–763.

Nash, G.B., Cooke, B.M., Marsh, K., Berendt, A., Newbold, C. and Stuart, J. (1992b). Rheological analysis of the adhesive interactions of red blood cells parasitized by *Plasmodium falciparum*. *Blood* **79**, 798–807.

Naumann, K.M., Jones, G.L., Saul, A. and Smith, R. (1991). A *Plasmodium falciparum* exo-antigen alters erythrocyte membrane deformability. *FEBS Letters* **292**, 95–97.

Newbold, C.I. (1999). Antigenic variation in *Plasmodium falciparum*: mechanisms and consequences. *Current Opinion in Microbiology* **2**, 420–425.

Newbold, C., Craig, A., Kyes, S., Berendt, A., Snow, R., Peshu, N. and Marsh, K. (1997a). PfEMP1, polymorphism and pathogenesis. *Annals of Tropical Medicine and Parasitology* **91**, 551–557.

Newbold, C., Warn, P., Black, G., Berendt, A., Craig, A., Snow, B., Msobo, M., Peshu, N. and Marsh, K. (1997b). Receptor-specific adhesion and clinical disease in *Plasmodium falciparum*. *American Journal of Tropical Medicine and Hygiene* **57**, 389–398.

Newbold, C., Craig, A., Kyes, S., Rowe, A., Fernandez-Reyes, D. and Fagan, T. (1999). Cytoadherence, pathogenesis and the infected red blood cell surface in *Plasmodium falciparum*. *International Journal for Parasitology* **29**, 927–937.

Nunomura, W., Takakuwa, Y., Parra, M., Conboy, J. and Mohandas, N. (2000). Regulation of protein 4.1R, p55 and glycophorin C ternary complex in human erythrocyte membrane. *Journal of Biological Chemistry* **275**, 24540–24546.

Ockenhouse, C.F., Ho, M., Tandon, N.N., Van Seventer, G., Shaw, S., White, N.J., Jamieson, G.A., Chulay, J.D. and Webster, H.K. (1991a). Molecular basis of sequestration in severe and uncomplicated *Plasmodium falciparum* malaria: differential adhesion of infected erythrocytes to CD36 and ICAM-1. *Journal of Infectious Diseases* **164**, 163–169.

Ockenhouse, C.F., Klotz, F.W., Tandon, N.N. and Jamieson, G.A. (1991b). Sequestrin, a CD36 recognition protein on *Plasmodium falciparum* malaria-infected erythrocytes identified by anti-idiotype antibodies. *Proceedings of the National Academy of Sciences of the USA* **88**, 3175–3179.

Ockenhouse, C.F., Tegoshi, T., Maeno, Y., Benjamin, C., Ho, M., Kan, K.E., Thway, Y., Win, K., Aikawa, M. and Lobb, R.R. (1992). Human vascular endothelial cell adhesion receptors for *Plasmodium falciparum*-infected erythrocytes: roles for endothelial leukocyte adhesion molecule 1 and vascular cell adhesion molecule 1. *Journal of Experimental Medicine* **176**, 1183–1189.

O'Connor, R.M., Lane, T.J., Stroup, S.E. and Allred, D.R. (1997). Characterization of a variant erythrocyte surface antigen (VESA1) expressed by *Babesia bovis* during antigenic variation. *Molecular and Biochemical Parasitology* **89**, 259–270.

O'Connor, R.M., Long, J.A. and Allred, D.R. (1999). Cytoadherence of *Babesia bovis*-infected erythrocytes to bovine brain capillary endothelial cells provides an *in vitro* model for sequestration. *Infection and Immunity* **67**, 3921–3928.

Oh, S., Chishti, A., Palek, J. and Liu, S. (1997). Erythrocyte membrane alterations in *Plasmodium falciparum* malaria sequestration. *Current Opinion in Hematology* **4**, 148–154.

Oh, S.S., Voigt, S., Fisher, D., Yi, S.J., LeRoy, P.J., Derick, L.H., Liu, S. and Chishti, A.H. (2000). *Plasmodium falciparum* erythrocyte membrane protein 1 is anchored to the actin–spectrin junction and knob-associated histidine-rich protein in the erythrocyte skeleton. *Molecular and Biochemical Parasitology* **108**, 237–247.

Oquendo, P., Hundt, E., Lawler, J. and Seed, B. (1989). CD36 directly mediates cytoadherence of *Plasmodium falciparum* parasitized erythrocytes. *Cell* **58**, 95–101.

Pasloske, B.L., Baruch, D.I., Van, S.M., Handunnetti, S.M., Aikawa, M., Fujioka, H., Taraschi, T.F., Gormley, J.A. and Howard, R.J. (1993). Cloning and characterization of a *Plasmodium falciparum* gene encoding a novel high-molecular weight host membrane-associated protein, PfEMP3. *Molecular and Biochemical Parasitology* **59**, 59–72.

Pasloske, B.L., Baruch, D.I., Ma, C., Taraschi, T.F., Gormley, J.A. and Howard, R.J. (1994). *PfEMP3* and *HRP1*: co-expressed genes localized to chromosome 2 of *Plasmodium falciparum*. *Gene* **144**, 131–136.

Paulitschke, M. and Nash, G.B. (1993). Membrane rigidity of red blood cells parasitized by different strains of *Plasmodium falciparum*. *Journal of Laboratory and Clinical Medicine* **122**, 581–589.

Perlmann, H., Berzins, K., Wahlgren, M., Carlsson, J., Björkman, A., Patarroyo, M.E. and Perlmann, P. (1984). Antibodies in malarial sera to parasite antigens in the membrane of erythrocytes infected with early asexual stages of *Plasmodium falciparum*. *Journal of Experimental Medicine* **159**, 1686–1704.

Petersen, C., Nelson, R., Magowan, C., Wollish, W., Jensen, J. and Leech, J. (1989). The mature erythrocyte surface antigen of *Plasmodium falciparum* is not required for knobs or cytoadherence. *Molecular and Biochemical Parasitology* **36**, 61–65.

Peterson, M.G., Crewther, P.E., Thompson, J.K., Corcoran, L.M., Coppel, R.L., Brown, G.V., Anders, R.F. and Kemp, D.J. (1988). A second antigenic heat shock protein of *Plasmodium falciparum*. *DNA* **7**, 71–78.

Pfeffer, S.R. and Rothman, J.E. (1987). Biosynthetic protein transport and sorting by the endoplasmic reticulum and Golgi. *Annual Review of Biochemistry* **56**, 829–852.

Podgorski, A. and Elbaum, D. (1985). Properties of red blood cell membrane proteins: mechanism of spectrin and band 4.1 interaction. *Biochemistry* **24**, 7871–7876.

Pologe, L.G. and Ravetch, J.V. (1986). A chromosomal rearrangement in a *P. falciparum* histidine-rich protein gene is associated with the knobless phenotype. *Nature* **322**, 474–477.

Pologe, L.G., Pavlovec, A., Shio, H. and Ravetch, J.V. (1987). Primary structure and subcellular localization of the knob-associated histidine-rich protein of *Plasmodium falciparum*. *Proceedings of the National Academy of Sciences of the USA* **84**, 7139–7143.

Pongponratn, E., Riganti, M., Punpoowong, B. and Aikawa, M. (1991). Microvascular sequestration of parasitized erythrocytes in human falciparum malaria: a pathological study. *American Journal of Tropical Medicine and Hygiene* **44**, 168–175.

Pouvelle, B., Spiegel, R., Hsiao, L., Howard, R.J., Morris, R.L., Thomas, A.P. and Taraschi, T.F. (1991). Direct access to serum macromolecules by intraerythrocytic malaria parasites. *Nature* **353**, 73–75.

Pouvelle, B., Gormley, J.A. and Taraschi, T.F. (1994). Characterization of trafficking pathways and membrane genesis in malaria-infected erythrocytes. *Molecular and Biochemical Parasitology* **66**, 83–96.

Pouvelle, B., Buffet, P.A., Lepolard, C., Scherf, A. and Gysin, J. (2000). Cytoadhesion of *Plasmodium falciparum* ring-stage-infected erythrocytes. *Nature Medicine* **6,** 1264–1268.

Rabilloud, T., Blisnick, T., Heller, M., Luche, S., Aebersold, R., Lunardi, J. and Braun-Breton, C. (1999). Analysis of membrane proteins by two-dimensional electrophoresis: comparison of the proteins extracted from normal or *Plasmodium falciparum*-infected erythrocyte ghosts. *Electrophoresis* **20**, 3603–3610.

Ramsey, E.M. and Donner, M.W. (1980). *Placental Vasculature and Circulation: Anatomy, Physiology, Radiology, Clinical Aspects: Atlas and Textbook*. Philadelphia: Saunders.

Raventos-Suarez, C., Kaul, D.K., Macaluso, F. and Nagel, R.L. (1985). Membrane knobs are required for the microcirculatory obstruction induced by *Plasmodium falciparum*-infected erythrocytes. *Proceedings of the National Academy of Sciences of the USA* **82**, 3829–3833.

Ravetch, J.V., Kochan, J. and Perkins, M. (1985). Isolation of the gene for a glycophorin-binding protein implicated in erythrocyte invasion by a malaria parasite. *Science* **227**, 1593–1597.

Read, D.G., Bushell, G.R. and Kidson, C. (1990). The effect of *Plasmodium falciparum* exo-antigens on the morphology of uninfected erythrocytes. *Parasitology* **100**, 185–190.

Reeder, J.C., Cowman, A.F., Davern, K.M., Beeson, J.G., Thompson, J.K., Rogerson, S.J. and Brown, G.V. (1999). The adhesion of *Plasmodium falciparum*-infected erythrocytes to chondroitin sulfate A is mediated by *P. falciparum* erythrocyte membrane protein 1. *Proceedings of the National Academy of Sciences of the USA* **96**, 5198–5202.

Ringwald, P., Peyron, F., Lepers, J.P., Rabarison, P., Rakotomalala, C., Razanamparany, M., Rabodonirina, M., Roux, J. and Lebras, J. (1993). Parasite virulence factors during falciparum malaria: rosetting, cytoadherence, and modulation of cytoadherence by cytokines. *Infection and Immunity* **61**, 5198–5204.

Roberts, D.D., Sherwood, J.A., Spitalnik, S.L., Panton, L.J., Howard, R.J., Dixit, V.M., Frazier, W.A., Miller, L.H. and Ginsburg, V. (1985). Thrombospondin binds falciparum malaria parasitized erythrocytes and may mediate cytoadherence. *Nature* **318**, 64–66.

Roberts, D.J., Craig, A.G., Berendt, A.R., Pinches, R., Nash, G., Marsh, K. and Newbold, C.I. (1992). Rapid switching to multiple antigenic and adhesive phenotypes in malaria. *Nature* **357**, 689–692.

Roberts, D.J., Pain, A., Kai, O., Kortok, M. and Marsh, K. (2000). Autoagglutination of malaria-infected red blood cells and malaria severity. *Lancet* **355**, 1427–1428.

Rodriguez, M.H. and Jungery, M. (1986). A protein on *Plasmodium falciparum*-infected erythrocytes functions as a transferrin receptor. *Nature* **324**, 388–391.

Rogerson, S.J., Reeder, J.C., Alyaman, F. and Brown, G.V. (1994). Sulfated glycoconjugates as disrupters of *Plasmodium falciparum* erythrocyte rosettes. *American Journal of Tropical Medicine and Hygiene* **51**, 198–203.

Rogerson, S.J., Chaiyaroj, S.C., Ng, K., Reeder, J.C. and Brown, G.V. (1995). Chondroitin sulfate A is a cell surface receptor for *Plasmodium falciparum* infected erythrocytes. *Journal of Experimental Medicine* **182**, 15–20.

Rogerson, S.J., Novakovic, S., Cooke, B.M. and Brown, G.V. (1997). *Plasmodium falciparum*-infected erythrocytes adhere to the proteoglycan thrombomodulin in static and flow-based systems. *Experimental Parasitology* **86**, 8–18.

Rothman, J.E. (1994). Mechanisms of intracellular protein transport. *Nature* **372**, 55–63.

Rothman, J.E. and Orci, L. (1992). Molecular dissection of the secretory pathway. *Nature* **355**, 409–415.

Rowe, A., Obeiro, J., Newbold, C.I. and Marsh, K. (1995). *Plasmodium falciparum* rosetting is associated with malaria severity in Kenya. *Infection and Immunity* **63**, 2323–2326.

Rowe, J.A., Moulds, J.M., Newbold, C.I. and Miller, L.H. (1997). *P. falciparum* rosetting mediated by a parasite-variant erythrocyte membrane protein and complement receptor 1. *Nature* **388**, 292–295.

Rowe, J.A., Rogerson, S.J., Raza, A., Moulds, J.M., Kazatchkine, M.D., Marsh, K., Newbold, C.I., Atkinson, J.P. and Miller, L.H. (2000). Mapping of the region of complement receptor (CR) 1 required for *Plasmodium falciparum* rosetting and demonstration of the importance of CR1 in rosetting in field isolates. *Journal of Immunology* **165**, 6341–6346.

Rowland, P.G., Nash, G.B., Cooke, B.M. and Stuart, J. (1993). Comparative study of the adhesion of sickle cells and malaria-parasitized red blood cells to cultured endothelium. *Journal of Laboratory and Clinical Medicine* **121**, 706–713.

Ruangjirachuporn, W., Udomsangpetch, R., Carlsson, J., Drenckhahn, D., Perlmann, P. and Berzins, K. (1991). *Plasmodium falciparum*: analysis of the interaction of antigen Pf155/RESA with the erythrocyte membrane. *Experimental Parasitology* **73**, 62–72.

Rubio, J.P., Thompson, J.K. and Cowman, A.F. (1996). The *var* genes of *Plasmodium falciparum* are located in the subtelomeric region of most chromosomes. *EMBO Journal* **15**, 4069–4077.

Salmon, M.G., De Souza, J.B., Butcher, G.A. and Playfair, J.H. (1997). Premature removal of uninfected erythrocytes during malarial infection of normal and immunodeficient mice. *Clinical and Experimental Immunology* **108**, 471–476.

Saul, A., Lawrence, G., Smillie, A., Rzepczyk, C., Reed, C., Taylor, D., Anderson, K., Stowers, A., Kemp, R., Allworth, A., Anders, R., Brown, G., Pye, D., Schoofs, P., Irving, D., Dyer, S., Woodrow, G., Briggs, W., Reber, R. and Sturchler, D. (1999). Human phase I vaccine trials of 3 recombinant asexual stage malaria antigens with montanide ISA720 adjuvant. *Vaccine* **17**, 3145–3159.

Schetters, T.P.M. and Eling, W.M.C. (1999). Can *Babesia* infections be used as a model for cerebral malaria? *Parasitology Today* **15**, 492–497.

Schrével, J., Deguercy, A., Mayer, R. and Monsigny, M. (1990). Proteases in malaria-infected red blood cells. *Blood Cells* **16**, 563–584.

Schulman, S., Roth, E.F.J., Cheng, B., Rybicki, A.C., Sussman, I.I., Wong, M., Wang, W., Ranney, H.M., Nagel, R.L. and Schwartz, R.S. (1990). Growth of *Plasmodium falciparum* in human erythrocytes containing abnormal membrane proteins. *Proceedings of the National Academy of Sciences of the USA* **87**, 7339–7343.

Secomb, T.W. and Skalak, R. (1982). A two-dimensional model for capillary flow of an asymmetric cell. *Microvascular Research* **24**, 194–203.

Sharma, Y.D. and Kilejian, A. (1987). Structure of the knob protein (*kp*) gene of *Plasmodium falciparum*. *Molecular and Biochemical Parasitology* **26**, 11–16.

Shear, H.L. (1993). Transgenic and mutant animal models to study mechanisms of protection of red blood cell genetic defects against malaria. *Experientia* **49**, 37–42.

Shear, H.L., Roth, E.J., Fabry, M.E., Costantini, F.D., Pachnis, A., Hood, A. and Nagel, R.L. (1993). Transgenic mice expressing human sickle hemoglobin are partially resistant to rodent malaria. *Blood* **81**, 222–226.

Shear, H.L., Grinberg, L., Gilman, J., Fabry, M.E., Stamatoyannopoulos, G., Goldberg, D.E. and Nagel, R.L. (1998). Transgenic mice expressing human fetal globin are protected from malaria by a novel mechanism. *Blood* **92**, 2520–2526.

Sherman, I.W. (1985). Membrane structure and function of malaria parasites and the infected erythrocyte. *Parasitology* **91**, 609–645.

Sherman, I.W. and Greenan, J.R. (1986). *Plasmodium falciparum*: regional differences in lectin and cationized ferritin binding to the surface of the malaria-infected human erythrocyte. *Parasitology* **93**, 17–32.

Sherman, I.W. and Jones, L.A. (1979). *Plasmodium lophurae*: membrane proteins of erythrocyte-free plasmodia and malaria-infected red blood cells. *Journal of Protozoology* **26**, 489–501.

Sherwood, J.A., Roberts, D.D., Marsh, K., Harvey, E.B., Spitalnik, S.L., Miller, L.H. and Howard, R.J. (1987). Thrombospondin binding by parasitized erythrocyte isolates in falciparum malaria. *American Journal of Tropical Medicine and Hygiene* **36**, 228–233.

Shirley, M.W., Biggs, B.A., Forsyth, K.P., Brown, H.J., Thompson, J.K., Brown, G.V. and Kemp, D.J. (1990). Chromosome 9 from independent clones and isolates of *Plasmodium falciparum* undergoes subtelomeric deletions with similar breakpoints *in vitro*. *Molecular and Biochemical Parasitology* **40**, 137–145.

Siano, J.P., Grady, K.K., Millet, P. and Wick, T.M. (1998). Short report. *Plasmodium falciparum*: cytoadherence to $\alpha_V\beta_3$ on human microvascular endothelial cells. *American Journal of Tropical Medicine and Hygiene* **59**, 77–99.

Silamut, K., Phu, N.H., Whitty, C., Turner, G.D., Louwrier, K., Mai, N.T., Simpson, J.A., Hien, T.T. and White, N.J. (1999). A quantitative analysis of the microvascular sequestration of malaria parasites in the human brain. *American Journal of Pathology* **155**, 395–410.

Sim, B.K.L., Chitnis, C.E., Wasnioska, K., Hadley, T.J. and Miller, L.H. (1994). Receptor and ligand domains for invasion of erythrocytes by *Plasmodium falciparum*. *Science* **264**, 1941–1944.

Simmons, D., Woollett, G., Bergin, C.M., Kay, D. and Scaife, J. (1987). A malaria protein exported into a new compartment within the host erythrocyte. *EMBO Journal* **6**, 485–491.

Smith, J.D., Chitnis, C.E., Craig, A.G., Roberts, D.J., Hudson-Taylor, D.E., Peterson, D.S., Pinches, R., Newbold, C.I. and Miller, L.H. (1995). Switches in expression of *Plasmodium falciparum var* genes correlate with changes in antigenic and cytoadherent phenotypes of infected erythrocytes. *Cell* **82**, 101–110.

Smith, J.D., Craig, A.G., Kriek, N., Hudson-Taylor, D., Kyes, S., Fagen, T., Pinches, R., Baruch, D.I., Newbold, C.I. and Miller, L.H. (2000). Identification of a *Plasmodium falciparum* intercellular adhesion molecule-1 binding domain: a parasite adhesion trait implicated in cerebral malaria. *Proceedings of the National Academy of Sciences of the USA* **97**, 1766–1771.

Stahl, H.D., Crewther, P.E., Anders, R.F., Brown, G.V., Coppel, R.L., Bianco, A.E., Mitchell, G.F. and Kemp, D.J. (1985a). Interspersed blocks of repetitive and charged amino acids in a dominant immunogen of *Plasmodium falciparum*. *Proceedings of the National Academy of Sciences of the USA* **82**, 543–547.

Stahl, H.D., Kemp, D.J., Crewther, P.E., Scanlon, D.B., Woodrow, G., Brown, G.V., Bianco, A.E., Anders, R.F. and Coppel, R.L. (1985b). Sequence of a cDNA encoding a small polymorphic histidine- and alanine-rich protein from *Plasmodium falciparum*. *Nucleic Acids Research* **13**, 7837–7846.

Stahl, H.D., Bianco, A.E., Crewther, P.E., Anders, R.F., Kyne, A.P., Coppel, R.L., Mitchell, G.F., Kemp, D.J. and Brown, G.V. (1986). Sorting large numbers of clones expressing *Plasmodium falciparum* antigens in *Escherichia coli* by differential antibody screening. *Molecular Biology and Medicine* **3**, 351–368.

Stahl, H.D., Crewther, P.E., Anders, R.F. and Kemp, D.J. (1987). Structure of the *fira* gene of *Plasmodium falciparum*. *Molecular Biology and Medicine* **4**, 199–211.

Stanley, H.A. and Reese, R.T. (1986). *Plasmodium falciparum* polypeptides associated with the infected erythrocyte plasma membrane. *Proceedings of the National Academy of Sciences of the USA* **83**, 6093–6097.

Stuart, J. (1985). Erythrocyte rheology. *Journal of Clinical Pathology* **38**, 965–977.

Stuart, J., Bull, B. and Juhan-Vague, I. (1984). Microrheological techniques for the measurement of erythrocyte deformability. In: *Investigative Microtechniques in Medicine and Biology* (J. Chayen and L. Bitensky, eds), pp. 297–326. New York: Marcel Dekker.

Su, X.Z., Heatwole, V.M., Wertheimer, S.P., Guinet, F., Herrfeldt, J.A., Peterson, D.S., Ravetch, J.A. and Wellems, T.E. (1995). The large diverse gene family *var* encodes proteins involved in cytoadherence and antigenic variation of *Plasmodium falciparum*-infected erythrocytes. *Cell* **82**, 89–100.

Swift, A. and Machamer, C. (1991). A Golgi retention signal in a membrane-spanning domain of coronavirus E1 protein. *Journal of Cell Biology* **115**, 19–30.

Tanabe, K. (1990a). Ion metabolism in malaria-infected erythrocytes. *Blood Cells* **16**, 437–449.

Tanabe, K. (1990b). *Plasmodium* and the infected erythrocyte: glucose transport in malaria infected erythrocytes. *Parasitology Today* **6**, 225–229.

Taylor, D.W., Parra, M., Chapman, G.B., Stearns, M.E., Rener, J., Aikawa, M., Uni, S., Aley, S.B., Panton, L.J. and Howard, R.J. (1987a). Localization of *Plasmodium falciparum* histidine-rich protein 1 in the erythrocyte skeleton under knobs. *Molecular and Biochemical Parasitology* **25**, 165–174.

Taylor, D.W., Parra, M. and Stearns, M.E. (1987b). *Plasmodium falciparum*: fine structural changes in the cytoskeletons of infected erythrocytes. *Experimental Parasitology* **64**, 178–187.

Thevenin, B.J. and Low, P.S. (1990). Kinetics and regulation of the ankyrin–band 3 interaction of the human red blood cell membrane. *Journal of Biological Chemistry* **265**, 16166–16172.

Thevenin, B.J.M., Crandall, I., Ballas, S.K., Sherman, I.W. and Shohet, S.B. (1997). Band 3 peptides block the adherence of sickle cells to endothelial cells *in vitro*. *Blood* **90**, 4172–4179.

Thompson, J.K., Rubio, J.P., Caruana, S., Brockman, A., Wickham, M.E. and Cowman, A.F. (1997). The chromosomal organization of the *Plasmodium falciparum var* gene family is conserved. *Molecular and Biochemical Parasitology* **87**, 49–60.

Trager, W., Rudzinska, M.A. and Bradbury, P.C. (1966). The fine structure of *Plasmodium falciparum* and its host erythrocytes in natural malarial infections in man. *Bulletin of the World Health Organization* **35**, 883–885.

Trelka, D.P., Schneider, T.G., Reeder, J.C. and Taraschi, T.F. (2000). Evidence for vesicle-mediated trafficking of parasite proteins to the host cell cytosol and erythrocyte surface membrane in *Plasmodium falciparum* infected erythrocytes. *Molecular and Biochemical Parasitology* **106**, 131–145.

Trenholme, K.R., Gardiner, D.L., Holt, D.C., Thomas, E.A., Cowman, A.F. and Kemp, D.J. (2000). *Clag9*: a cytoadherence gene in *Plasmodium falciparum* essential for binding of parasitized erythrocytes to CD36. *Proceedings of the National Academy of Sciences of the USA* **97**, 4029–4033.

Treutiger, C.J., Hedlund, I., Helmby, H., Carlson, J., Jepson, A., Twumasi, P., Kwiatkowski, D., Greenwood, B.M. and Wählgren, M. (1992). Rosette formation in *Plasmodium falciparum* isolates and anti-rosette activity of sera from Gambians with cerebral or uncomplicated malaria. *American Journal of Tropical Medicine and Hygiene* **46**, 503–510.

Treutiger, C., Heddini, A., Fernandez, V., Mulle, W. and Wählgren, M. (1997). PECAM-1/CD31, an endothelial receptor for binding *Plasmodium falciparum*-infected erythrocytes. *Nature Medicine* **3**, 1405–1408.

Triglia, T., Stahl, H.D., Crewther, P.E., Scanlon, D., Brown, G.V., Anders, R.F. and Kemp, D.J. (1987). The complete sequence of the gene for the knob-associated histidine-rich protein from *Plasmodium falciparum*. *EMBO Journal* **6**, 1413–1419.

Triglia, T., Stahl, H.D., Crewther, P.E., Silva, A., Anders, R.F. and Kemp, D.J. (1988). Structure of a *Plasmodium falciparum* gene that encodes a glutamic acid-rich protein (garp). *Molecular and Biochemical Parasitology* **31**, 199–201.

Turner, G.D.H., Morrison, H., Jones, M., Davis, T.M.E., Looareesuwan, S., Buley, I.D., Gatter, K.C., Newbold, C.I., Pukritayakamee, S., Nagachinta, B., White, N.J. and Berendt, A.R. (1994). An immunohistochemical study of the pathology of fatal malaria — evidence for widespread endothelial activation and a potential role for intercellular adhesion molecule-1 in cerebral sequestration. *American Journal of Pathology* **145**, 1057–1069.

Tyler, J., Reinhardt, B. and Branton, D. (1980). Associations of erythrocyte membrane proteins. Binding of purified bands 2.1 and 4.1 to spectrin. *Journal of Biological Chemistry* **255**, 7034–7039.

Udomsangpetch, R., Lundgren, K., Berzins, K., Wåhlin, B., Perlmann, H., Troye-Blomberg, M., Carlsson, J., Wahlgren, M., Perlmann, P. and Björkman, A. (1986). Human monoclonal antibodies to Pf155, a major antigen of malaria parasite *Plasmodium falciparum*. *Science* **231**, 57–59.

Udomsangpetch, R., Aikawa, M., Berzins, K., Wahlgren, M. and Perlmann, P. (1989a). Cytoadherence of knobless *Plasmodium falciparum*-infected erythrocytes and its inhibition by a human monoclonal antibody. *Nature* **338**, 763–765.

Udomsangpetch, R., Carlson, J., Wåhlin, B., Holmquist, G., Ozaki, L.S., Scherf, A., Mattei, D., Mercereau-Puijalon, O., Uni, S., Aikawa, M., Berzins, K. and Perlmann, P. (1989b). Reactivity of the human monoclonal antibody 33G2 with repeated sequences of three distinct *Plasmodium falciparum* antigens. *Journal of Immunology* **142**, 3620–3626.

Udomsangpetch, R., Wåhlin, B., Carlson, J., Berzins, K., Torii, M., Aikawa, M., Perlmann, P. and Wahlgren, M. (1989c). *Plasmodium falciparum*-infected erythrocytes form spontaneous erythrocyte rosettes. *Journal of Experimental Medicine* **169**, 1835–1840.

Udomsangpetch, R., Brown, A.E., Dahlem, S.C. and Webster, H.K. (1991). Rosette formation by *Plasmodium coatneyi*-infected red blood cells. *American Journal of Tropical Medicine and Hygiene* **44**, 399–401.

Udomsangpetch, R., Thanikkul, K., Pukrittayakamee, S. and White, N.J. (1995). Rosette formation by *Plasmodium vivax*. *Transactions of the Royal Society of Tropical Medicine and Hygiene* **89**, 635–637.

Udomsangpetch, R., Chivapat, S., Viriyavejakul, P., Riganti, M., Wilairatana, P., Pongponratin, E. and Looareesuwan, S. (1997). Involvement of cytokines in the histopathology of cerebral malaria. *American Journal of Tropical Medicine and Hygiene* **57**, 501–506.

Urban, B.C., Ferguson, D.J., Pain, A., Willcox, N., Plebanski, M., Austyn, J.M. and Roberts, D.J. (1999). *Plasmodium falciparum*-infected erythrocytes modulate the maturation of dendritic cells. *Nature* **400**, 73–77.

Van Dijk, M.R., Waters, A.P. and Janse, C.J. (1995). Stable transfection of malaria parasite blood stages. *Science* **268**, 1358–1362.

Van Schravendijk, M.R., Wilson, R.J. and Newbold, C.I. (1987). Possible pitfalls in the identification of glycophorin-binding proteins of *Plasmodium falciparum*. *Journal of Experimental Medicine* **166**, 376–390.

Van Schravendijk, M., Rock, E.P., Marsh, K., Ito, Y., Aikawa, M., Neequaye, J., Ofori, A.D., Rodriguez, R., Patarroyo, M.E. and Howard, R.J. (1991). Characterization and localization of *Plasmodium falciparum* surface antigens on infected erythrocytes from west African patients. *Blood* **78**, 226–236.

Van Schravendijk, M., Pasloske, B., Baruch, D., Handunnetti, S. and Howard, R. (1993). Immunochemical characterization and differentiation of two approximately 300-kD erythrocyte membrane-associated proteins of *Plasmodium falciparum*, PfEMP1 and PfEMP3. *American Journal of Tropical Medicine and Hygiene* **49**, 552–565.

Van Wye, J., Ghori, N., Webster, P., Mitschler, R.R., Elmendorf, H.G. and Haldar, K. (1996). Identification and localization of Rab6, separation of Rab6 from Erd2 and implications for an 'unstacked' Golgi, in *Plasmodium falciparum. Molecular and Biochemical Parasitology* **83**, 107–120.

Vazeux, G., Le Scanf, C. and Fandeur, T. (1993). The *RESA-2* gene of *Plasmodium falciparum* is transcribed in several independent isolates. *Infection and Immunity* **61**, 4469–4472.

Vernot-Hernandez, J.P. and Heidrich, H.-G. (1984). Time-course of synthesis, transport and incorporation of a protein identified in purified membranes of host erythrocytes infected with a knob-forming strain of *Plasmodium falciparum. Molecular and Biochemical Parasitology* **12**, 337–350.

Vernot-Hernandez, J.P. and Heidrich, H.-G. (1985). The relationship to knobs of the 92,000 D protein specific for knobby strains of *Plasmodium falciparum. Zeitschrift für Parasitenkunde* **71**, 41–51.

Voigt, S., Hanspal, M., LeRoy, P.J., Zhao, P.S., Oh, S.S., Chishti, A.H. and Liu, S.C. (2000). The cytoadherence ligand *Plasmodium falciparum* erythrocyte membrane protein 1 (PfEMP1) binds to the *P. falciparum* knob-associated histidine-rich protein (KAHRP) by electrostatic interactions. *Molecular and Biochemical Parasitology* **110**, 423–428.

Wahlgren, M., Fernandez, V., Scholander, C. and Carlson, J. (1994). Rosetting. *Parasitology Today* **10**, 73–79.

Wåhlin, B., Wahlgren, M., Perlmann, H., Berzins, K., Björkman, A., Patarroyo, M.E. and Perlmann, P. (1984). Human antibodies to a M_r 155,000 *Plasmodium falciparum* antigen efficiently inhibit merozoite invasion. *Proceedings of the National Academy of Sciences of the USA* **81**, 7912–7916.

Wåhlin, B., Sjolander, A., Ahlborg, N., Udomsangpetch, R., Scherf, A., Mattei, D., Berzins, K. and Perlmann, P. (1992). Involvement of Pf155-RESA and cross-reactive antigens in *Plasmodium falciparum* merozoite invasion *in vitro*. *Infection and Immunity* **60**, 443–449.

Waitumbi, J.N., Opollo, M.O., Muga, R.O., Misore, A.O. and Stoute, J.A. (2000). Red cell surface changes and erythrophagocytosis in children with severe *Plasmodium falciparum* anemia. *Blood* **95**, 1481–1486.

Waller, K.L., Cooke, B.M., Nunomura, W., Mohandas, N. and Coppel, R.L. (1999). Mapping the binding domains involved in the interaction between the *Plasmodium falciparum* knob-associated histidine-rich protein (KAHRP) and the cytoadherence ligand *P. falciparum* erythrocyte membrane protein 1 (PfEMP1). *Journal of Biological Chemistry* **274**, 23808–23813.

Waller, R.F., Reed, M.B., Cowman, A.F. and McFadden, G.I. (2000). Protein trafficking to the plastid of *Plasmodium falciparum* is via the secretory pathway. *EMBO Journal* **19**, 1794–1802.

Waterkeyn, J.G., Wickham, M.E., Davern, K.M., Cooke, B.M., Coppel, R.L., Reeder, J.C., Culvenor, J.G., Waller, R.F. and Cowman, A.F. (2000). Targeted mutagenesis of *Plasmodium falciparum* erythrocyte membrane protein 3 (PfEMP3) disrupts cytoadherence of malaria-infected red blood cells. *EMBO Journal* **19**, 2813–2823.

Waters, M. and Pfeffer, S. (1999). Membrane tethering in intracellular transport. *Current Opinion in Cell Biology* **11**, 453–459.

Weber, J.L. (1988). Interspersed repetitive DNA from *Plasmodium falciparum. Molecular and Biochemical Parasitology* **29**, 117–124.

Weidekamm, E., Wallach, D.F., Lin, P.S. and Hendricks, J. (1973). Erythrocyte membrane alterations due to infection with *Plasmodium berghei. Biochimica et Biophysica Acta* **323**, 539–546.

Weisz, O., Machamer, C. and Hubbard, A. (1992). Rat liver dipeptidylpeptidase IV contains competing apical and basolateral targeting information. *Journal of Biological Chemistry* **267**, 22282–22288.

Wellems, T.E. and Howard, R.J. (1986). Homologous genes encode two distinct histidine-rich proteins in a cloned isolate of *Plasmodium falciparum*. *Proceedings of the National Academy of Sciences of the USA* **83**, 6065–6069.

Wellems, T.E., Walliker, D., Smith, C.L., do Rosario, V.E., Maloy, W.L., Howard, R.J., Carter, R. and McCutchan, T.F. (1987). A histidine-rich protein gene marks a linkage group favored strongly in a genetic cross of *Plasmodium falciparum*. *Cell* **49**, 633–642.

Wickramasinghe, S.N. and Abdalla, S.H. (2000). Blood and bone marrow changes in malaria. *Baillière's Best Practice and Research. Clinical Haematology* **13**, 277–299.

Wickramasinghe, S.N., Phillips, R.E., Looareesuwan, S., Warrell, D.A. and Hughes, M. (1987). The bone marrow in human cerebral malaria: parasite sequestration within sinusoids. *British Journal of Haematology* **66**, 295–306.

Winograd, E. and Sherman, I.W. (1989). Characterization of a modified red cell membrane protein expressed on erythrocytes infected with the human malaria parasite *Plasmodium falciparum*: possible role as a cytoadherent mediating protein. *Journal of Cell Biology* **108**, 23–30.

Winograd, E., Greenan, J.R. and Sherman, I.W. (1987). Expression of senescent antigen on erythrocytes infected with a knobby variant of the human malaria parasite *Plasmodium falciparum*. *Proceedings of the National Academy of Sciences of the USA* **84**, 1931–1935.

Wiser, M.F., Lanners, H.N., Bafford, R.A. and Favaloro, J.M. (1997). A novel alternate secretory pathway for the export of *Plasmodium* proteins into the host erythrocyte. *Proceedings of the National Academy of Sciences of the USA* **94**, 9108–9113.

Wright, I.G. (1972). An electron microscope study of intravascular agglutination in the cerebral cortex due to *Babesia argentina* infections. *International Journal for Parasitology* **2**, 209–215.

Wright, I.G., Goodger, B.V. and Clark, I.A. (1988). Immunopathophysiology of *Babesia bovis* and *Plasmodium falciparum* infections. *Parasitology Today* **4**, 214–218.

Wu, Y.M., Sifri, C.D., Lei, H.H., Su, X.Z. and Wellems, T.E. (1995). Transfection of *Plasmodium falciparum* within human red blood cells. *Proceedings of the National Academy of Sciences of the USA* **92**, 973–977.

Wu, Y.M., Kirkman, L.A. and Wellems, T.E. (1996). Transformation of *Plasmodium falciparum* malaria parasites by homologous integration of plasmids that confer resistance to pyrimethamine. *Proceedings of the National Academy of Sciences of the USA* **93**, 1130–1134.

Yayon, A., Cabantchik, Z.I. and Ginsburg, H. (1984). Identification of the acidic compartment of *Plasmodium falciparum*-infected human erythrocytes as the target of the antimalarial drug chloroquine. *EMBO Journal* **3**, 2695–2700.

Yuan, J., Bunyaratvej, A., Fucharoen, S., Fung, C., Shinar, E. and Schrier, S.L. (1995). The instability of the membrane skeleton in thalassemic red blood cells. *Blood* **86**, 3945–3950.

Yuthavong, Y. and Limpaiboon, T. (1987). The relationship of phosphorylation of membrane proteins with the osmotic fragility and filterability of *Plasmodium berghei*-infected mouse erythrocytes. *Biochimica et Biophysica Acta* **929**, 278–287.

Schistosomiasis in the Mekong Region: Epidemiology and Phylogeography

S.W. Attwood

Wolfson Wellcome Biomedical Laboratories, Department of Zoology, The Natural History Museum, London, SW7 5BD, UK

ADVANCES IN PARASITOLOGY VOL 50
0065–308X $30.00

ABSTRACT

An account is given of progress made over the last 20 years in the study of Mekong schistosomiasis, causative agent *Schistosoma mekongi* (Trematoda: Digenea). Emphasis is given to the discussion of work concerning the origin and subsequent dispersal of *S. mekongi* and related taxa, including relevant snails. The role of such phylogeographical data in schistosomiasis control and the prediction of areas at risk is examined. New palaeogeographical models are reviewed in relation to traditional explanations for the biogeographic deployment of Southeast Asian *Schistosoma* and their intermediate hosts. The demographics and molecular ecology of *Neotricula aperta* (Gastropoda: Pomatiopsidae), the snail host of *S. mekongi*, are reviewed with particular reference to new models for the life cycle of this species and their importance in snail control. The use of population genetic data in the limitation of *N. aperta* populations is evaluated and strategies suggested for schistosomiasis control efforts directed against the intermediate host. Developments in the taxonomy of *N. aperta*, and related taxa, and changes in nomenclature are covered. The direction of future investigations into the problem of Mekong schistosomiasis is also discussed.

1. INTRODUCTION

Since the discovery of schistosomiasis in the lower Mekong Basin in 1957 (Figure 1), the disease has continued to pose a serious public health problem in the region. Over 150 000 persons live in areas where the transmission of *Schistosoma mekongi* Voge, Bruckner and Bruce, 1978 is endemic, and in 1990 over 80 000 of these were actually infected (Gang, 1991; Stich *et al.*, 1999). The disease causes severe morbidity in southern Laos and deaths due to ascites, jaundice or gastrointestinal bleeding are not uncommon (Gang, 1991). All of the areas surveyed so far lie along the Mekong river within three provinces, together these cover parts of Cambodia and southern Laos. The year 1980 saw the publication of *The Mekong Schistosome* (Bruce *et al.*, 1980), a comprehensive volume of contributions from researchers covering all aspects of the biology of *S. mekongi* as well as the biology and ecology of the intermediate host, the caenogastropod snail *Neotricula aperta* (Temcharoen, 1971). Since 1980, much has been learnt regarding the epidemiology and control of the parasite, its origins, distribution, relations with sister taxa, and the ecology and systematics of the intermediate host. Over the same period there have been numerous changes in nomenclature, which reflect our better understanding of the taxa involved. After nearly a decade of mass chemotherapy and education, the number of persons infected has fallen to around 7000

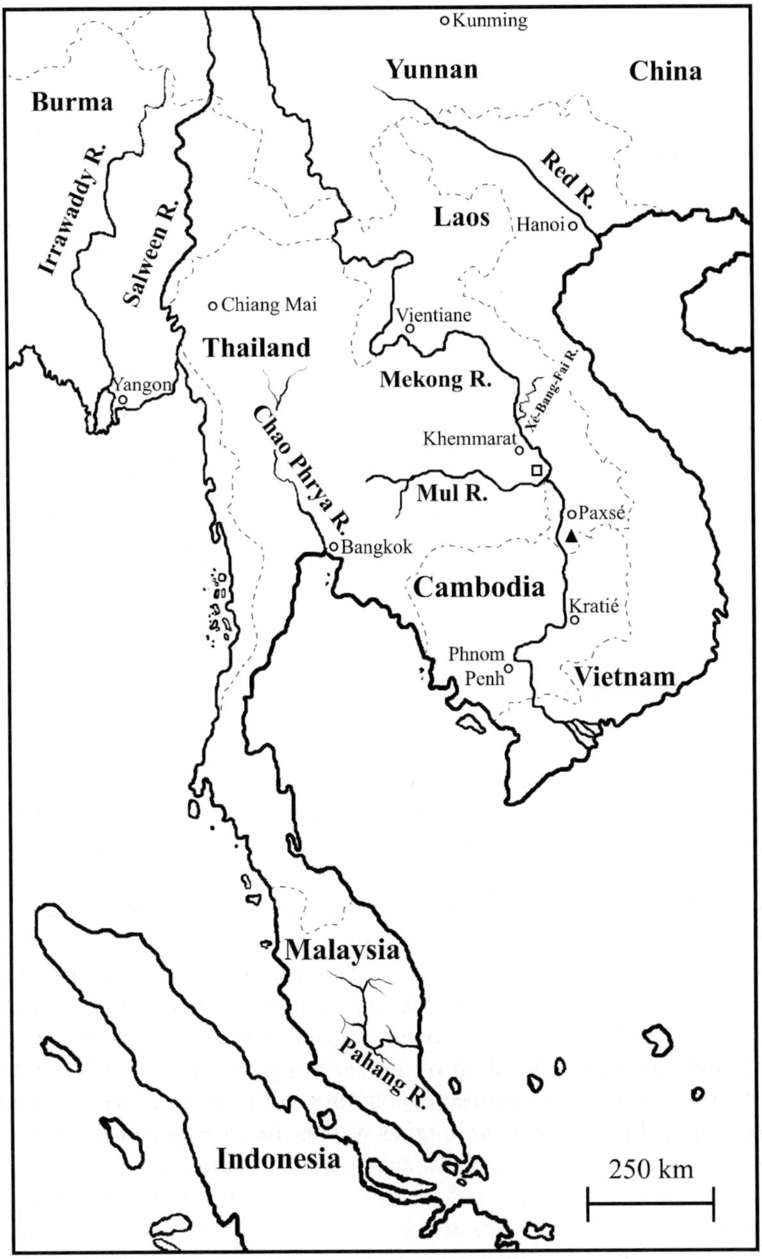

Figure 1 The middle and lower Mekong Basin showing some of the more important rivers and selected tributaries. The Pak-Mul dam (Khong-Chiam), □, and Khong Island, ▲, are also indicated. International boundaries and scale are approximate.

(Stich *et al.*, 1999); however, even such prolonged and intensive control efforts have been unable to break transmission of the human infection in any of the provinces affected. In addition, other rivers and territories are now being recognized as at risk from Mekong schistosomiasis. Unfortunately, little work has been done on the biology of the schistosome itself, which researchers have assumed to be little different from that of the related *Schistosoma japonicum* Katsurada, 1904.

This review provides an account of the current position of research into Mekong schistosomiasis and discusses the past two decades of studies into the biology of the disease and its transmission. The focus is on schistosomiasis control and the phylogeography of *Schistosoma mekongi* and closely related taxa, these being areas into which most research has been directed and most advances made. In particular, the status of *Schistosoma malayensis* and *Schistosoma sinensium* is considered in relation to *S. mekongi*, and the radiation of *Schistosoma* throughout Southeast Asia. The value of a phylogeographical study of the relevant snail faunas to our understanding of the evolution, dispersal and colonization history of *Schistosoma* is shown. Further, the molecular ecology of *N. aperta* is discussed and its relevance to snail control investigated. Davis (1979, 1980, 1992) argued for a Gondwanan origin of *Schistosoma*. The radiation of the *S. japonicum* group of schistosomes is considered to have occurred after entry into southern China off the Indian Plate, following the collision of the latter with mainland Asia during the Miocene. Davis's hypotheses still provide a useful foundation for research into the systematics of these taxa; however, more recent palaeogeographical models (see Hutchinson, 1989) call for revision of earlier ideas. A new phylobiogeographical model is described here, developing that of Davis (1979) to accommodate our changing views on the evolution of rivers such as the Mekong and Salween.

Field work underlying studies of Mekong schistosomiasis has often been performed in inaccessible and insecure areas; this, together with difficulties in the transport and laboratory maintenance of *Neotricula*, has been a deterrent to those considering work in this area. Consequently, it is hoped that this review will stimulate research into this important problem and facilitate communication between public health workers and research scientists. A presentation of the approaches and findings of both fields of endeavour in a single account will help guide future biomedical research; the role of such research in the formulation of strategies for epidemiological surveillance and disease control must also be appreciated. Sections two to four below describe the epidemiological situation, history of control, and continuing public health implications of Mekong schistosomiasis. Sections five and six outline our current understanding of the biology of *Schistosoma mekongi* and its intermediate host, as well as the ecology of transmission. The final sections develop phylogeographical models for *S. mekongi* and related taxa, based on updated palaeogeographical models for Southeast Asia and reciprocal illumination through a consideration of the origins and dispersal history of the snails involved in their transmission. The value of such models in future disease control programmes and in facilitating further research is outlined.

2. THE HISTORY OF MEKONG SCHISTOSOMIASIS

Towards the close of the 1950s a patchy distribution of highly focal human schistosomiasis was discovered on the Southeast Asian mainland. The disease was apparently restricted to the lower Mekong Basin (Figure 1), that is to Thailand, Laos and Cambodia (Dupont *et al.*, 1957; Harinasuta and Kruatrachue, 1962; Audebaud *et al.*, 1968; Sornmani, 1969). The first cases of Mekong schistosomiasis were reported in Paris among a number of residents who originated from Laos; the disease was initially diagnosed by Dupont (Dupont *et al.*, 1957) and then by Barbier (1966), together recognizing six cases. A number of reports of schistosomiasis in southern Vietnam have been received (Iijima and Garcia, 1967); however, these require substantiation.

2.1. Laos

Prior to 1962 the only well-documented focus of Mekong schistosomiasis was along the lower Mekong river at Khong Island (Figure 2) in Champassac Province, southern Laos, some 25 km north of the border with Cambodia. Khong Island is the largest of the Mekong islands. The 1969 epidemiological survey at Khong Island, conducted by a Smithsonian Institute–Mahidol University team (Sornmani *et al.*, 1971; Harinasuta *et al.*, 1972) revealed the shallow water near the market at Ban Xieng-Wang, Khong Town (14°6′30″N; 105°51′45″E) to be a site of intense transmission of schistosomiasis. The overall prevalence was 14·4% in humans, with the peak of 63·3% in the 7–15-year-old cohort, and 11·0% in dogs. More recently, the prevalence in the 7–14-year-old cohort was estimated to be 30·2% (Sleigh, 1989) with the overall prevalence equal to approximately 10% (Stürchler, 1988). The persistence of this endemic focus of human schistosomiasis in apparent isolation was attributed to the local hydrology, the use of this part of the river both as a public bathing place and as a latrine, and to the high levels of human traffic to and from the market (Sornmani *et al.*, 1980). The market at Khong was popular with Thai and Vietnamese people, as well as those of southern Laos, until the political upheaval of the 1970s. The many islets that lie off the eastern shore of Khong Island are observed, during the low-water period (February to May), to interrupt or capture sections of the river as shallow pools or streams.

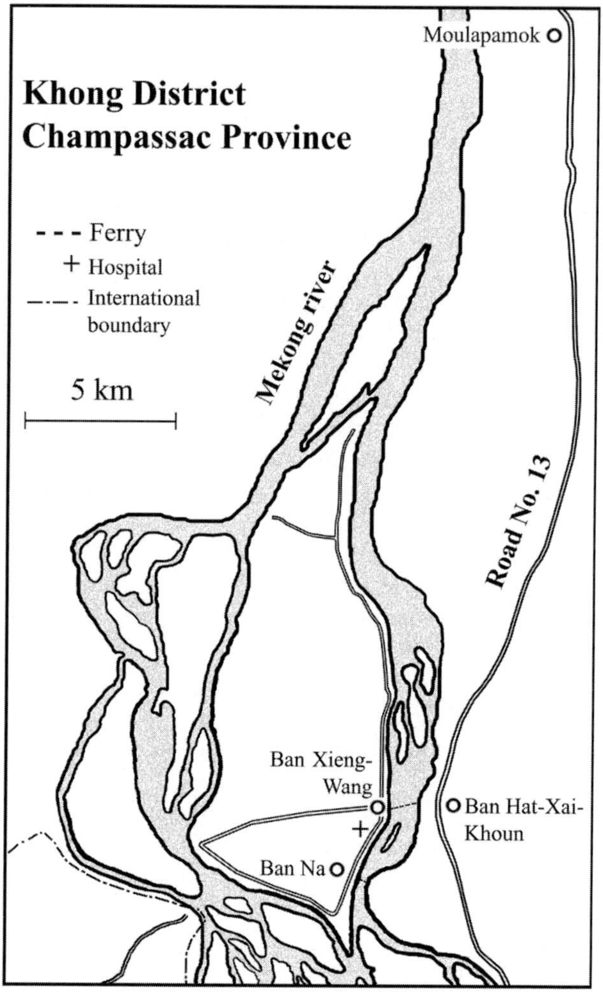

Figure 2 The Mekong river around Khong Island, Champassac Province, southern Laos.

These shallow regions form ideal habitats for aquatic snails (the intermediate hosts for schistosomiasis) and their food, such as diatoms and filamentous green algae (Attwood, 1995a). The existence of a second focus in Laos, around Vientiane and Luang-Prabang (the Laotian cities of the northwest) as evidenced by Wittes *et al.* (1984) has not been confirmed; however, transmission in these areas is unlikely as the Mekong river provides a less suitable habitat for the intermediate host north of Khemmarat (see Figure 1).

2.2. Cambodia

Schneider (1976) discussed the evidence for a focus of human schistosomiasis at Kratié in Kratié Province of northeastern Cambodia (12°27′10″N; 106°1′45″E), 170 km downstream of the Lao–Cambodian border and Khone falls (Figure 3). In 1968 a high prevalence (47·0%) of schistosomiasis was recorded among the ethnic Vietnamese communities of the floating villages then common around Kratié (Jolly *et al.*, 1970a,b). Initial surveys by the Royal Cambodian Health Service in July 1968 had detected eggs of *Schistosoma* in 10·5% of stool samples from 661 members of these villages (Biays *et al.*, 1999). Iijima (1970) showed, using an intradermal antigen test against *Schistosoma japonicum*, that although schistosomiasis was most prevalent in Kratié Province during 1968 and 1969, the disease was also present in several other provinces, namely Kampong Cham, Stung Treng, and areas along the Vietnamese border (Figure 3). The prevalence of infection was found to be 13·6% by the antigen test (sample size 448) and 3·6% (of 55) by stool

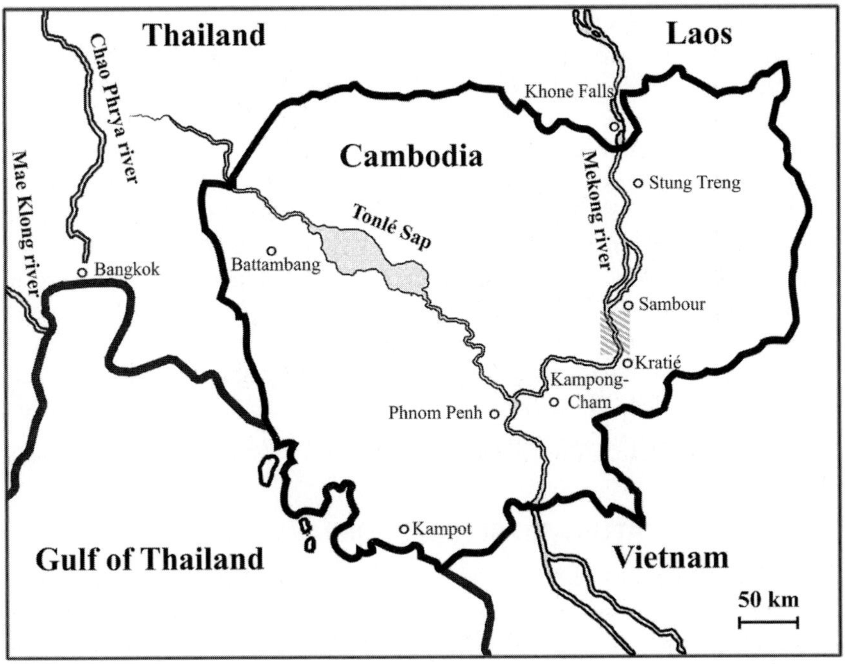

Figure 3 The Mekong river in Cambodia. The shaded area south of Sambour indicates those riparian communities involved in the Médecins Sans Frontières schistosomiasis control programme (1994–1999).

examination; this may be compared with prevalences of 35·9% (of 563) and 33·6% (of 119), respectively, within Kratié itself. The findings also suggest that the antigen test was more sensitive than stool examination. The overall prevalence at Kratié between 1968 and 1970 was reported as 7–10% in fishermen and 14–22% in the 1–14-year-old cohort (Iijima *et al.*, 1973). During the 1970s and 80s the political situation in the region prevented further surveys. However, Maunoury *et al.* (1990) provided indirect evidence for ongoing transmission of schistosomiasis in Cambodia; these authors detected the disease in five Cambodian refugees presenting at a hospital in northern France. Similar reports were received from hospitals in the USA (Cuesta *et al.*, 1992).

2.3. The Aetiology of Mekong Schistosomiasis

It was assumed (Barbier, 1966; Iijima *et al.*, 1971; Sornmani *et al.*, 1971) that the parasite in the lower Mekong was *S. japonicum*, the causative agent of schistosomiasis on the Chinese mainland and in Japan. Barbier (1966) speculated that the Mekong schistosome may have been introduced by Japanese troops during World War II. However, the snail intermediate hosts of *S. japonicum*, subspecies of *Oncomelania hupensis* Gredler, 1881 (Gastropoda: Pomatiopsidae), are not known from Indochina. Iijima *et al.* (1971) identified worms collected from patients at Khong Island as *S. japonicum*; however, subsequent investigations revealed the epidemiological, morphological and biological peculiarities of the adult worms that led to their distinction as a new species, *Schistosoma mekongi* Voge, Bruckner and Bruce, 1978. It was also at Khong that Viroj Kitikoon (Kitikoon *et al.*, 1973; Sornmani *et al.*, 1973) succeeded in identifying the intermediate host of *S. mekongi* despite fruitless attempts by others (Brandt, 1968, 1970; Temcharoen, 1971) including the 1968/69 World Health Organization (WHO) team (Iijima *et al.*, 1971; Lo *et al.*, 1971). These were not oncomelanids, as had been expected, but a little known species of triculine snail (Pomatiopsidae: Triculinae) originally named *Lithoglyphopsis aperta* Temcharoen, 1971. *Tricula aperta* was later transferred to *Neotricula* on the basis of differences in reproductive anatomy (Davis *et al.*, 1986).

3. CURRENT STATUS AND SCHISTOSOMIASIS CONTROL ACTIVITIES

3.1. Cambodia

Reports of hepatosplenomegaly and ascites among young adults from Sambour hospital in the north of Kratié Province (Figure 3) were initially attributed to dengue haemorrhagic fever. However, a Medécins Sans Frontières (MSF) physician later correctly returned a diagnosis of schistosomiasis (see Biays *et al.*, 1999), and in 1992 the Cambodian Ministry of Public Health established an anti-schistosomiasis group with the task of identifying the species responsible. An associated study performed by MSF estimated the prevalence of schistosomiasis to be as high as 84% in primary school children (Goubert *et al.*, 1994). Stich *et al.* (1999) described a well-established schistosomiasis focus at Kratié with a peak burden of morbidity and infection among the 10–15-year-old cohort. The presence of *N. aperta* at Kratié had been considered highly probable (Schneider, 1976; Harinasuta, 1984); the first published report of the snail at Kratié was provided by Attwood *et al.* (1998). Prior to 1994 up to 40% of the admissions to Kratié hospital were due to schistosomiasis, and deaths due to oesophageal bleeding were common. Biays *et al.* (1999) attributed the severity of the problem in Kratié, which local people stated had arisen within the previous 20 years, to changes effected by the Khmer Rouge (1975–1979). During this period much of the population was forced into traditional agriculture, which involved increased human water contact and the use of human faeces as fertiliser in rice paddy.

In view of the severity of the public health problem, a baseline survey of schistosomiasis was conducted by MSF along the Mekong river in Kratié Province between December 1994 and April 1995. The total population at risk was an estimated 60 000 with around 17 000 people infected. The surveys were based on two-slide examinations of single stool samples using the Kato–Katz thick smear technique (Katz *et al.*, 1972). The investigation focused on the two northernmost districts of Kratié Province, Kratié and Sambour, populated by some 32 000 people (in 29 villages) mostly living on the Mekong river (Figure 3). The MSF project was divided into two surveys: the first was of households in villages selected for a high intensity of infection (1396 people), whilst the second involved the 6–16-year-old cohort covering all 20 of the schools in the two provinces (2391 children). Prior to treatment (December 1994) the overall prevalence was 49·3% in households and 40·0% in schools. The peak prevalence of 72% occurred in the 10–14-year-old cohort (Stich *et al.*, 1999). These data indicated that transmission had remained at high levels since the report of Jolly *et al.* (1970b), and demonstrated an increase in prevalence relative to the samples of Iijima *et al.* (1973), who reported a prevalence of around 22%. The intervention comprised mass treatment with a single oral dose of praziquantel (40 mg kg^{-1} body weight). The follow up survey in April 1995, 5 months after treatment, showed that the overall prevalence in schools had fallen to 14% (Stich *et al.*, 1999), although only a fraction of the original number of schools was resampled.

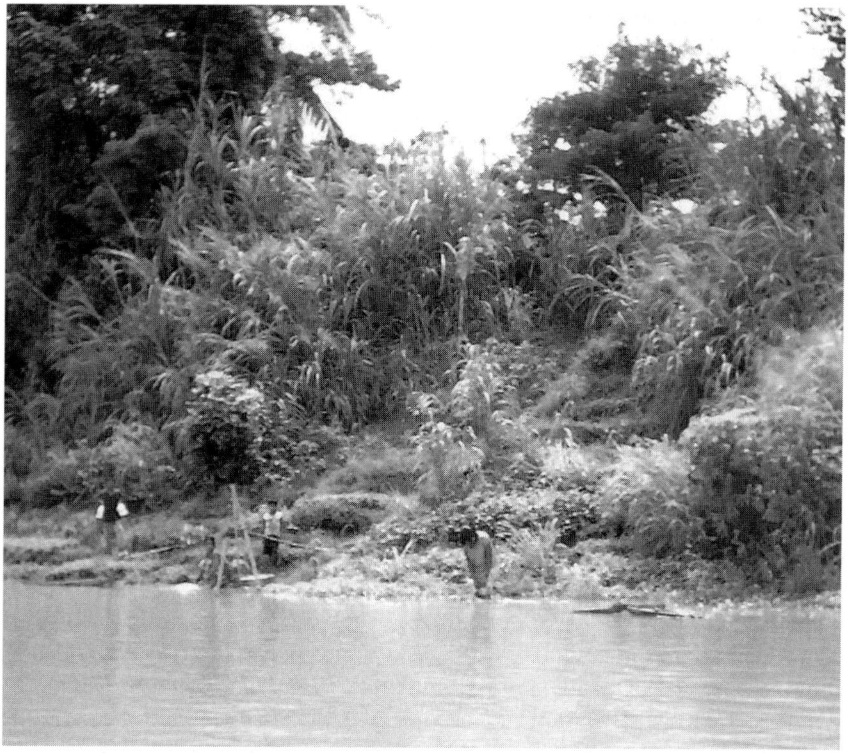

Figure 4 The laundry area at Ban Hat-Xai-Khoun, Khong District, southern Laos. In spite of control efforts this site remains an endemic focus of *Schistosoma mekongi* transmission. The photograph was taken in early May 2000, at the start of the high-water period that year.

3.2. Laos

Schistosomiasis control in the Lao Peoples' Democratic Republic (PDR) began in 1989, some 6 years before the start of control efforts in Cambodia, and focused on Khong District (Champassac Province) in southern Laos, including Khong Island and outlying villages. The estimated population at risk was 60 000 with 7500 of these living in the four communes of Khong Island. The control programme was initiated by the Ministry of Health, Laos, with funding and technical assistance from WHO. The baseline prevalence in children was 50·7%, again based on Kato–Katz faecal smear examination. Administration of praziquantel (single oral dose of $40\,\mathrm{mg\,kg^{-1}}$ body weight) began immediately after the baseline survey in October 1989, when coverage reached 88% of the target (child) population, and continued until November 1995. The final round of mass treatment was performed in May 1998 and covered all endemic districts. Follow-up surveys in June 1999 were encouraging in that the prevalence in school children had fallen to 0·8%. However, in spite of the low overall prevalence, that in one village, Hat-Xai-Khoun (Figures 2 and 4) on the east bank of the Mekong river, remained high (26·8% in children and 12·6% in pigs; WHO, Geneva, personal communication). In addition, Attwood *et al.* (2001) have demonstrated an infection rate for *S. mekongi* in *N. aperta* at Hat-Xai-Khoun of 0·22%; this suggests that in spite of 9 years of chemotherapy, molluscan infection rates have changed little from the 0·3% reported by Kitikoon *et al.* in 1973.

The control of *N. aperta* is likely to prove effective in a combined anti-schistosomiasis programme with chemotherapy of villagers in endemic areas. However, such control has been evaluated on only one occasion, this was by a WHO team on Khong Island at Ban Xieng-Wang. The small-scale trial took place in May 1991 during the low-water period of the Mekong river; this time is also recognized as that of maximum snail population density (Yasuraoka, 1992). Beginning a little over 20 m from the shore, 20 sacks, each containing 1 kg of niclosamide, were suspended across the Mekong river near the district hospital (see Figure 2); this achieved an approximate concentration of 0·5 p.p.m. downstream after 2 h. On the day following treatment the *N. aperta* population density 10 m downstream had fallen to only 2 m^{-2}, around 1% of the initial density. The population density 150 m downstream fell to zero from an initial 1·9 m^{-2}. Less encouragingly, 5 days after treatment the density 10 m downstream rose to 2400% of its original value and then fell to its pre-treatment value over the next 4 days. The density 150 m downstream rose to only 280% of initial levels after 5 days; however, there were increases to over 1200% of pre-treatment values at this station by day 10. These less than satisfactory results were attributed to an insufficient level of niclosamide and a greater influence of the river's current than first thought (Yasuraoka, 1992). The overall effects of the molluscicide trial appear to have been a marked increase in snail population density in areas of initial paucity, with little effect on original high-density foci. It is likely that local extirpation of snails left vacant habitats that were particularly vulnerable to recolonization from outside the treatment area; this may be due to an epilithic algal bloom, or growth of some other food item, in the vacant habitats (Attwood, 1996a). Habitats in which the snail population density was initially high are probably never fully cleared of snails and therefore did not achieve such a 'bloom'. As the 1991 trial was small scale and of only 10 days' duration, it is not possible to determine the long-term effects of such snail control methods and therefore more extensive trials are required.

4. THE FUTURE OF SCHISTOSOMIASIS CONTROL IN THE LOWER MEKONG

4.1. Epidemiology

Although Stich *et al.* (1999) demonstrated a reduction in overall prevalence from 40 to 14% in Kratié Province after the administration of praziquantel, the short interval between treatment and follow-up (December to April) must be considered. Transmission of Mekong schistosomiasis occurs mainly during April when river levels are lowest, snails are most abundant, and human water contact is most frequent (Kitikoon *et al.*, 1973). Consequently there would be a limited chance of reinfection by the time of the follow-up survey. Stich *et al.* (1999) highlighted the need for longer-term monitoring of the situation and plans for this over the next few years have been made by MSF. It is probable that the prevalence will soon return to its original levels once intervention is stopped, unless a serious attempt is made to change patterns of human water contact.

Biays *et al.* (1999) provided data on the efficacy of praziquantel treatment in 20 cases of clinically advanced schistosomiasis during the 1995 intervention at Kratié Province. Treatment comprised oral doses of praziquantel ($60\,mg\,kg^{-1}$) and 200 mg mebendazole per day for 3 days, with follow-up after 30 months. The clinical efficacy of treatment was inconsistent with mortality in five cases, no change in three cases, temporary improvement in five cases, and distinct improvement in only five cases. The remaining two patients could not be contacted at follow-up. Similarly, Gang (1991) reported that 12·3% of children at Khong Island showing intensities >100 epg (eggs per gram of faecal material examined) remained stool positive after treatment. The persistence of infection at Ban Hat-Xai-Khoun after 9 years of treatment also suggests that Mekong schistosomiasis cannot be controlled completely by such methods alone. As there was generally little opportunity for reinfection over the course of these studies, it may be concluded that treatment failed to remove all parasites from those originally most heavily infected; thus a reservoir of infection can be assumed to remain after treatment. The findings in Laos also suggested that chemotherapy in regions of low overall initial prevalence achieved only slight further reductions. The data set, collected by the WHO team at Khong District (Gang, 1991), itself must be interpreted with caution as the follow-up sample sizes were often much smaller than those of the pre-treatment samples, in some cases only 20% of the original number was resampled. In addition, direct faecal smears without concentration methods can yield up to 20 negative smears even though the patient may be passing over 4000 eggs per day (see Jordan and Webbe, 1969). Low infection intensities are particularly difficult to detect and egg production may decline with age of infection, possibly accentuating any peak of infection in younger cohorts (Hagan *et al.*, 1998). Such problems with detection of infection make the monitoring and control of residual infection even more of a problem.

In both the MSF and WHO studies the peak prevalence of infection was in 10–14-year-olds. In contrast, a peak-shift toward the 30–50-year-old cohort has been reported for *S. japonicum* in China (Cross, 1976; Ross *et al.*, 1997). Gang (1991) suggested that future intervention should focus on adults rather than children, reasoning that the relatedness between *S. japonicum* and *S. mekongi* would lead to similar patterns of infection. However, the ecologies of the snails involved in transmission differ greatly, in particular *O. hupensis* is amphibious and occurs mostly in rice fields, a habitat frequented more by adults than children. Nevertheless, age-dependent differences in infection appear highly reproducible across quite different schistosome species (e.g., *S. haematobium* and *S. mekongi*). In cases where children experience lower levels of exposure than adults, the low levels of infection and reinfection in the latter may be attributed to innate and/or acquired immunity (Hagan *et al.*, 1998). The peak of infection tends to shift toward the younger age classes where the intensity of transmission is greatest or parasite longevity is reduced (Maizels *et al.*, 1993), but these do not appear to be significant factors in the case of *S. japonicum* and *S. mekongi*. In any case, there does not seem to be a strong argument for concentrating attack phase intervention on adults, except in the treatment of individuals with severe symptoms (who tend to be fishermen).

4.2. Snail Control

The question remains as to the most effective approach in the future control of Mekong schistosomiasis. Pholsena (in press) concluded that although human schistosomiasis in Khong District has now been controlled from a public health perspective, re-emergence of the disease is likely unless future control measures are implemented. As 9 years of chemotherapy failed to stop transmission even at the culmination of the programme, this method alone is unlikely to be effective. Snail control through molluscicidING is the most obvious choice of combined control strategy and will be discussed in this section.

The main problem facing any snail control programme appears to be the colonization potential of *N. aperta*; this is evidenced by findings of Attwood (1994), who reported colonization rates exceeding 90 snails $m^{-2} h^{-1}$ for *N. aperta* (γ-strain) in the Mekong river in May. In addition, the range of *N. aperta*, which until recently had been thought restricted to the Mekong and Mul rivers (Schneider, 1976; Attwood, 1995b), is now known to include several Mekong river tributaries in Laos and probably also Cambodia. The present author has recently collected *N. aperta* in tributaries draining the Annam mountains of Khammouanne and Savannakhet Provinces, Laos (Figure 5). Any programme of snail control in endemic areas such as Khong Island must include possible source populations in upstream Mekong tributaries. That recolonization of the Mekong from such streams is an ongoing process is suggested by the genetic distances, as high as 1·01 (Nei's 1978 minimum standard genetic distance), reported by Attwood *et al.* (1998) between Mekong river populations separated by only 200 km. Such genetic distances could not arise by random drift alone over the time scales involved.

Clearly, a Mekong river habitat left vacant in March or April following snail control is particularly vulnerable to rapid recolonization by snails from source populations in Mekong river tributaries; this may then result in population densities exceeding pre-control levels through overgrowth of the algal epilithon (see Section 3.2). The problem is particularly serious in that snails from potential source populations have been found to exhibit greater compatibility with *S. mekongi* than some Mekong river strains (Attwood and Upatham, 1999). In addition, there is the possibility that source populations also harbour *S. mekongi* and could introduce the parasite to previously unaffected areas of the Mekong river, particularly if snail control is conducted in a blanket fashion. Snail control directed against source populations in Mekong river tributaries may lead to effective and longer lasting control when used in combination with Mekong river intervention. Snail populations are often denser in source tributaries and the life cycle in such populations may precede that in the Mekong river; this appears to be a result of the lower water levels and relatively minor flooding found in the tributaries, which provide ideal habitats for *N. aperta*. Consequently a malacological survey, covering the Mekong river tributaries of Khammouanne, Savannakhet and Champassac Provinces of southern Laos, is a prerequisite for any reliable programme of disease control. The timing of the life cycle in the various tributaries must also be determined so that the main periods of snail migration are identified. Screening for *Schistosoma* is also necessary. Ideally, mitochondrial DNA sequence data should also be collected for the samples taken, in order to infer the history of migration and colonization among these stocks. Work along these lines is already underway in this laboratory and aims to provide data of use in the design of future control programmes.

The molluscan fauna of the lower Mekong river includes an extensive endemic (monophyletic) fauna of 11 triculine genera and over 90 described species (see Davis, 1979). A similar endemic fauna is found among the fish species occupying the river around Khong Island (Pantulu, 1998). Protection of this fauna presents an additional challenge in the design of an appropriate control strategy. The most promising approach lies in the temporal and spatial localization of a molluscicide, especially to avoid snails such as *Hydrorissoia, Jullienia* and *Paraprososthenia* spp. (Triculinae) which complete their life cycles ahead of *N. aperta* (see Attwood, 1995b). Yasuraoka (1990) did not

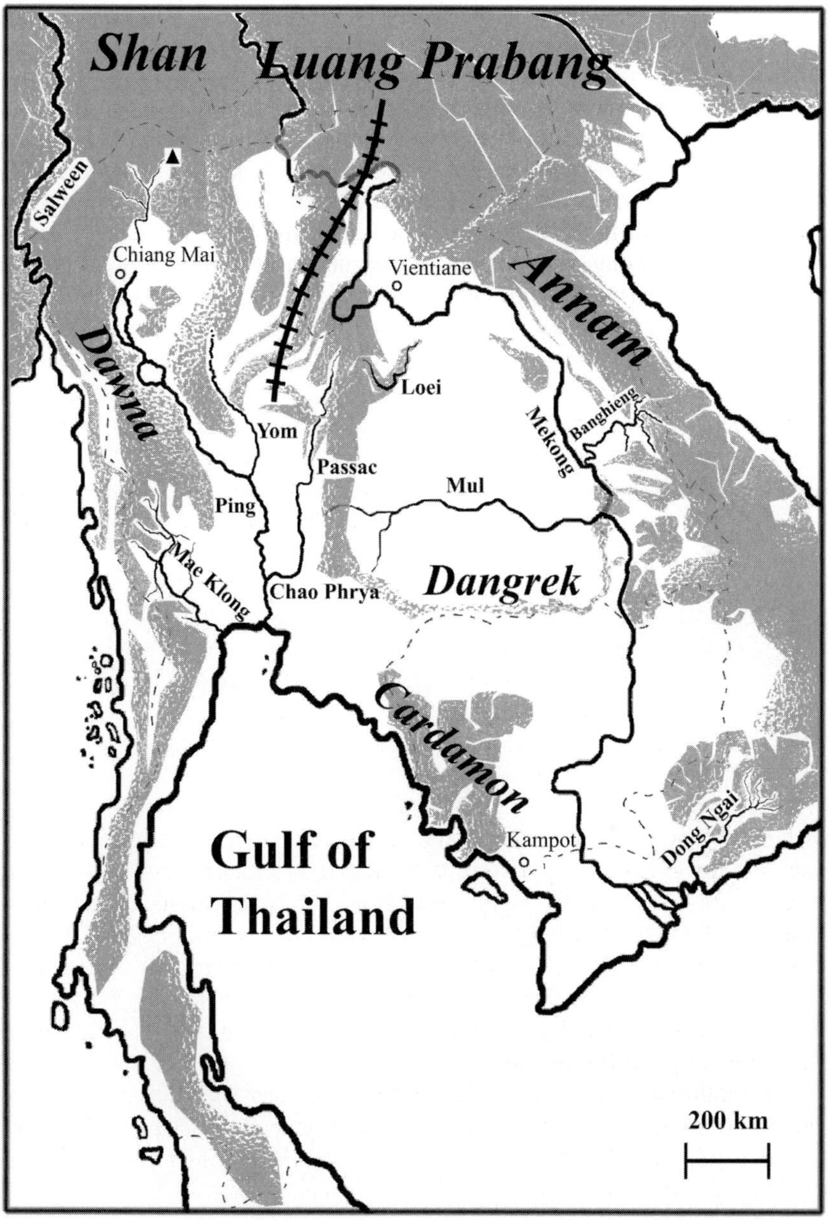

Figure 5 The Mekong region. Major mountain ranges are depicted as shaded areas. The Uttaradit suture, formed around 200 million years ago by the closing of the Tethys Ocean, is shown as a thick, crossed line (after Hutchinson, 1982). Certain rivers are omitted to facilitate draughting.

regard the piscicidal activity of niclosamide as a likely source of conflict with local fishing communities; however, the present author found that some fishermen on Khong Island (in May 1991) attributed allegedly diminished fish catches to the activities of the WHO team. Focusing control on key tributaries of the Mekong river may have the added benefit of reducing the ecological impact. These tributaries tend to have less diverse faunas and present smaller volumes of water for treatment than the main river itself.

There has been much discussion concerning the role of water impoundment along the Mekong river (dam construction, weirs, etc.) in the spread of schistosomiasis. A number of authors have suggested that the construction of dams such as that at Pak-Mul (Figure 6), on the Mul river close to its juncture with the Mekong in Northeast Thailand, could lead (or even has led) to the establishment of *S. mekongi* in Thailand (for example, see Woodruff and Upatham, 1992 and papers cited therein). However, no evidence has been provided for the transmission of *S. mekongi* in Northeast Thailand, although it would be difficult to distinguish infections acquired across the border in southern Laos

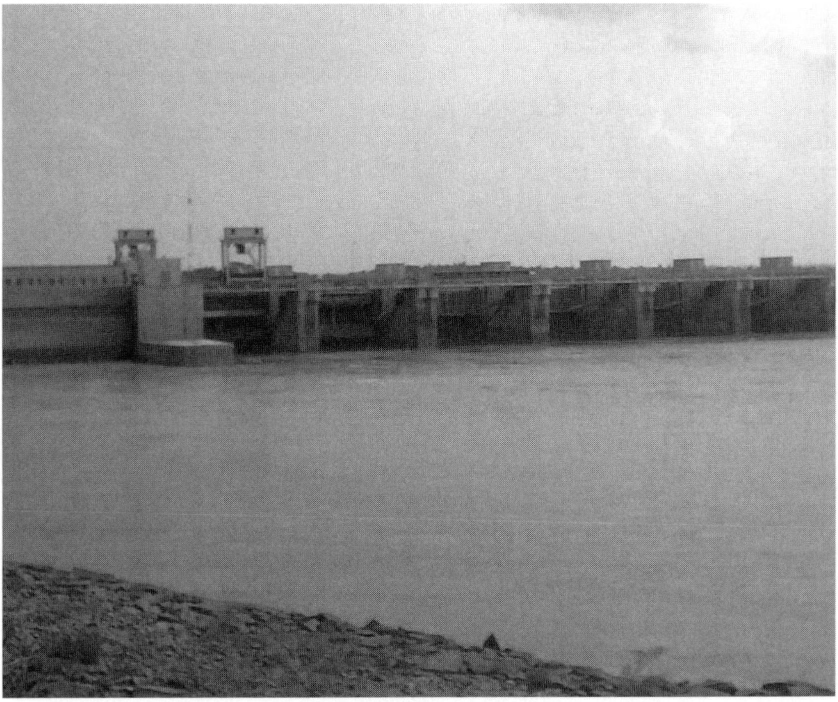

Figure 6 The Pak-Mul dam on the Mul river of Northeast Thailand (viewed from downstream).

from local transmission. The tendency to regard *Neotricula* as having the same responses to impoundment as those snails transmitting schistosomiasis in Africa or South America must be avoided. The pulmonate snails transmitting *Schistosoma haematobium* and *Schistosoma mansoni* differ markedly in biology and ecology from the caenogastropod snails responsible for the transmission of *S. mekongi*. In contrast to the African and South American pulmonate snails, available ecological data (Davis *et al.*, 1976; Attwood, 1995b) suggest that *N. aperta* will not thrive in the deeper, slower flowing and more turbid waters associated with water impoundment. Populations of the β-strain of *N. aperta* above Pak-Mul have increased only slightly since operation of the dam began in 1994 (see Attwood, 1996b), and it is not yet clear if this is to be a sustained trend. It has been suggested that slower flowing water would enhance miracidial success but this is likely to be offset by a decline in snail population density. On the other hand, new habitats may be created for *N. aperta* in the shallower waters found downstream of the dams. The matter is an important one however, and requires further investigation as several mainstream dams are now planned along the lower Mekong river.

An additional tool that may soon become available in the control of human schistosomiasis is that of a vaccine conferring protective immunity. Almost all research to date on Asian schistosomiasis has focused on *S. japonicum*. A number of recombinant antigen vaccines have been tested in several animal models. The schistosome-derived glutathione *S*-transferase (GST) family enzymes have proven good target molecules in vaccine production. The GSTs have a role against host immune responses and are expressed in the worm's tegument. Such GST-based vaccines achieved a 53·5% reduction in liver egg burden in pigs and similar reductions in water buffaloes infected with *S. japonicum* (see Liu *et al.*, 1995, 1997). The glycolytic enzyme triosephosphate isomerase (TPI) has also been evaluated as it is commonly expressed in the surface membranes of newly transformed schistosomula (Harn *et al.*, 1985). Biochemically purified TPI, from Chinese strain *S. japonicum*, has been tested and achieved significant (57–60%) reductions in egg burdens; however, only slight reductions in worm burdens were achieved (Miao *et al.*, 1998). A recombinant form of *S. japonicum* TPI is now being developed and is showing promising results (Sun *et al.*, 1999). A third likely target is the invertebrate myofibrillar protein paramyosin; this is common in the muscle layer of cercariae, lung stage and adult *S. japonicum*, within the postacetabular glands of cercariae, and, most importantly, within the tegument matrix of lung schistosomula (Gobert *et al.*, 1997). Laboratory models using the mouse and a Chinese strain of *S. japonicum* showed reductions in worm burdens of around 30% with both recombinant and biochemically purified protein (McManus *et al.*, 1998; Pearce *et al.*, 1988, respectively). Protection seems to last for at least 12 months in cattle. Although no vaccine is likely to achieve the complete elimination of the worms from the definitive host it is thought that a reduction of worm burdens by 50% or more would greatly reduce the morbidity associated with human schistosomiasis (McManus, 2000). Unlike *S. japonicum*, the transmission of *S. mekongi* does not involve a strong zoonotic element and so this disease should be more readily controlled by vaccination. However, the populations at risk from *S. mekongi* in each endemic country are much smaller than those in China and it may be difficult to justify the cost of vaccine development and testing. Fortunately, the production of recombinant forms of the antigenic proteins has now reduced such costs considerably. No specific vaccine development programme for *S. mekongi* has as yet been established. However, some background research towards the development of a recombinant vaccine has been undertaken, for example the determination of an *S. mekongi* GST-gene sequence by Vichasri-Grams *et al.* (1997).

4.3. The Current Range of *Schistosoma mekongi*

It is now becoming clear that *Neotricula aperta*, and probably also *Schistosoma mekongi*, is more widespread than first reported by Schneider (1976). Current phylogeographical hypotheses (see Hutchinson, 1989 and Section 7.2) lead us to expect that these taxa will be found in the streams draining the Laotian highlands of Champassac, Khammouanne and Savannakhet provinces, many of which are tributaries of the Mekong. Indeed, it is probable that *N. aperta* is more common outside the Mekong river than within it, and we should look for new foci of Mekong schistosomiasis beyond the main river itself. Other areas are indicated by our phylogeographical models as at risk from schistosomiasis; these include the elevated streams draining the Ping or Loei river valleys, the Cardamon highlands in Cambodia, and the Dong Ngai drainage in Vietnam including the region westwards to the border with Cambodia (see Figure 5). As mentioned below, human schistosomiasis has already been reported from the Ping river valley and *N. aperta* is found in higher-gradient rivers of Khammouanne and Savannakhet Provinces in Laos (Attwood and Upatham, 1999). The predictions for Cambodia also appear to be supported. The WHO team of 1968/69 reported a prevalence based on antigen tests of 61% in the area of Kampong Cham, which is about 50 km downstream of Kratié towards Phnom Penh (see Figure 3; Iijima, 1970; Iijima *et al.*, 1973). More recently Stich *et al.* (1999) reported that such tests have detected human schistosomiasis along the Mekong river and its tributaries in Stung Treng Province, as far north of Kratié as the border with Laos. In addition, Harinasuta (1984) reported an overall prevalence of 0·34% from Battambang Province with most cases originating from the western side of Tonlé lake, a tributary of the Mekong some 300 km west of Kratié. Together these observations suggest that schistosomiasis in Cambodia is more widespread than first apparent. Consequently, future surveys and subsequent control measures should be extended to include all these regions.

5. *SCHISTOSOMA MEKONGI* AND RELATED TAXA

5.1. Taxonomic Studies

Voge *et al.* (1978) compared the Mekong strain of *Schistosoma 'japonicum'*, from humans and dogs at Khong Island, with samples of Chinese, Japanese, Philippine and Taiwanese strains of *S. japonicum*. Morphological characters suggested that the Mekong schistosome was indeed a member of the *S. japonicum* group: the egg possessed a minute lateral spine, there were seven testes compressed into a single column, the male was long and narrow (allotype, 15 mm long and up to 410 μm wide) and the female vitellaria filled only the posterior 40% of the body. The pomatiopsid intermediate host and biogeographic deployment were also consistent with the *S. japonicum* group. Unlike *S. haematobium* and *S. mansoni*, the tegument of the Mekong schistosome is free of tubercles with only minute spines on the suckers and gynecophoric canal. As in the other strains of *S. japonicum*, the habitat in the definitive host was the superior mesenteric and portal veins and the eggs were passed in the faeces.

Voge *et al.* (1978) were able to identify only two reliable characters (in addition to snail specificity) distinguishing the Mekong schistosome from *S. japonicum* and these were the basis for elevating the Mekong strain to species status. First, the embryonated eggs of *Schistosoma mekongi* were consistently smaller than those of *S. japonicum* (70 × 60 μm compared with 80 × 70 μm; Shekhar, 1987), although this can vary with host these comparisons were all made within the mouse model. Second, the prepatent period in the mouse was consistently longer in *S. mekongi* (by 7–8 days) than in *S. japonicum*. In *S. mekongi* no eggs were found in the liver at 26 or 30 days, but eggs were found after 35 days. In *S. japonicum* eggs are found *in utero* and in the host liver by day 26, at which time the ovary of *S. mekongi* is small and barely outlined. Iijima *et al.* (1971) reported that the ovary was larger in the Mekong strain; however, characters such as body size, and size of gonads and suckers are not reliable in taxonomy and may vary with host species, age of infection, crowding or fixation techniques. Sobhon and Upatham (1990) reported three major differences in tegumental structure between *S. japonicum* and *S. mekongi*. First, *S. mekongi* lacks the long parallel ridges found in *S. japonicum* and instead shows tall, irregular, highly branched and perforated ridges, which may form microvilli posteriorly. Second, in addition to the three different kinds of sensory papillae found on *S. japonicum*, *S. mekongi* also possesses other surface projections, described as pleomorphic (non-sensory) papillae and concentrated in the mid-region of the body (especially the male). Third, the spines on the surface of male *S. mekongi* are shorter and less numerous than those of male *S. japonicum*.

Other distinctive characters of *S. mekongi* relate to the life cycle or fecundity. In keeping with other members of the *S. japonicum* group, overall productivity appears quite low in *S. mekongi*. The output of a single snail per day may be up to 1500 cercariae with *S. mansoni* and 2000 with *S. haematobium* (see Jourdane and Théron, 1987). In contrast, an *S. mekongi* line in the β-strain of *N. aperta* (see below) produced an average of 42 cercariae per day over a 12-week period (Lohachit *et al.*, 1980b). Such comparisons are, however, highly dependent on factors such as initial miracidial dose, age and duration of the parasitic process sampled, and local variations in host–parasite compatibility. Nevertheless, the productivity of *S. mekongi* appears significantly lower than that of *S. mansoni* and *S. haematobium*. It is possible that the greater population densities of *N. aperta* (see Attwood, 1995b) and cercarial success compensate for the lower productivity in *S. mekongi*. The fecundity of the Mekong schistosome also appears lower, in that an estimated 95 eggs per day (per worm) were released into the stools or rectal mucosa; this may be compared with the 250 eggs per day produced on average by *S. japonicum* (see Byram and Von Lichtenberg, 1980).

The duration of cercariogenesis in *S. mekongi* is typical of *Schistosoma* in general and the process lasts for over 32 weeks (Jourdane and Théron, 1987); approximately 50% of the production in *S. mekongi* is achieved within the first 12–22 weeks (Lohachit *et al.*, 1980b). The emergence of cercariae follows a circadian rhythm, beginning at sunrise (6 a.m.) and falling almost to zero by 10 a.m. (Lohachit *et al.*, 1980b). This pattern is probably timed to coincide with the period of maximum human water contact (as people bathe, launder clothes and collect water before the heat of the day) and implies a different epidemiological pattern from *S. japonicum*, in which emergence generally peaks at 11 a.m. and falls to zero around 3 p.m. (Pesigan *et al.*, 1958). Adults working in rice paddy are therefore most likely to be exposed to *S. japonicum*. In common with other schistosomes, natural infection rates of *S. mekongi* are quite low; for example, 0·3% in *N. aperta* at Khong Town (Kitikoon *et al.*, 1973). This further supports the idea that snail population density and greater human water contact support endemic schistosomiasis in southern Laos in the face of apparently reduced parasite fecundity. In addition, laboratory infection rates are higher in *S. mekongi*, with rates of over 20% recorded for *N. aperta*. This may be compared with only 5% in some *S. japonicum*–*O. hupensis* associations (see Section 6.3). *S. mekongi* is closely related to *Schistosoma malayensis* Greer, Ow-Yang and Yong, 1988, a species transmitted in Pahang state of peninsular Malaysia by the snail *Robertsiella kaporensis* (Pomatiopsidae: Triculinae) and affecting the Orang Asli people of the region. The two species differ in terms of life cycle and biogeography, and morphological differences have not proved reliable taxonomic characters in this case.

5.2. Molecular Systematic Studies

Until recently there had been relatively few studies of genetic variation among the *S. japonicum* group taxa. Yong *et al.* (1985) examined variation at 11 allozyme loci and found that *S. japonicum* shared alleles with *S. malayensis* at only a single locus. The same authors also found that *S. japonicum* showed fixed differences at all 11 loci when compared with *S. mekongi*. In contrast, *S. malayensis* and *S. mekongi* differed at only five of the loci. Fletcher *et al.* (1981) observed that different strains of *S. mansoni* show an average Nei's (1978) genetic distance (*D*) of 0·06 by allozyme electrophoresis. In contrast, *S. japonicum* appears more variable, with Woodruff *et al.* (1987) reporting relatively large genetic distances between Chinese and Philippine strains, *D* ranging from 0·45 to 1·10, and Fletcher *et al.* (1980) reporting $D = 0{\cdot}45$. The greater variation within *S. japonicum* may reflect a history of greater environmental instability, with the intermediate hosts entering a variety of new habitats, all within the early Miocene, or a more recent radiation of *S. mansoni* (see Section 8.4). Bowles *et al.* (1993) examined sequence variation for internal transcribed spacer regions of the nuclear *rRNA* gene family and for mitochondrial cytochrome oxidase *c* subunit I (COI); these authors did not report evolutionary distances but summarised the variation as percentage sequence-similarities. Their *S. japonicum* and *S. mansoni* sequences differed by 24%, whilst the *S. japonicum* and *S. mekongi* samples differed by only 13%, which corresponds to *D* of around 0·4. Blair *et al.* (1997) extended these analyses to include *S. malayensis* and the findings again supported the relationships described above on the basis of allozyme and morphological variation (Le *et al.*, 2000c). Since these reports Le and his co-workers (2000b) have obtained near complete DNA sequences for the coding regions of the mitchondrial genome of *S. japonicum* and *S. mekongi*, although these data have yet to be utilized fully in phylogenetic analysis. In addition to the data obtained by Bowles and Blair (above), Sørensen *et al.* (1998, 1999a,b) have published COI and NADI mitochondrial DNA sequences for *S. japonicum* field isolates covering six Chinese provinces; these authors found very low levels of variation among these populations. However, by utilizing a single-strand conformation polymorphism (SSCP) approach, Bøgh *et al.* (1999) were able to reveal useful levels of interpopulation variation for these regions of the mitochondrial genome. Sørensen *et al.* (1999b) have also demonstrated the potential value of the presence (or absence) of a restriction site marker in the mitochondrial NADI gene in the delineation of *S. japonicum* cohorts. Recent work by Le *et al.* (2000a) highlights the phylogenetic importance of mitochondrial-gene-order differences between the major clades of *Schistosoma*. In summary, the genetic studies indicate that *S. mekongi* is a distinct species of the *S. japonicum* group and is most closely related to *S. malayensis*. However, the studies of DNA sequence variation have mostly been based on aged laboratory lines and samples of limited scope. As access to field sites becomes easier, more comprehensive studies based on well-defined populations, stocks and taxa will be possible (see also Section 8.3).

6. THE INTERMEDIATE HOST

6.1. Ecology and Demographics

Neotricula aperta is the natural intermediate host of *S. mekongi* responsible for transmitting schistosomiasis in the lower Mekong Basin (Figure 7). The total known range of *N. aperta* is from Khemmarat in Northeast Thailand, down the Mekong river to Kratié in Cambodia, a distance of some 480 km (see Figure 1). *Neotricula aperta* is assigned to the Pomatiopsidae, a family of conservative rissooidean snails, in that there is a relationship between a bursa copulatrix, seminal receptacle and a bipartite pallial oviduct (see Figure 8). The Pomatiopsidae are most readily distinguished from taxa of the European Hydrobiidae, with which there is considerable convergence, by the nature of the central tooth and the observation that, in the pomatiopsid female, sperm enter the bursal complex via a spermathecal duct (Davis, 1980). There are two pomatiopsid subfamilies: the Pomatiopsinae, to which *Oncomelania* is assigned, and the Triculinae, which includes *Neotricula*. The modern Triculinae are entirely Southeast Asian and southern Chinese in distribution. In the lower Mekong river of Laos, Thailand and Cambodia, the Triculinae represent a remarkable adaptive radiation of 11 genera and over 90 recognised species within a single clade, the tribe Pachydrobiini. A second tribe, the Triculini, shows a similar radiation in southern China (Davis, 1992). These major adaptive radiations are considered by Davis (1982) to have occurred during the Miocene. Davis (1979, 1982) proposed that these snails had kept pace with the evolution of the main rivers of Asia as they cut their way to the sea following their inception at the time of the Himalayan orogeny. Adaptive radiation would have been driven by rapid change in the aquatic environment and the occurrence of new and vacant habitats, which fractionated populations and drove speciation.

N. aperta is almost exclusively epilithic, grazing diatoms and filamentous green algae from the substratum (Attwood, 1996a,c); there is also evidence that this snail can utilize fermentable organics taken up from solution (Attwood, 1995a). The snails are generally found in well-oxygenated,

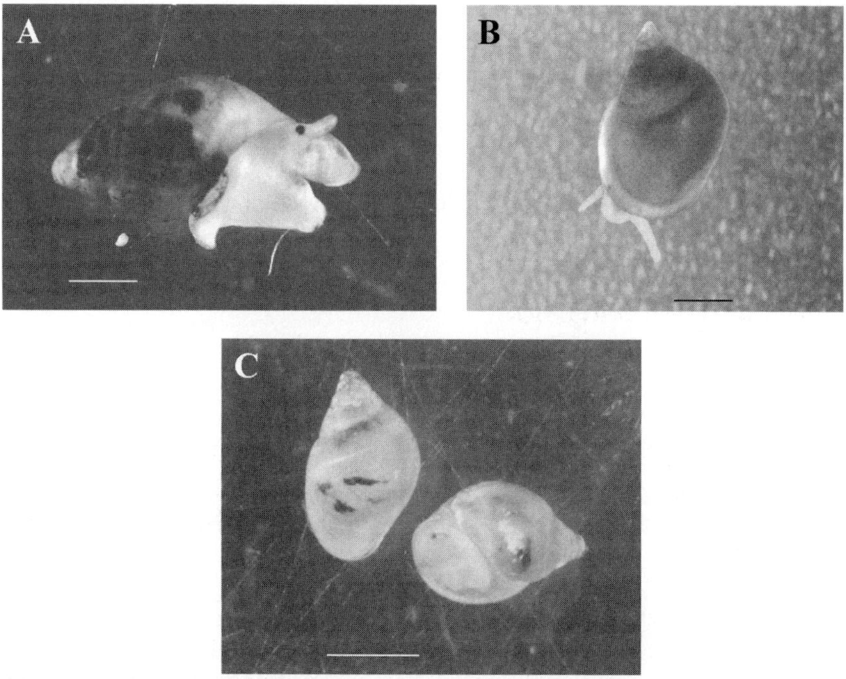

Figure 7 The three strains of *Neotricula aperta* as described by Davis *et al.* (1976). A. α-strain showing diffuse pigmentation across the mantle; this is particularly dense over the ctenidia and kidney. B. β-strain showing a relatively unpigmented mantle and globose shell. C. γ-strain showing an ovate-conic shell with four pigment spots on the mantle under the body whorl. Scale bar 1 mm.

fast-flowing fresh waters at depths of 0·5–3 m. The stream flow of the Mekong and its tributaries shows marked seasonal variations. Generally, the river rises following the onset of the southwest monsoon in mid-May and the maximum level is achieved in September or October; there is considerable snail mortality during the spate (Attwood, 1995b). *N. aperta* is dioecious and apparently amphimictic (Staub *et al.*, 1990); the eggs take 4–5 weeks to hatch and longevity is generally 15 months (Liang and Kitikoon, 1980; Lohachit *et al.*, 1980a).

The life cycle of *N. aperta*, which cannot be observed directly due to the annual spate in the Mekong river, has been the subject of some debate. The life cycle is, however, an important factor in models of schistosomiasis transmission and in the design of snail control measures. Consequently, our current understanding of the demographics and bionomics of *N. aperta* is reviewed in this section. The first hypothesis, for which an attempt had been made to fit

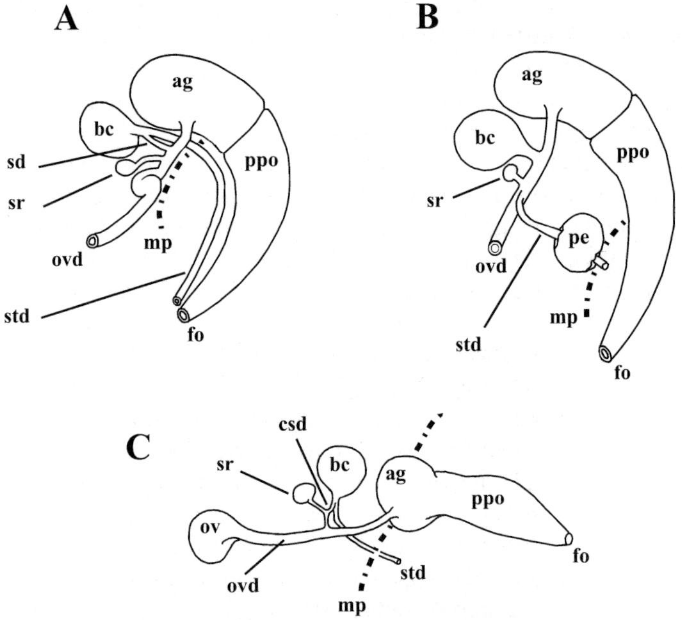

Figure 8 Differences in reproductive anatomy between the pomatiopsine and triculine female. A. Pomatiopsinae: Pomatiopsini, the spermathecal duct (std) extends to the anterior edge of the mantle cavity, and a sperm duct (sd) connects the spermathecal duct and bursal duct to the oviduct (ovd) (based on Davis, 1979). B. *Tricula bollingi* (Triculinae: Triculini), the spermathecal duct enters the pericardium (pe) and is short, terminating at the posterior limit of the mantle cavity (mp). C. *Neotricula aperta* (Triculinae: Pachydrobiini), spermathecal duct runs direct to the posterior edge of the mantle cavity, the duct of the bursa copulatrix (bc) runs into that of the seminal receptacle (sr) as a U-shaped common sperm duct (csd), a slender sperm duct connects the common sperm duct to the oviduct, and there is no loop or twist in the gonadal oviduct. Albumen gland, ag; anterior opening of oviduct, fo; ovary, ov; posterior pallial oviduct, ppo. Drawings not to scale.

epidemiological data, was proposed by Bruce and Schneider (1976) and developed by Upatham *et al.* (1980). This model, known as the 'egg survival hypothesis' (Upatham *et al.*, 1980) and denoted here as H1, proposes that *N. aperta* is unable to tolerate spate conditions and the associated ecological trauma. Under H1 the adults all die in July and August with the population being continued in the form of eggs that undergo delayed development. The eggs are assumed to hatch in March or April, after the restoration of low-water conditions, with the F_1 generation reaching maturity by June or July. However, Attwood (1995b) regarded the evidence for H1 as weak and based on ambiguities or inconsistent observations. For example, laboratory studies failed to demonstrate delayed egg development and there were conflicting reports in the literature regarding the time of oviposition in *N. aperta*. Most authors suggested oviposition between January and March of the second year (Davis *et al.*, 1976; Kitikoon and Schneider, 1976; Davis, 1979), but some inferred pre-spate oviposition (Lohachit *et al.*, 1980a; Upatham *et al.*, 1980). Similarly, one group of researchers suggested that peak mortality of adult snails occurs in early high water (July to August) (Upatham *et al.*, 1980), while most indicated a peak mortality between January and March of the second year (Davis *et al.*, 1976; Davis, 1979; Lohachit *et al.*, 1980a).

Attwood (1995b) proposed an alternative life-cycle model of post-spate survival (H2). The main evidence for H2 was as follows and also serves to highlight the inadequacies of egg survival. The maximum mean shell length for *N. aperta* in the Mekong river at Khemmarat occurred during October to December 1991; this is not concordant with H1, which implies a maximum in July. The Gini coefficient (G) was used to detect, within a single sample, the presence of individuals drawn from two or more statistical populations (see Sen, 1973), in this case on the basis of shell length. G values were found to be greatest in March; this implies the existence of at least two cohorts at that time. A sudden fall in mean shell length was observed in April 1992 with a concomitant increase in population uniformity; this was assumed to represent the loss (death) of the larger, presumably older, snails from the population. The mortality was accompanied by a proportional rise in the coefficient of variation, as might be expected where one substitutes a population of nascent juveniles for a population of adults. Further, Davis *et al.* (1976) reported collecting thousands of empty *N. aperta* shells from Khemmarat in early March but no new young were found until April; these authors assumed that the ensuing spate conditions would have pulverised any empty shells deposited in November or December, and that the shells found in March must have represented a recent mortality. Davis (1979) also reported finding rotting specimens of adult *N. aperta* at Khemmarat in February.

In view of the above, H2 was proposed as follows: there is protandry with the males maturing in May and the females maturing fully in late June to early November, the period of high water and also the proposed time of copulation. Oviposition was considered to be delayed and to occur from January until the end of March. The eggs would then hatch between February and the end of April. The remaining adults were assumed to die in late March as a result of exhaustion following a period of prolonged oviposition. Anatomical features, such as the large bursa copulatrix of female *N. aperta*, further supported the case for H2. The large bursa may serve to manage the sperm store over the high-water period, as supported by dissection of snails collected in late June (Davis *et al.*, 1976). H2 was later refined by Attwood (1999), see Section 7.1 and Figure 9, using molecular genetic data. Clearly an understanding of the life cycle is important as it relates to questions of the location and timing of molluscicide applications in schistosomiasis control, the potential for host snail dispersal and colonization, and the interpretation of molecular systematic data. Consequently, further population genetic studies are necessary in order to understand fully the bionomics of this species.

6.2. The Polytypic Nature of *Neotricula aperta*

Temcharoen (1971) originally described *Lithoglyphopsis aperta* from Laos. Three strains (α, β and γ; see Figure 7) were originally described for *L. aperta* at Khemmarat in Northeast Thailand and in southern Laos (Davis *et al.*, 1976) and all are to varying degrees ($\gamma >> \beta > \alpha$) capable of transmitting schistosomiasis, although the γ-strain alone is epidemiologically significant (Attwood *et al.*, 1997). Davis *et al.* (1976) described two strains of *N. aperta* from the Mekong (α and γ) and one strain (β) from the Mul river, all from Northeast Thailand. The three strains are distinguished on the basis of shell (sculpture, shape and size), mantle pigment patterns, ecology and minor aspects of anatomy; these include differences in radula characters and the number and size of gill filaments. The strains differ in size ($\alpha > \beta > \gamma$) and in the shape of the body whorl and aperture. The mantle of the α-strain (Figure 7A) shows a light dusting of melanin in bands corresponding to the line of the ctenidia, whilst the β-strain (Figure 7B) lacks pigmentation. The γ-strain (Figure 7C) shows a conspicuous pattern of melanin spots; there are usually four spots although variants are common. The strains are not well understood owing to difficulties in laboratory culture, and attempts at breeding rarely succeed beyond the F_1 generation (no interstrain hybrids have been demonstrated). The snails are relatively small, with mean (maximum) shell length ranging from 1·8 mm, γ-strain, to 3·5 mm, α-strain; this has led to technical difficulties in allozyme and ecological studies. Interstrain differences in habitat have been recognized; whilst the β- and γ-strains are fluviatile, found in the Mul (a tributary of the Mekong) and Mekong rivers respectively, the α-strain is restricted to ephemeral pools along the banks and islands of the Mekong river. Davis (1980) referred *L. aperta* to *Tricula* on the basis of both shell and radula characters. *Tricula aperta* was later transferred to *Neotricula* on the basis of differences in reproductive anatomy (Figure 8; Davis *et al.*, 1986).

6.3. Infection Rates with *Schistosoma mekongi*

Attwood *et al.* (1997) reported laboratory infection rates of 3·0%, α-strain; 6·0%, β-strain; and 20·5%, γ-strain, for *N. aperta*, with the greater infectivity to the γ-strain, over both the α- and β-strains, representing a statistically significant difference ($P < 0{\cdot}001$, χ^2-test). These findings are in marked contrast to those of Sornmani (1976) and Lohachit *et al.* (1980b), who reported that infection rates in the β-strain of *N. aperta* were highest among the three strains (being 50–60%). Results suggesting that the β-strain is most susceptible seem paradoxical considering that schistosomiasis has not become established in parts of the lower Mul river, where the β-strain is found at very high population densities (Attwood, 1996b) and where ecological and socio-economic conditions are similar to those in southern Laos. One possible explanation for the observation of greater compatibility with the β-strain is that the schistosome isolate used was routinely passaged in the β-strain, which is generally easier to maintain in the laboratory. There is evidence that populations of snails from a given area may vary in their susceptibility to an allopatric strain of the parasite (see Manning *et al.*, 1995; Morand *et al.*, 1996). Consequently, the greater susceptibility of the β-strain may be due to prolonged use of this snail as a laboratory host. The *Schistosoma mekongi* isolate (from Kratié) used by Attwood *et al.* (1997) was a recent one (collected in 1996), and so the greater infectivity with the γ-strain may reflect the natural transmission process. However, it is also possible that the differences were due to the use of a different (Laotian) *S. mekongi* isolate in the earlier studies. No other published reports concerning the infectivity of different strains of *S. mekongi* to the molluscan host are available. Shekhar (1987) reported interstrain variations in compatibility with *S. malayensis* in the mouse; these variations covered many aspects of the parasitological process.

The overall infection rates for *S. mekongi* in *N. aperta* agree with those for other associations within the *S. japonicum* group; laboratory rates of up to 4·7% have been reported for Philippine *S. japonicum* in the snail *Oncomelania hupensis quadrasi* (see Pesigan *et al.*, 1958). In the *S. mansoni* group higher rates, of 40–70% (Chernin and Dunavan, 1962) and 25–30% (Chernin and Antolics, 1975), have been reported for the *S. mansoni–Biomphalaria* association. Natural infection rates of *S. mekongi* are much lower than those achieved in the laboratory, probably because of additional barriers to the location of hosts by miracidia; this is typical of schistosomes in general. Natural infection rates for the γ-strain at Khong Island were reported to be 0·30% (Kitikoon *et al.*, 1973). Consequently, the results of laboratory experiments can serve only to indicate a potential for parasite transmission and to distinguish further between the strains of *N. aperta*.

6.4. Relationships with Other Triculinae

Neotricula aperta was first reported from the Mekong river around Khong Island in Laos. Re-examination of the holotype suggested the α-strain, and the type locality was recorded as Ban Na on Khong Island, Laos (Davis *et al.*,

1976) (see Figure 2). However, no definitive anatomical descriptions were provided and shell (photographic) and radula data do not suggest *N. aperta*; therefore it is unclear which of the three original strains (α, β and γ), if any, was involved (Attwood, 2001). The presence of the α-strain at Khong Island has not been substantiated, although the γ-strain is common there. In addition, the types deposited by Temcharoen (shells only) are in poor condition and reportedly difficult to distinguish from sympatric species such as *Manningiella conica* Temcharoen, 1971. *Manningiella* Brandt, 1970 is no longer a valid genus and most species have been transferred to *Hubendickia* and *Halewisia* (see Davis, 1980); unfortunately *M. conica* is anatomically unknown. Consequently, and for reasons of convenience, the γ-strain of *N. aperta* from Khong Island is used to represent *N. aperta* in systematic studies until the taxonomic history has been clarified. The molluscan fauna at Khong Island must be resampled and the taxon originally called *M. conica* reassessed. It is important that the taxonomy of *N. aperta* be clarified as, for example, the α-strain of *N. aperta* is much less compatible with *S. mekongi* than the other strains. It is similarly important to determine if any other species, particularly those with different ecological characteristics, are involved in transmission. Such data are central to the matter of schistosomiasis control. Other related aspects of disease transmission, such as the existence of 'decoy' snails for miracidia in *N. aperta* habitats, also require investigation.

7. PHYLOGENIES FOR *NEOTRICULA APERTA*

7.1. The *Neotricula aperta* Complex

There have been relatively few investigations into the genetic basis of polytypy in *N. aperta*. The difficulties may be attributed to the instability of the Mekong river as a habitat for snails, which has a marked effect on population structure, and a lack of information in the past on the life cycle of these snails (Attwood, 1999). Allozyme-based studies (Attwood *et al.*, 1998) revealed significant multilocus genetic distances between the three strains of *N. aperta* from Khemmarat, Northeast Thailand (Nei's, 1978 *D*, 0·6–1·2) and between the γ-strain from Thailand and southern Laos ($D = 1{\cdot}5$). In marked contrast, Staub *et al.* (1990) reported only minor genetic distances between the Thai α- and γ-strains (average $D = 0{\cdot}01$). The genetic distance between the β-strain and the α- and γ-strains *pooled* was 0·66. Staub *et al.* (1990) also reported two cryptic taxa from the Mekong river at Khemmarat, and each of these taxa included *both* α- and γ-strain snails. The 1990 team were able to obtain significant multilocus distances only after re-sorting their samples (strains), a posteriori, into four new groupings with *D* values ranging from 0·2 to 0·9;

these new taxa had no morphological basis. Again in contrast to the 1990 findings, Attwood *et al.* (1998) did not detect a pair of cryptic taxa that each included both α- and γ-strain individuals.

In view of the lack of taxonomic data and inconsistency of the allozyme results, a polymerase chain reaction (PCR)-based restriction fragment length polymorphism (RFLP) analysis of *N. aperta* was performed (Attwood, 1999). Variation at the internal transcribed spacers flanking the 5·8S rRNA gene was examined in this study. In keeping with the 1998 study, the RFLP analysis included the α-, β- and γ-strains from Khemmarat, Northeast Thailand, the γ-strain populations from Khong Island and Kratié and a γ-strain-like taxon from the Xé Bang-Fai river (XBF) of highland central Laos, which flows into the Mekong in Thailand about 120 km upstream of Khemmarat (see Figure 1). The XBF-strain was previously unknown and represented the first report of *N. aperta* in a mountain (minor) river and outside the Mekong–Mul system (Attwood and Upatham, 1999). The differences between taxa were reported as Nei and Miller's (1990) genetic distance × 100 (*D*).

Attwood *et al.* (1998) found the α-strain of *N. aperta* to be heterogeneous (*D* within the strain = 0·22), and this variation was reduced by re-sorting the sample into two subtaxa (Alph-I and -II). RFLP patterns for Alph-I most closely resembled the pattern for the γ-strain, whereas those for Alph-II suggested a grouping with the XBF-strain. The γ-strain, sampled at Khemmarat, also showed two subtaxa (*D* = 0·69), namely TG-I and TG-II; these subtaxa do not, however, correspond to those of Staub *et al.* (1990) as they do not include individuals of both α- and γ-strain phenotypes. In further contrast to Staub *et al.* (1990), the genetic divergence within the original α- and γ-strain samples found by Attwood (1999) is similar to that between populations and therefore unlikely to reflect the existence of sibling species. For example, distances (*D*) among γ-strain populations sampled ranged from 0·68 to 1·51 (*F* = similarity (Nei and Li, 1979) = 0·84−0·93); these values are little greater than the *D*-value observed within the γ-strain, which was 0·69. Attwood (1999) found the β-strain to be most genetically diverged from the other taxa; the distance between the β-strain and the α-strain was 3·68 ± 1·20, and that between the β-strain and all γ-strain populations ranged from 4·03 to 5·49. The work of Attwood (1999) has been repeated by Attwood and Johnston (2001) using COI DNA sequences. The COI phylogeny was found to be much the same as that estimated from the RFLP data (see Figure 10) except that the XBF-strain was found on the branch leading to TG-II.

Recent palaeogeographical models suggest that the *N. aperta* complex diverged as recently as the late Pleistocene (see Section 8.1.3). In view of this, the genetic distances reported by Attwood *et al.* (1998) and Attwood (1999) appear rather large. However, as mentioned above, speciation in the Triculinae probably occurred rapidly throughout the Cenozoic. Spolsky *et al.* (1996) studied the evolution of *Oncomelania h. hupensis* on the Chinese mainland using sequence divergence for the mitochondrial cytochrome *b* gene. These authors reported *F* values of 0·96 between populations from Sichuan and Yunnan Provinces (separated by approximately 400 km). Again such values imply low levels of divergence when compared with those for *N. aperta* populations. Hope and McManus (1994) examined the same *Oncomelania* taxa as did Spolsky *et al.* (1996) but reported genetic distances similar to those of Attwood (1999). Hope and McManus considered such levels of divergence as indicating the presence of sibling species, as did Woodruff *et al.* (1999). On this basis the β- and XBF-strains in the RFLP studies might be considered as sibling species of *N. aperta* (γ-strain). However, once one takes into account the 'background' level of expected interpopulation variation, the case for sibling species becomes much weaker.

High levels of interpopulation variation in *N. aperta* may be attributed to low dispersal rates linked to an inability to aestivate and survive desiccation or transport out of water. The severe annual flood in the Mekong river also has an effect, as habitats are regularly destroyed and populations reduced or eliminated. Recovery from the annual flood may be through recruitment in diminished yet surviving populations, leading to population bottlenecks that heighten the impact of genetic drift, or though the extinction and recolonization (turnover) of local populations between years (i.e. metapopulation dynamics; Hanski, 1994). The long-term persistence of *N. aperta* in the Mekong river as a metapopulation would imply rapid differentiation of populations through recurrent founder effects. Snail dispersal between local populations may have a homogenizing effect within the metapopulation. However, the severe conditions in the lower Mekong could limit gene flow by regularly destroying neighbouring populations and thereby isolating breeding groups. Consequently, the high genetic distances observed between populations by Attwood (1999) could have been more a result of population dynamics rather than of low vagility per se. Indeed, Attwood (1994) demonstrated that the colonization potential of *N. aperta* can be high during the low-water period. The expected fixation time for new (neutral) mutations, assuming Wright–Fisher demography, is a number of generations roughly proportional to the population size (Kingman, 1982; Tajima, 1983); this implies that fixation by genetic drift alone would require over 1 million years for most *r*-selected annual populations (i.e. species with a high innate capacity for population increase). As *N. aperta* probably colonized its present range during the Pleistocene, the geographic discontinuity of genetic variants observed is most probably due to some population level effect along the lines of the metapopulation process described above (Attwood, 1999). Habitats left vacant in the Mekong river at Khemmarat each year (by extinct local populations) could be recolonized by snails originating in tributaries of the Mekong, such as the Xé Bang-Fai river, and washed downstream on twigs or leaves. The disappearance of *N. aperta* from certain stretches of the Mekong river, with reappearance in subsequent years, has been observed in Northeast Thailand; these local populations appear to cover at least 2500 m^2.

One possible explanation for the genetic subdivision of the γ-strain at Khemmarat in Northeast Thailand, as reported by Attwood (1999), is as a colonization event. Snails arising in one or more of the smaller rivers draining the highlands of central Laos may have colonized the Mekong river and hybridized with part of the γ-strain population at Khemmarat to produce taxon TG-II, with its closer affinity to the XBF-strain. Attwood (1999) noted that the average shell length of TG-II was significantly greater than that of TG-I ($P < 0{\cdot}01$) and that the two taxa occurred at Khemmarat (in 1997) in the ratio of 1 : 3, respectively. Taxon TG-I, with less genetic heterogeneity, would therefore represent the 'pure' γ-strain endemic in Northeast Thailand. Clearly, as the TG-II polymorphism was not identical to that of the snails from the XBF sample, the source of the colonists was probably not the Xé Bang-Fai but more probably a river such as the Banghieng, which flows into the Mekong just north of Khemmarat (see Figure 5). Indeed, the present author has found a γ-strain population in the Banghieng river of southern Laos. That the source of the colonists at Khemmarat is a tributary in Laos is further supported by the observation that the substrata are more eroded and the waters more turbulent in the Mekong river north of Khemmarat (conditions unfavourable to *N. aperta*).

Attwood (1999) proposed a mechanism by which a population structure such as that described above may occur. The mechanism assumes that some adult *N. aperta* are able to survive the annual flood that occurs in the Mekong river and its tributaries. Figure 9 summarizes this model, in which *N. aperta* may mature and copulate either before (May/June) or after (late January) the spate; this produces two cohorts, one hatching in late January and the other in March. These 'early' and 'late' cohorts represent TG-II and TG-I respectively, and occur at a ratio of about 1 : 3, with this ratio evening out in years of only mild flooding. The two cohorts were detected in the Mekong river of Northeast Thailand in both the 1992 and 1997 samples. The cohorts differ in their opportunity to mate with colonists from other rivers and it is this that would explain the genetic differences between them. The spate is less severe in minor rivers such as the Xé Bang-Fai and the majority of *N. aperta* in such habitats will have copulated by June. Consequently, females swept downstream and arriving in the Mekong in January will be equivalent to early cohort individuals as found in the Mekong river. The descendants of the colonists would, in subsequent years, hybridize primarily with early-cohort local snails; this would explain the greater shell length of TG-II and its affinity with snails such as the XBF-strain. The greater shell length of TG-II may be explained by the fact that the life cycle in Mekong tributaries is generally ahead of that in the Mekong river (as a result of shallower waters and a shorter spate period). The greater heterogeneity of TG-II in the present study probably occurs because the colonists from Laos originate in a constellation of

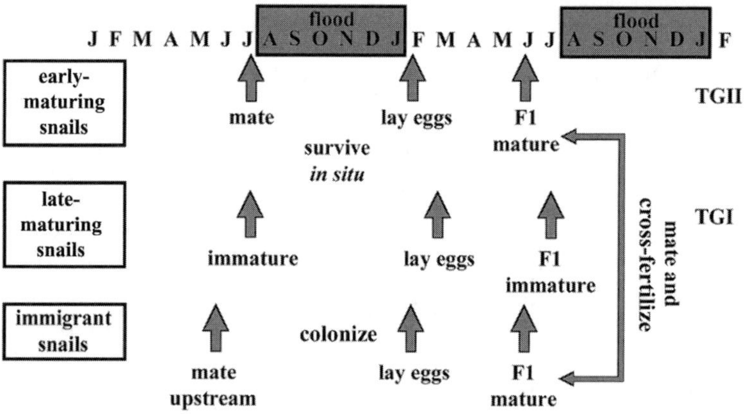

Figure 9 The life cycle of *Neotricula aperta*, γ-strain, in the Mekong river of Northeast Thailand. TGI refers to the 'late' cohort with its smaller shell as observed in April or May. TGII is the 'early' cohort, which has a greater chance of mating with snails colonizing the Mekong river from tributaries in central Laos. A timescale in months is shown along the top of the diagram.

populations and streams. Late-cohort individuals mature too late in the year to mate with colonists or local snails originating in the early cohort. The model also agrees with H2 and the demographic data collected by Attwood (1995b), as described in Section 6.1. Additional data involving more rapidly evolving molecular markers (such as microsatellites or mitochondrial D-loop DNA sequences) are vital in order to distinguish the relative roles of recruitment and colonization in the persistence and spread of *N. aperta* in the lower Mekong Basin.

7.2. Phylogeography of *Neotricula aperta*

A phylogeny involving the four strains of *N. aperta* and based on RFLP patterns (Attwood, 1999) is given in Figure 10. The Fitch tree for these taxa suggests a phylogeography involving colonization progressively downstream from Khemmarat southwards to Kratié Province in Cambodia (see Figure 1). The genetic clustering of the epidemiologically significant populations in Cambodia and southern Laos is consistent with this cline and may be relevant in the future control of Mekong schistosomiasis. As detailed in Section 8.1.3, the Mekong river is unlikely to have assumed its present course along the eastern border of the Khorat Plateau (Figure 11) and on to Kratié until the late Pleistocene (Hutchinson, 1989), making the diversification of *N. aperta*

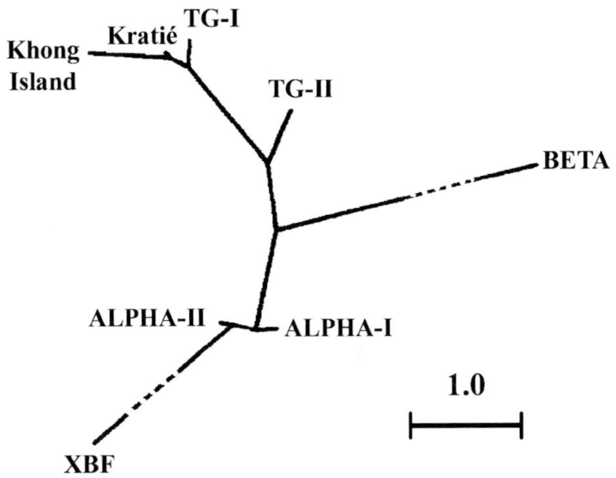

Figure 10 An unrooted Fitch tree for *Neotricula aperta* based on Nei and Miller's (1990) genetic distance for RFLP data. Line lengths are proportional to branch lengths. Broken lines reflect uncertainty due to large standard errors in the distance estimates (after Attwood, 1999).

appear a rather rapid event. *Neotricula aperta* populations south of Khong Island cannot be much more than 500 000 years old, and those at Kratié little over 10 000 years old. Snail populations around Khemmarat, in Northeast Thailand, are likely to be the oldest of the Mekong river populations. In addition, prior to the mid-Pleistocene uplift of the western margin of the Khorat Plateau (strictly a basin), it is likely that the Mul river flowed west towards the current location of the Chao Phrya river headwaters (Hutchinson, 1989). The zoogeography of *N. aperta* is further complicated by the probable occurrence of extensive lava flows in southern Laos approximately 800 000 years ago; these flows extended the central (Annam) highlands of Laos southwards to produce the Bolovens Plateau and hills of Champassac Province (see Figure 12) and to cover the mouth of the Mul river, severing its connexion with the Mekong (Workman, 1977).

Palaeogeographical models are not yet sufficiently developed as to afford a complete history of the early Cenozoic rivers of Southeast Asia. However, the data so far available suggest that colonization of the lower Mekong by ancestors of *N. aperta* began within the last 1 million years. The α- and XBF-strains appear to be the basal taxa in the phylogeny represented by Figure 10, and it is likely that the ancestral character of *N. aperta* resembled that of the α-strain today. The pre-Mekong river could have introduced α-strain-like snails to the hills of central Laos in the late Pliocene. These snails may then be in a position to colonize the eastern margin of the Khorat Plateau (i.e. Northeast Thailand),

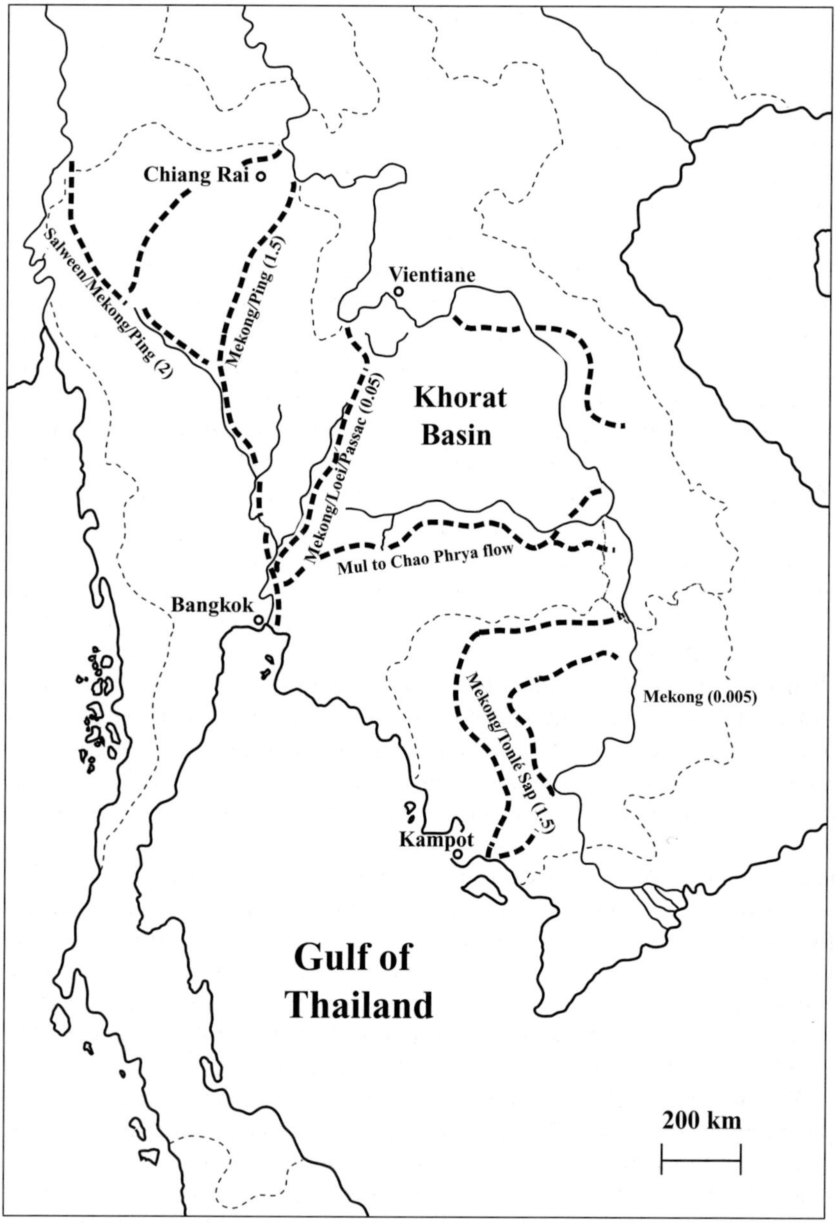

Figure 11 Major course changes along the Mekong river during the late Cenozoic. Prehistoric river courses are shown as broken lines; the names of the captured rivers are shown along with the approximate times of capture ($\times 10^{-6}$ years) in parentheses. Based on the palaeogeographical maps of Gregory (1925) and Hutchinson (1989).

after the tilting of the basin in Thailand, which could easily have effected the necessary flow reversals (see Gibling and Ratanasthien, 1980). The accompanying elevation of the hills in southern Laos would then lead to the evolution of the γ-strain, through XBF-strain intermediates, in rivers such as the Xé Bang-Fai and Xé Banghieng. The γ-strain would be better suited to the more fluviatile conditions which formed as the uplift progressed in Laos. The colonization of Northeast Thailand by early γ-strain-like taxa would have begun after the Mekong river assumed its present course along the east of the Khorat Plateau toward Paxsé. Block faulting throughout Northeast Thailand, at the close of the Tertiary, no doubt produced numerous dams and lakes from the evolving pre-Mekong. The α-strain of *N. aperta* is adapted to life in shallow pools and backwaters and may have evolved this ability after becoming trapped in the lentic habitats created as the river cut south to Khemmarat.

A parsimonious hypothesis for the β-strain of *N. aperta* considers its evolution from the same antecedent form as the present α-strain, entering the Mekong river at about the same time. The β-strain is basal to the lineage bearing the γ-strain populations of southern Laos and Cambodia and perhaps arose when ancestral *N. aperta* became isolated in the fast-flowing headwaters of the Mul river, which at that time apparently flowed west towards central Thailand. The β-strain would have remained a geographical isolate throughout the mid-Pleistocene, until the Mul river flow had reversed and found a channel across the lava flows at its junction with the Mekong; this isolation would explain the large genetic distances observed with the other strains of *N. aperta* (see Attwood, 1999). The lava flows that occurred in southern Laos 800 000 years ago have provided many of the habitats occupied by modern *N. aperta*, with extensive stretches of shallow rapids, rock outcrops and minor water falls. It is most likely that major colonization of the lower Mekong by the γ-strain of *N. aperta* occurred after these habitats became available. Similarly, the β-strain would have colonized its present range only after new fluviatile habitats became available in the form of these lava flows; this ecological requirement also explains the absence of the β-strain from the middle Mul river (or Chao Phrya river) and its apparent isolation at the mouth of the Mul. Support for this theory would be gained if surveys of the present day Mul river headwaters revealed snails resembling *N. aperta*.

The above hypothesis involving a highland origin for *N. aperta* is supported by observations of other generalized Triculinae. Snails such as *Gammatricula, Jinhongia, Neotricula* and *Tricula* occupy similar fast-flowing, but relatively stable, highland streams and minor rivers, and not the major rivers with which they are associated. This observation reflects the hypothesized origin of the clade in the mountain streams of northern Burma (Davis *et al.*, 1992). The differences between the α-strain and the other members of the *N. aperta* complex may therefore be due to recent selection on the latter during the invasion of a large river. The rapid diversification leading to the

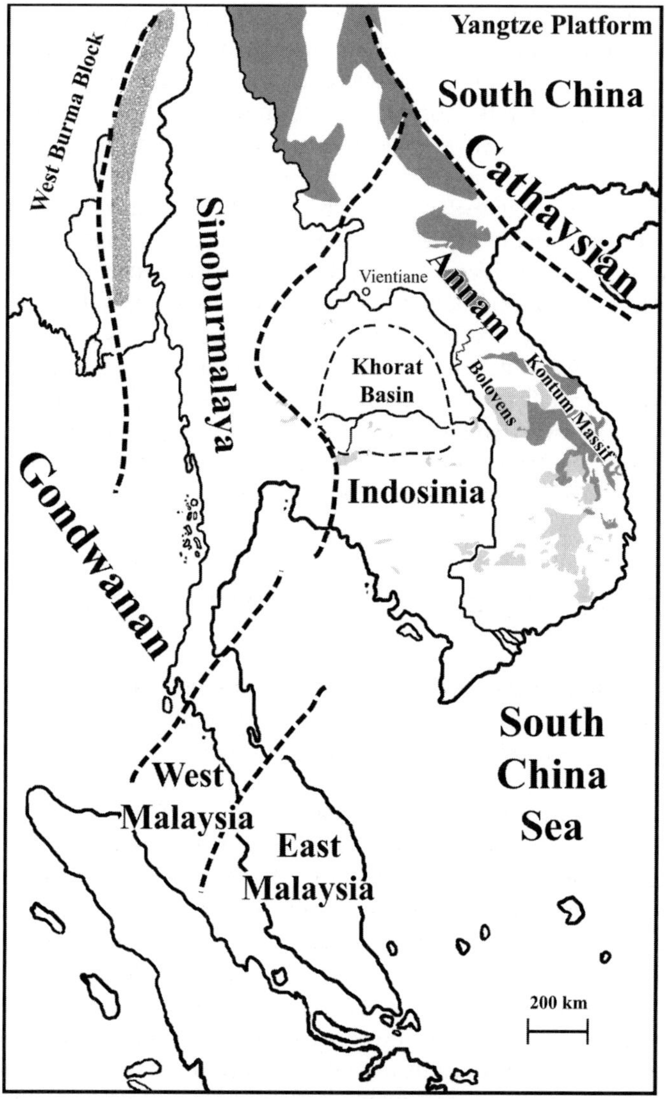

Figure 12 Western Sundaland showing geological provinces. Palaeozoic (or earlier) mountain ranges are shaded dark grey, whereas local Quaternary (more recent) orogenies are shaded light grey. Volcanism in the Pleistocene around the Bolovens Plateau is likely to have had a profound effect on the biogeography of *Neotricula aperta*. The Yangtze Platform of South China is Cathaysian in origin, whereas all terranes shown to the southwest are Gondwanan (e.g. Indosinia, Sinoburmalaya). The shaded area parallel to the margin of the West Burma Block represents the Burman volcanic arc, which was active throughout the Tertiary (based on Bunopas and Vella, 1983, and Hutchinson, 1989). Scale approximate.

three main strains of *N. aperta* (occurring between 1 million and 10 000 years ago) was probably the result of the stochastic nature of the young Mekong river and the absence of competitors, such as pulmonate snails, from the newly emerging habitats. The evolution of compatibility with *Schistosoma* remains a question if the α-strain is considered to represent the ancestral form of *N. aperta*. The α-strain is least compatible with *S. mekongi*; however, it is possible that this strain evolved resistance to the parasite in response to the greater parasite pressure expected in snail populations confined to small pools and flooded gullies. It is conceivable that the ancestral form of *N. aperta* was compatible with *S. mekongi* and was involved in the colonization of the lower Mekong by this parasite. The above model is provided as a useful working hypothesis which is able to explain the current biogeographical deployment of these taxa in the light of data available to date. DNA sequence data for *N. aperta* populations, and those of *S. mekongi* where present, will help assess such hypotheses. These data would allow us to clarify the route of colonization and to confirm the ancestral form of *N. aperta*.

8. THE PHYLOGEOGRAPHY OF SOUTHEAST ASIAN *SCHISTOSOMA*

8.1. Palaeogeography and Late Cenozoic Instability

8.1.1. *The Need for Revised Hypotheses*

The consensus view of the evolution and colonization history of the Southeast Asian schistosomes has been based largely on the ideas presented in papers such as those by Davis (1979, 1980, 1981, 1982, 1992). These hypotheses exploit the reciprocal illumination gained by an examination of phylogenies for both the parasites and their intermediate hosts. The hypotheses presented by Davis were based on an extensive set of characters for a large number of Pomatiopsidae (e.g. see Davis *et al.*, 1994) and provided well-supported predictions regarding the colonization of Southeast Asia and southern China by *Schistosoma* and relevant snails. However, these traditional hypotheses were based on the concept of a relatively stable Southeast Asian geology throughout the Cenozoic and this no longer appears to be the case. Consequently, revision is necessary in order to accommodate more recent developments in Southeast Asian palaeogeography, such as those presented by Hutchinson (1989), Hall (1998) and Lacassin *et al.* (1998). A revised hypothesis, incorporating these new palaeogeographical models, is developed in this section. The main tenets of Davis's hypotheses remain; however, changes in the timing of events are proposed and new potential routes of colonization are described. A timescale is also presented for the colonization of the lower rivers. A more serious challenge to the traditional hypothesis has arisen from recent molecular data concerning schistosome evolution (Snyder and Loker, 2000) and these findings are discussed in Section 8.4.

8.1.2. *The Conventional View*

The Pomatiopsidae have a Pangaean distribution; however, that of the Pomatiopsinae is Gondwanan with extant taxa showing a 'southern continental' (vicariant) distribution (Davis, 1979). A Gondwanan origin was thus proposed for *Schistosoma* with the ancestors of *S. mansoni* and *S. haematobium* being isolated on the African Plate. The African and South American taxa were thereby separated from the ancestors of the *S. japonicum* and *S. indicum* groups as Gondwana broke up in the late Mesozoic (Davis, 1979, 1980) (Figure 13). The present distribution of the *S. japonicum* and *S. indicum* groups would then be a result of their divergence on the Indian Plate during the period of rafting northwards toward Eurasia (90–50 million years ago). Colonization of mainland Southeast Asia began after the collision with the Indian Plate (about 40 million years ago) and the onset of the Tibetan uplift, which initiated the main rivers of Asia (Hutchinson, 1989). Fossils resembling *Oncomelania* are known from the early Miocene of India (Davis 1982). Davis (1979) suggested that the main route of colonization was via the Northwest Burma–Brahmaputra corridor, which opened approximately 18 million years ago. The biogeography of extant snails suggested that the mid-Miocene was also the point at which pre-*S. japonicum* became established in amphibious Pomatiopsinae of the Yangtze river drainage in southern China. As precursors of *S. japonicum* entered the Yangtze, pre-*S. mekongi/malayensis* became isolated in Triculinae of the evolving Mekong and (perhaps) Salween river systems. The *S. indicum* group, characterized by an egg bearing a subterminal spine, was thought to have dispersed on the Indian Plate in pulmonate snails. Colonization of the Southeast Asian mainland by this group was most probably associated with human activity in the Holocene (Barker and Blair, 1996); the current biogeography of these taxa does not appear to be vicariant on a pattern of riparian colonization as seen in the distribution of the *S. japonicum* group. Separation of the Yangtze and Mekong river systems was believed to have occurred in the late Miocene during the period of lake lowering in Yunnan, China, and the disruption of connexions between the two rivers (Davis, 1979). This would have isolated the Mekong river Pachydrobiini (including *N. aperta*) from the Pomatiopsinae in Yunnan; therefore, according to this model, pre-*S. japonicum* and pre-*S. mekongi* have been geographically separated for around 12 million years.

The above hypothesis also leads to predictions regarding phylogenetic constraint and the ability to transmit schistosomiasis (Davis, 1992). Transmission

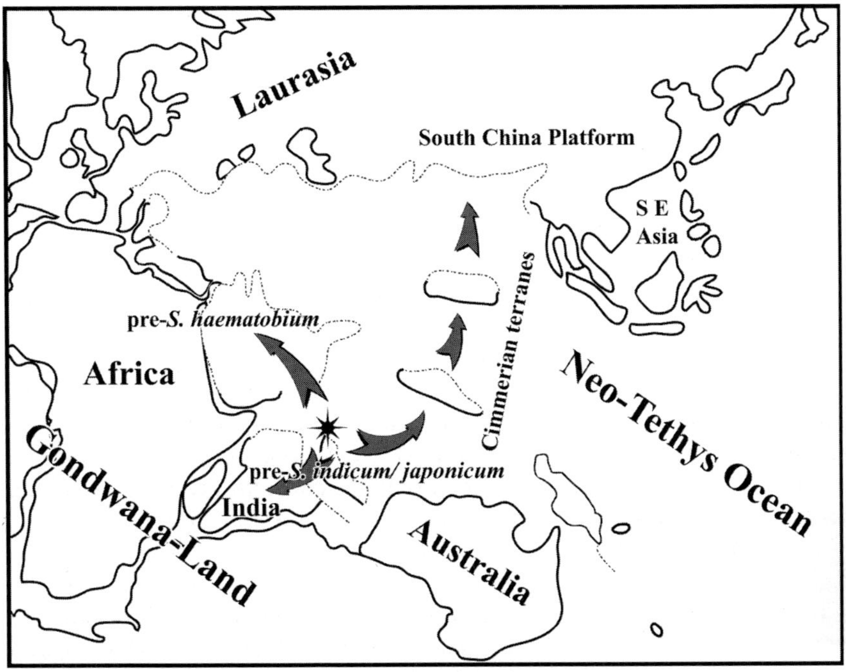

Figure 13 The break up of Gondwana throughout the Cretaceous and the origin and dispersal of early *Schistosoma*. The schematic follows Davis (1979) in that *Schistosoma* is shown to arise in Gondwana with subsequent rafting to Southeast Asia on the Indian Plate. Here, however, *Schistosoma* is considered to have arisen on one of the Cimmerian fragments (denoted by a star) destined to collide with Asia at any time during the Mesozoic but prior to the accretion of India. Consequently, the initial radiation of *Schistosoma* in Asia may have been essentially isochronous with that in Africa/India (rather than subsequent to the latter). The African radiation may have involved a common ancestral form that entered India before the separation of the fragment. The arrows show possible routes of migration and diversification. The broken lines represent surfaces of collision and accretion (based on Smith *et al.*, 1981 and Hall, 1998).

of *S. mekongi* and *S. malayensis* is restricted to the *Neotricula* clade. *Robertsiella*, host of *S. malayensis* in West Malaysia, and *Neotricula* appear to be derived from progenitors resembling the latter, and show affinity with the Salween and Mekong drainages (respectively); these rivers were thought to have separated from the Yangtze about 5 million years ago, on the assumption of a stable Cenozoic geography. *Jinhongia jinhongensis* (Guo and Gu, 1985) is reported to transmit an unknown species of *Schistosoma* in Yunnan (Davis *et al.*, 1992); this may be a relative of *S. mekongi* as it is transmitted by a member of the *Neotricula* clade and is associated with the Mekong river.

The so-called *Schistosoma 'sinensium'* of northern Thailand is likely to be a species distinct from that described as *S. sinensium s.s.* (Bao, 1958) from Sichuan Province, China (see also Pao, 1959). This Thai schistosome is unlikely to be *S. sinensium* (for reasons given in Section 8.3) and will be referred to as *Schistosoma* n. sp. throughout this chapter. Under the conventional hypothesis the Thai schistosome appears relictual in northern Thailand, reflecting a colonization event in northern Burma some 6 million years ago, and remains associated with the tract of the extended Brahmaputra–Irrawaddy drainage. In addition, *Schistosoma* n. sp. of Thailand is transmitted by conserved Triculini, namely *Tricula bollingi* Davis, 1968. In the laboratory *N. aperta* is weakly susceptible to *S. malayensis* and the new taxon (see Davis, 1992). Further, *Pomatiopsis lapidaria* (Pomatiopsidae: Pomatiopsinae) of North America can be experimentally infected with *S. japonicum*, even though their respective ancestors were separated over 150 million years ago at the break up of Gondwana (Davis, 1979). The conclusion to be drawn is that *S. japonicum*-group parasites have a general ability to utilize pomatiopsid hosts and that there may be little pressure upon snails to develop resistance. *Schistosoma* does not appear to have invaded those Triculinae which have diverged into lotic, main river, habitats and this may be more a result of low miracidial success than of adaptations among snails to exclude parasites. *Neotricula aperta* is lotic but is *r*-selected and achieves much higher population densities than other lotic Triculinae; this may foster transmission, especially during the low-water period, and reduce parasite pressure on these populations. Consequently, there is some phylogenetic constraint imposed by the isolation of snails into different river systems; however, one cannot expect compatibility to be seen in all taxa of a susceptible clade (because of differences in snail ecology).

Figure 14 shows a 'river-based' cladogram for Southeast Asian *Schistosoma* constructed according to the conventional phylogeographic hypothesis above; the dates of divergence of taxa are based on the timing of isolating events linked to the evolution of the main rivers of Asia (i.e. the time at which the rivers separated). The cladogram is in effect a summary of predictions based on the conventional hypothesis. Figure 14 agrees well with phylogenetic hypotheses based on current, albeit limited, DNA sequence data for several of these schistosomes (e.g., Blair *et al.*, 1997). Also in keeping with the traditional hypothesis, Hall (1998) adopts the general view that the India–Asia collision would have driven dispersal from Gondwana to Southeast Asia via India, with later speciation centred on Sundaland (see Figure 12). Davis (1979) suggested that overland colonization of Southeast Asia would only be possible via the northeast tip of the Indian Plate, the northwest being an area of extreme volcanism; this volcanism, a result of subduction ahead of the hard collision with mainland Asia, is still a feature of more recent tectonic models (see Hutchinson, 1989). However, the conventional account

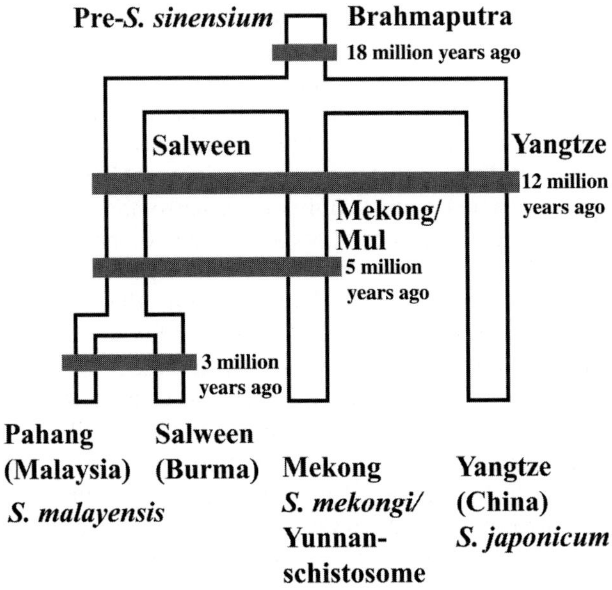

Figure 14 A river-based cladogram for Southeast Asian *Schistosoma* summarizing the traditional phylogeographical model (see text). The dates shown are predicted divergence times based on the isolation of taxa in the main river systems as these evolved in a linear fashion down to the sea. The taxa now found in each river are given at the base of the diagram. This simple phylogeographical model for *Schistosoma* is no longer considered to be adequate.

of phylogeographical events following the initial introduction of taxa is incongruent with modern palaeogeographical models and new hypotheses must be developed and tested.

8.1.3. *A New Phylogeographical Model*

The first departure from the conventional picture of the colonization of mainland Southeast Asia by the precursors of the *Schistosoma japonicum* group involves the timing of the separation of the main rivers of the region. It now appears likely that connections between the upper Mekong and Yangtze rivers were broken in the late Miocene (7–5 million years ago) rather than the mid-Miocene (12 million years ago). It has become clear that Tibet may have had mountains of moderate stature prior to the collision with India, similar to those of northern Sinoburmalaya (see Figure 12) in which *Tricula bollingi* is found today (Mitchell, 1981). Such hilly terrain would have been particularly suitable for colonization by triculine snails dispersing from Northeast India. Following the initial orogeny, to an average elevation of 2500 m, the Tibetan Plateau is thought to have experienced a second uplift in the Pliocene to achieve the average 5000 m observed today (Xu, 1981). The second uplift probably initiated the separation of the upper Yangtze from the other major rivers of Southeast Asia, such as the Irrawaddy and Mekong, as the faster waters cut deeper channels into the plateau and across Yunnan. As the climatic changes associated with the second uplift would have been intolerable, any pomatiopsid snails present must have dispersed separately into the middle reaches of their respective rivers in Yunnan before the Pliocene elevation. Consequently, the progenitors of *S. japonicum* and *S. sinensium* (i.e. Yangtze river taxa) and those of *S. malayensis*, *S. mekongi* and *Schistosoma* n. sp. of Thailand (i.e. Mekong river taxa) were separated no later than 5 million years ago. The explosive radiation of the Pachydrobiini in the Mekong river around Khong Island was considered to have begun in the late Miocene (Davis *et al.*, 1985). However, such hypotheses were based on the concept of a stable Cenozoic geology in the region and it is by no means certain that all colonization was via Tibet. Other routes of colonization were likely to have been available and these are discussed in Section 8.2. Southeast Asia experienced extensive tectonic activity with marked changes in drainage configuration throughout the Cenozoic (Gordon, 1882; Gregory, 1925; later developed and evidenced by Tapponier *et al.*, 1982, 1986; Lacassin *et al.*, 1998). Further, many of the mountains formed within Sundaland during the Quaternary are likely to be linked to activity along strike-slip faults and therefore geologically short lived (Hall, 1998). This view of regional geology is inconsistent with traditional models for the colonization of Southeast Asia by *Schistosoma*, which is considered to be in a linear fashion, southwards from Southwest China, with schistosomes and relevant snails colonizing new habitats available as the nascent river systems cut their way down to the sea (Davis and Greer, 1980). Triculine snails were thought to have colonized Northeast Thailand and Laos as the Mekong river cut its way across the Khorat Plateau (Davis and Greer, 1980); however, as already stated, the Mekong is unlikely to have been a major river in southern Indochina until the mid-Pleistocene.

During the Pliocene the Mekong appears to have flowed due south from Chiang Rai (see Figure 11), down what is today the Ping river valley, to enter the Gulf of Thailand via the present Chao Phrya river delta (Hutchinson, 1989). This may explain the finding of Thai *Schistosoma 'sinensium'* and *Tricula* in association with the Ping river system around Chiang Dao, Northwest Thailand. Late Cenozoic faulting along the Uttaradit suture (see Figure 5) next diverted the Mekong eastwards along its present course towards Vientiane (see Figure 11). Later in the Pleistocene the Mekong once again flowed toward the present Chao Phrya delta, however, this time via the valley of the Loei/Passac river (see Figures 5 and 11) (Hutchinson, 1989); the finding of

Neotricula burchi (Davis, 1968) in Loei Province, Northeast Thailand, may also reflect the introduction of pachydrobiine snails to the region by the pre-Mekong river. After extending its course southwards to the location of the present Mul–Mekong river junction, the Mekong river appears to have undergone further course changes. The channel now occupied by the Mekong south of Khong Island probably originated a little over 5000 years ago (Hutchinson, 1989). Indeed, the 'Mekong' may have flowed westwards in the late Pliocene, just south of the mountains along the Cambodian–Thai border, or down the present Tonlé-Sap and into the Gulf of Thailand near Kampot (Figure 15).

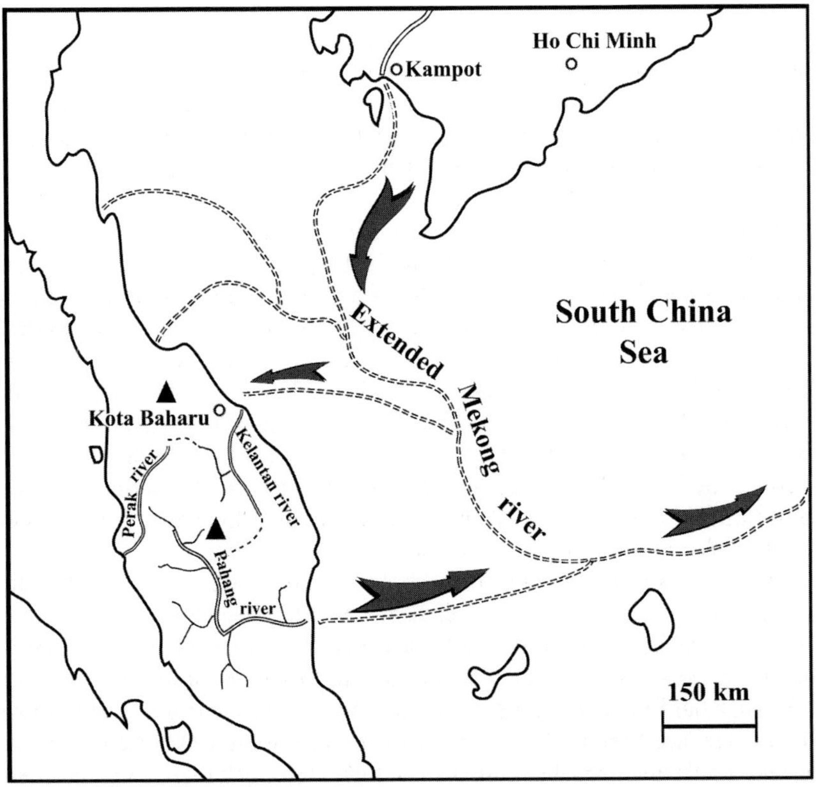

Figure 15 The extension of the Mekong river from Cambodia to peninsular Malaysia during the Pliocene. The broken lines represent extended river basins and the arrows the predominant direction of flow and potential routes of faunal dispersal (based on Rainboth, 1996). The black triangles show areas where *Schistosoma malayensis* has been found. As the Perak and Pahang rivers were once conterminous, *S. malayensis* may have diverged from *S. mekongi*-like taxa following their introduction to the Pahang river from the extended Mekong of Cambodia. Scale approximate.

The current Mekong delta would have been occupied solely by the Dong Ngai river, which drains the eastern slopes of the Vietnamese highlands and shares a delta with the Mekong today (Workman, 1977). In view of these recent course changes, the *N. aperta* complex in Northeast Thailand would have diverged well within the last million years, making this event even more rapid than previously thought (Attwood, 1999). Low sea levels associated with the Pleistocene glacial periods would have allowed the pre-Mekong river to flow directly from the present coast of Cambodia to the Malay Peninsula (Hall, 1998). Consequently, *S. malayensis* in the Pahang river drainage of West Malaysia probably diverged from *S. mekongi* after its introduction from Cambodia, via the extended Mekong river during the Pleistocene (Figure 15).

8.2. Routes of Colonization

The geographical point of origin of *Schistosoma mekongi* and *Neotricula* remains unresolved. Samples have been difficult to collect across the disparate and often inaccessible areas involved and recent zoogeographical patterns have been hard to interpret. A fundamental problem has been the exact mechanism by which ancestral pomatiopsid snails and schistosomes became isolated in the upper reaches of the Mekong and Yangtze rivers, the process suggested by Davis (1979) in explanation of current biogeographical patterns. The upper rivers present a harsh, cold, climate in which hydrobioid snails are unlikely to have flourished. Fortunately, improvements in the understanding of the geological history of Asia now shed some light on the colonization of the region. These new data afford the possibility of the direct colonization of Thailand by antecedent Triculinae and *Schistosoma* from Burma (originally from India), rather than via China and the upper Mekong as proposed by Davis *et al.* (1994).

One scenario is that the ancestors of both 'Yangtze' and 'Mekong' *Schistosoma* (see Section 8.1.3), and Triculinae, dispersed throughout northern Burma and Tibet until 5 million years ago. Indeed, Swan (1981) described the capture of the upper Irrawaddy by rivers now draining into the Brahmaputra and this would have provided a colonization route from India. Isolation of the Yangtze and Mekong taxa would then occur during the Pliocene orogeny. For example, taxa may have dispersed separately into the upper and lower Irrawaddy rivers (Yangtze taxa to the upper river), which then existed as two separate drainages (Hutchinson, 1989) (Figure 16A). Precursors of *Schistosoma* n. sp. and *S. mekongi* could then disperse into Thailand via the lower Irrawaddy and the extended Mekong–Salween river, which flowed together during the Pleistocene (around 1·5 million years ago, see Figure 11). Subsequent introductions from Burma into northern Yunnan (Yangtze river) were probably prevented by the ongoing elevation of the West Burma Block (see Hutchinson, 1989) (see Figure 12). A second possible scenario is one in which pre-*S. japonicum* and/or pre-*S. sinensium* entered southern China much earlier (in the Miocene) off one of the Tibetan (Cimmerian) blocks which collided with Asia before the Indian Plate (see Figure 16B and Section 8.4). This would permit the direct colonization of the upper Yangtze in Tibet by early *Schistosoma* and Pomatiopsidae, which then dispersed southwards into the Sichuan Basin (Figure 16B). The Yangtze platform basin has remained quite stable over the last 600 million years, and the course of the Yangtze has changed relatively little throughout its history (Hutchinson, 1989). In addition, the mountains of southern Yunnan, northern Laos and northern Vietnam are likely to have provided a barrier to dispersal over the last 200 million years (see Figure 12). The absence of *Oncomelania* and *S. japonicum* from mainland Southeast Asia is evidence for this barrier. This hypothesis of an independent origin for Yangtze taxa (off a Cimmerian block) and Mekong taxa (in northern India and Burma) implies that the ancestors of *S. sinensium* from Sichuan and of *Schistosoma* n. sp. from Northwest Thailand (Yangtze and Mekong taxa respectively) were separated some 200 million years ago; this is in contrast to the 5 million years suggested by scenario one. Clearly, the relationships between these two taxa are important in distinguishing between phylogeographies for Southeast Asian *Schistosoma*. Both these scenarios can explain the presence of a *Schistosoma* sp. on the Lao border in southern Yunnan (transmitted by the snail *Jinhongia*), the presence of *Schistosoma* and Triculinae in the Ping river valley of Thailand, the absence of *Neotricula* from the upper Mekong river, the absence of *S. japonicum* and *Oncomelania* from mainland Southeast Asia, and the observation of Davis *et al.* (1992) that the most conserved taxa of the Triculinae are found closest to the rivers of northern Burma. However, the introduction of *S. sinensium/S. japonicum* to China via one of the smaller Cimmerian fragments also implies a divergence time of 50–100 million years for the *S. mekongi* and *S. japonicum* lineages. Fortunately, comparative DNA sequence data for all the Asian taxa (when available) will greatly facilitate our decisions between the alternative models described above.

The possible dispersal of *Schistosoma* and snails along the 900 km Red river fault from southern Yunnan to northern Vietnam must also be investigated. As mentioned above, the Kontum Massif would have formed a barrier to taxa dispersing southwards into Indochina since the Palaeozoic. The Red river fault, however, also provides a channel permitting dispersal from Yunnan to Vietnam (Figure 16A). *Neotricula* and precursors of *S. mekongi* may have followed the Red river from Yunnan into Indochina; this would have become possible during the Pliocene after volcanic activity along the fault began to subside (see Allen *et al.*, 1984). Recent surveys by the present author suggested that *N. aperta* may be more common in the minor rivers of central/southern Laos and eastern Cambodia than in the Mekong river itself.

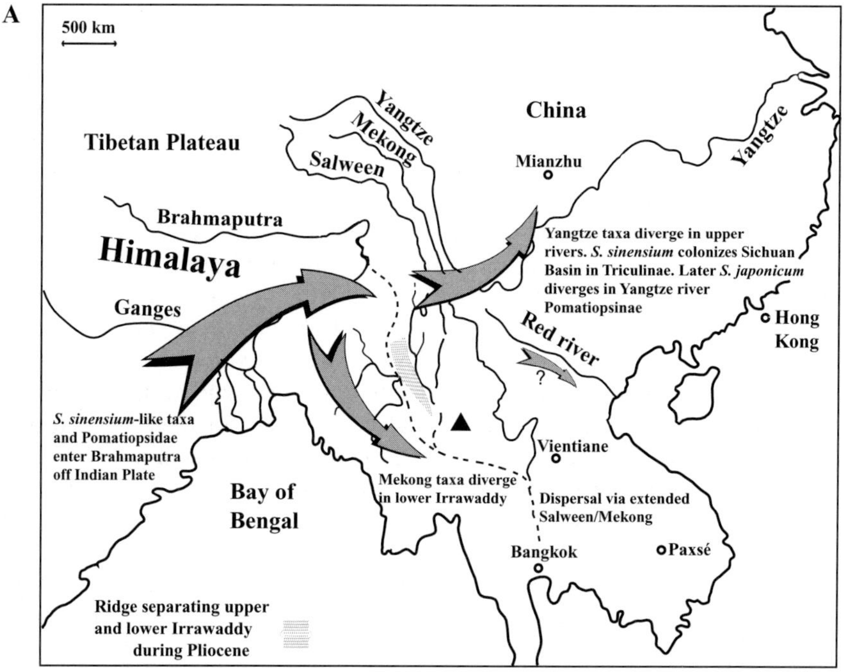
A
500 km
Tibetan Plateau
Yangtze
Mekong
Salween
China
Mianzhu
Yangtze
Brahmaputra
Himalaya
Ganges
Yangtze taxa diverge in upper rivers. S. sinensium colonizes Sichuan Basin in Triculinae. Later S. japonicum diverges in Yangtze river Pomatiopsinae
Hong Kong
Red river
?
S. sinensium-like taxa and Pomatiopsidae enter Brahmaputra off Indian Plate
Vientiane
Bay of Bengal
Mekong taxa diverge in lower Irrawaddy
Dispersal via extended Salween/Mekong
Bangkok
Paxsé
Ridge separating upper and lower Irrawaddy during Pliocene

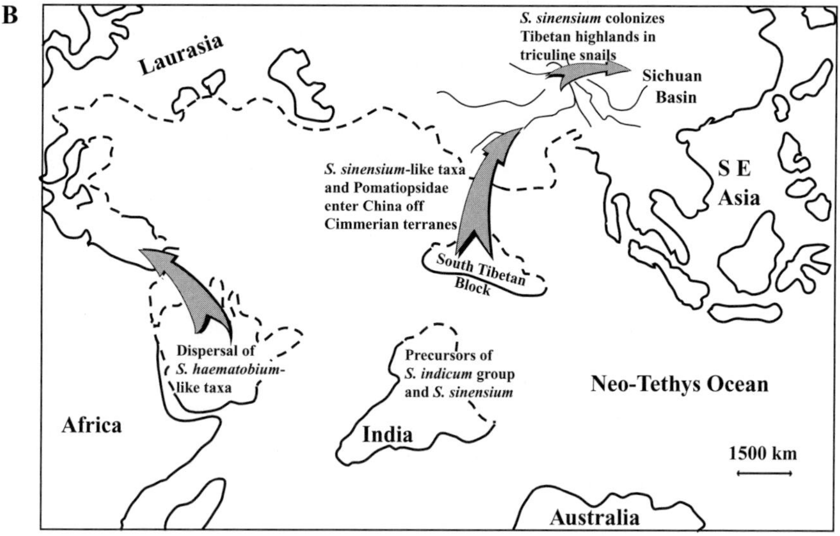
B
Laurasia
S. sinensium colonizes Tibetan highlands in triculine snails
Sichuan Basin
S. sinensium-like taxa and Pomatiopsidae enter China off Cimmerian terranes
S E Asia
South Tibetan Block
Dispersal of S. haematobium-like taxa
Precursors of S. indicum group and S. sinensium
Neo-Tethys Ocean
Africa
India
1500 km
Australia

If *N. aperta* had been introduced to these Annam chain drainages via the Red river fault one would expect to find triculine snails (probably also *Schistosoma*) in the rivers of the eastern, as well as the western, slopes of these mountains. Although many of the Annam mountains are pre-Mesozioc, there has been some movement along parts of the chain during the Quaternary. The extinction of a prehistoric river system running North–South in Vietnam is postulated but as yet uncorroborated (Workman, 1972).

There is still a long way to go in understanding this aspect of Southeast Asian zoogeography. Attempts at reconstructions have been thwarted by two major obstacles. First, the last period of glacial history may have had a far greater influence on patterns than the Neogene or even Palaeogene. In particular, fluctuations in climate and rainfall are likely to have been most extreme since the Pleistocene, as these are probably linked to changes in oceanic circulation patterns (Huang *et al.*, 1997; Hall, 1998). Second, the rapid industrialization of Thailand has done much to obscure patterns through habitat destruction; this factor is additional to changes in depth, flow and turbidity occurring throughout the Quaternary as rivers in the region stabilized and began to cut deeper channels. The impact of industrialization may also be seen in the observation that the habitats of extant Triculinae in Thailand tend to lie in inaccessible or international border areas where development has been limited. The apparent restriction of the *S. sinensium*-like taxon of Northwest Thailand to a single stream running close to the Thai–Burmese border may be explained in this manner. The Thai schistosome may in fact be widely distributed in northern Burma; however, the Burmese fauna has yet to be examined. If the Mekong river once shared a channel with the Mae Klong (see Figure 5), Ping and Passac rivers, one may expect to find Triculinae (and even *Schistosoma*) in the headwaters of these rivers, that is, throughout eastern and northern Thailand. It is not clear whether the failure to find more species of schistosomes and/or Triculinae in these regions is due to habitat destruction or a paucity of surveys. Reports made between 1964 and 1973 of human

---

Figure 16 Semi-schematic illustrating two possible scenarios for the radiation of *Schistosoma* across China and Southeast Asia. A. Isochronous colonization by ancestors of Yangtze taxa (*S. sinensium/S. japonicum* and Pomatiopsidae) and Mekong taxa (*Schistosoma* n. sp., *S. mekongi/malayensis* and Triculinae) during the Pliocene. The type locality of *Schistosoma* n. sp. is shown by a black triangle. Prehistoric river courses are denoted by broken lines. B. Heterochronous colonization during the Cretaceous and late Tertiary. The ancestor of *Schistosoma* n. sp. (and other Mekong taxa) enters Southeast Asia, from Burma, after the Indian Plate collides with Asia, having arisen in India from *S. indicum*-like taxa able to utilize triculine snails. The Mekong taxa thus colonize Southeast Asia during the Pliocene much later than the ancestors of the Yangtze taxa, which colonize southern China after rafting northwards on one of the Cimmerian terranes accreted during the Cretaceous. Scale and palaeogeographical features approximate.

schistosomiasis in Pitsanalouke of northern Thailand (close to the Ping river) must be reinvestigated, particularly as the intermediate host and species of *Schistosoma* are unknown (Harinasuta, 1984). Faunal remnants of a prehistoric river in Vietnam (as mentioned above) may be expected to persist in the Dong Ngai river of southern Vietnam and the drainages of the mountains of southeastern Cambodia (see Figure 5). The finding of Triculinae in the drainages of the eastern slopes of the Annam chain in Vietnam would be significant, as the faunas of this region are otherwise expected to show affinity with those of East Asia rather than Southeast Asia (Banarescu, 1972). Consequently, a search for *Neotricula* in the rivers of central and southern Vietnam, the drainages of the mountains of Southeast Cambodia, and the Dong Ngai river system would be informative. The Red river itself has yet to be surveyed thoroughly for *Schistosoma* and Pomatiopsidae.

8.3. Relationships among Taxa

The main points in the revision of Davis (1979, 1980, 1992) and the phylogeographical model for Southeast Asian *Schistosoma* may be summarized as follows. The time of divergence between pre-*S. japonicum* and pre-*S. mekongi* may be 100 million years ago or as little as 2 million years ago, depending on whether one adopts a Tibetan or Burmese origin for *S. japonicum*. *S. mekongi* and *S. malayensis* appear to have diverged as recently as the Pleistocene (1.6 million to 10 000 years ago), rather than the 5 million years or so that would be expected for a Salween to Pahang river route of colonization. In addition, the time of divergence between Thai *Schistosoma* n. sp. and *S. mekongi* is probably around 1·5 million years ago, not the 7–12 million years ago implied if the former were a relic of the colonization of southern China. The divergence between Pomatiopsinae (e.g., *Oncomelania*) and Triculinae (e.g., *Neotricula*) may similarly be considered as an early Pliocene event associated with the Irrawaddy river. As both *Neotricula* and *Tricula* are found in the Ping river valley *and* the lower Mekong river, their divergence must have taken place before the late Pliocene (>1·5 million years ago), with the *N. aperta* complex diverging in the Pleistocene (<1 million years ago).

A number of testable predictions concerning relationships arise from the above model. It is likely that *N. aperta* is more closely related to *N. burchi* than its other congeners. Phylogeography suggests that Thai *Tricula* will be more closely related to *N. aperta* and *N. burchi* than other *Tricula* from Hunan, Shanxi and Yunnan, China. It would be useful to know if Thai *Tricula* show an affinity with Mekong river *Tricula* from Yunnan (e.g., *T. gregoriana*, *T. hudiequanensis*, *T. xianfengensis*) relative to Hunanese *Tricula* (e.g., *T. gredleri*, *T. maxidens*, *T. odonta*), which are part of the extensive radiation of Triculini in the Yangtze. As scenario one suggests an independent origin for Chinese and Thai/Lao *Neotricula* within the last 2 million years, it may be important to assess the congeneric status of these taxa (currently based on anatomical characters) using molecular genetic techniques. Interestingly, *N. aperta* is conserved relative to *Neotricula* spp. of the mid-Yangtze river (Davis *et al.*, 1992). The status of *Tricula* from Yunnan, described as *T. bollingi* (see Davis *et al.*, 1992), must also be evaluated using DNA sequence data in order to rule out possible convergence and clarify the role of the Mekong river in colonization of mainland Southeast Asia by *Schistosoma*. The question of *Robertsiella* remains; this snail was probably present in peninsular Malaysia well before the introduction of pre-*S. malayensis*, as *Robertsiella* is highly derived anatomically relative to *Neotricula* (see Davis *et al.*, 1992). If these ideas are correct then the transmission of *S. malayensis* represents a recent change of intermediate host, perhaps to a snail better suited to the predominant habitats of the new region colonized (i.e. the flooded forests and woodland streams of West Malaysia). Molecular data will help clarify the phylogeography of *Robertsiella*, and DNA sequence data already collected for *S. malayensis* indicate that it is indeed most closely related to *S. mekongi* (see Blair *et al.*, 1997).

The revised model suggests that the closest relative to *S. mekongi*, aside from *S. malayensis*, would be the Thai schistosome described as *S. sinensium* by Greer *et al.* (1989); however, the conspicuous lateral spine on the egg of the latter led Baidikul *et al.* (1984) to regard this taxon as intermediate between the *S. indicum* and *S. japonicum* groups (see Rollinson and Southgate, 1987). In contrast, the present author recently isolated an apparently new *Schistosoma* species from *T. bollingi* in Chiang Mai Province, Northwest Thailand (see Figure 1, and see Section 8.1.2), and the egg of this taxon has a minute hook-shaped lateral spine; this egg is similar to that of *S. mekongi* in size but more ovate in outline (Figure 17). *Schistosoma* n. sp. differs from that described by Greer *et al.* (1989), also from the same stream in Chiang Mai Province, in several respects. The female worm is wider, the ventral sucker is larger in both sexes, the preacetabular distance is greater, reunion of the gut caeca is in a more anterior position, the testes and ovary are shaped differently, and the number of eggs found *in utero* is much greater than that reported by Greer and his co-workers. As the worms and eggs described by Greer *et al.* were recovered from field-trapped rodents, it is possible that these worms were not transmitted by *T. bollingi*. Baidikul *et al.* (1984) also provide photographs of eggs from naturally infected rodents. The egg photographed from a laboratory mouse by these authors does resemble *S. sinensium s.s*; however, this egg was from a laboratory infection based on Chinese material. A common schistosome infecting rodents in Thailand, and which also produces an egg bearing a subterminal spine, is *Schistosoma incognitum* Chandler, 1926, and possible intermediate hosts (*Lymnaea* or *Radix* spp.) were found in the stream in Chiang Mai. It is, however, unlikely that Greer *et al.* (1989) would have

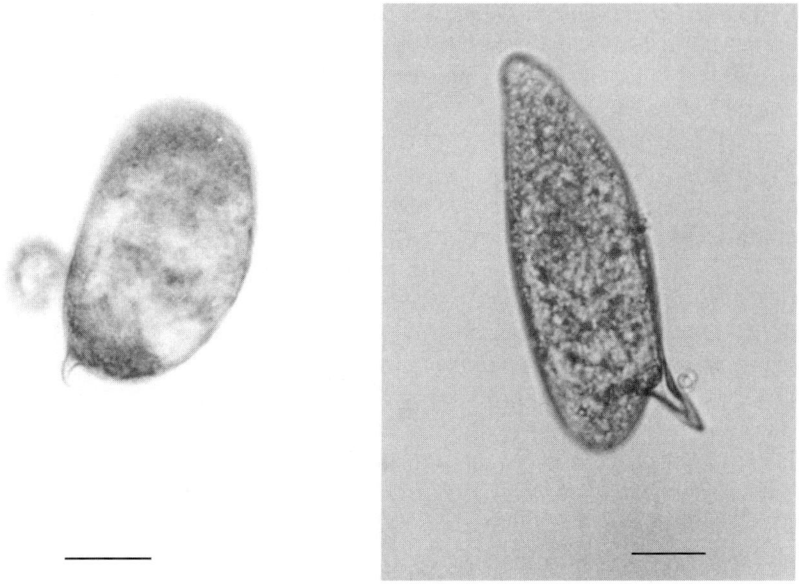

Figure 17 The egg of *Schistosoma* n. sp., Chiang Mai (Thailand), left, and *S. sinensium*, from Sichuan, right. Scale bar 20 μm.

overlooked the differences between these taxa. One explanation might be that two species of *Schistosoma* are transmitted by *T. bollingi* at one site, and that each research group found only one of these species. The new Thai schistosome, which was sampled and cultured from naturally infected *T. bollingi*, also differs from *S. sinensium* of Sichuan as described by Bao (1958). The male of the Chiang Mai taxon is larger in terms of both length and width but is a more slender worm (relative to its body length). The female is also larger but is a relatively less slender worm. The postacetabular constriction is less pronounced in both sexes and, in keeping with the Thai worm being larger overall, the diameter of the oral and ventral sucker is greater. The testes are larger and number 6 or 7 (rather than 8 or 9 as in *S. sinensium*). The vitellaria occupy a lesser proportion of the posterior fraction of the female worm; that is, the vitellaria are proportionally shorter in terms of body length. The ovary is larger and the number of eggs found *in utero* much greater. Consequently, it is likely that the Thai schistosome is a species distinct from *S. sinensium s.s.* of Sichuan; indeed the two parasites have been separated for at least 5 million years. Both taxa are transmitted by species of *Tricula*; however, the snail in Sichuan is an unknown species and is not *T. bollingi*. The present author has submitted a paper describing *Schistosoma* n. sp. from Northwest Thailand

Table 1 Biogeographical indicators and the phylogeography of Southeast Asian *Schistosoma*. The term 'taxa' here refers to *Schistosoma* and/or Triculinae.

Observation	Palaeogeographical feature indicated
Taxa in lower Salween/Irrawaddy river system of Burma	Salween–Mekong/Ping river colonization route opened into Thailand
Taxa in Mekong/Chao Phrya headwaters	Pre-Mekong flowed through Chao Phrya river valley during Pliocene
Taxa in drainage of Cardamon mountains in Cambodia	Pre-Mekong flowed into Gulf of Thailand at Kampot carrying taxa
Taxa in Red river	Red river fault acted as colonization route into Indochina
Taxa in Dong Ngai river headwaters and SE Cambodian highlands	Prehistoric river carried taxa south along eastern seaboard of Indochina
Lower Irrawaddy palaeolakes contain fossil Triculinae but not Pomatiopsinae	Pre-*Oncomelania* isolated from pre-*Tricula* during the Pliocene
Palaeolakes[a] associated with modern Ping and Salween valley contain fossil Triculinae	Taxa may have entered Thailand via extended Salween, along the Mekong/Ping river in the early Pleistocene

[a] Quaternary tilting of sedimentary basins along the Thai–Burma border, and fossil lacustrine molluscs, suggest the extinction of many lakes lying between the Salween, Chao Phrya and Mekong rivers (Gibling and Ratanasthien, 1980; Hutchinson, 1989).

(see Figure 18). *S. sinensium s.s.* is found in association with the Yangtze river drainage and the isolating mechanism that allowed *S. japonicum* to diverge from precursors of *S. sinensium* (or vice versa) is unclear, as both parasites are transmitted in similar habitats (irrigation channels and ditches around rice paddies or kitchen gardens). It is possible that the pomatiopsine intermediate host utilized by *S. japonicum* is not available to *S. sinensium* (see Section 8.5). Other testable predictions arise from the revised phylogeographical model and these are summarized in Table 1. The importance of data on the nature of the hydrobioid snail fauna and *Schistosoma* of the Burmese mountains to our understanding of schistosome phylogeography is apparent from the table, unfortunately such data are as yet unavailable.

8.4. An Asian Origin for *Schistosoma*?

A more fundamental challenge to the traditional view regarding the origin of *Schistosoma* has recently been made. Snyder and Loker (2000) used DNA sequences from the 28S rRNA gene for 10 of the 13 genera of Schistosomatidae to infer an Asian origin for *Schistosoma*; their study included *S. japonicum, S. mansoni* and *S. haematobium* but no other *Schistosoma* spp. The outgroup taxa comprised one member of each of the Sanguinicolidae and the Spirorchiidae (Platyhelminthes: Digenea), these taxa being considered representative of antecedent Schistosomatidae (the latter being a sister group to the Spirorchiidae; Brooks *et al.*, 1985). Phylogenies based on maximum likelihood and maximum parsimony analyses were congruent and indicated two major clades. The first clade comprised mostly avian schistosomes (e.g., *Dendritobilharzia, Gigantobilharzia, Ornithobilharzia*) but also involved the mammalian parasites *Heterobilharzia* and *Schistosomatium*, although the node joining this latter pair to rest of the avian clade was weak. The second clade comprised mammalian schistosomes only, namely *Schistosoma* and *Orientobilharzia*. The two basal groups in the mammalian clade were *S. japonicum* and *Orientobilharzia turkestanicum*; as both have an Asian distribution the authors concluded that *Schistosoma* (including *Orientobilharzia*) may have arisen in Asia rather than in Gondwana as previously thought (Davis, 1979, 1980).

The case for an Asian origin of *Schistosoma* deserves serious consideration and additional evidence for this is likely to accumulate over the next few years. Snyder and Loker (2000) support their case by pointing out that *Biomphalaria* did not occur in Africa before 1 million years ago, which implies that *S. mansoni* could not have existed before then. Further, Barker & Blair (1996) provided evidence that the *S. indicum* group may have arisen from African *Schistosoma*, with the colonization of Asia via domestic livestock brought from Africa by early humans. Snyder and Loker (2000) propose that descendants of the Asian schistosome lineage moved from Asia to Africa about 1 million years ago, where they underwent an extensive radiation and became exclusive parasites of Planorbidae (Pulmonata). The marked differences in mitochondrial DNA sequence order between *S. haematobium* and a cluster including *S. japonicum* and species of *Echinococcus*, *Fasciola* and *Taenia*, observed by Le *et al.* (2000a), also appear to agree with an Asian origin. The lesser interstrain variation in *S. mansoni*, when compared with *S. japonicum* (Section 5.2), may be the result of a recent colonization event. *Schistosoma* is considered to have reinvaded Asia in the Holocene. Snyder and Loker's proposal involves the origin of *Schistosoma* in prosobranchs (Caenogastropoda) or pulmonates of the mid-Miocene, presumably on the Indian Plate. The discussions in Section 8.1 suggest that had *Schistosoma* arisen in Cathaysian Asia (see Figure 12), the nascent taxa would have been bounded by high mountains, volcanism in the west and cold arid conditions to the north. In view of the incongruence between the hypothesis of an Asian origin and phylogeographical data, alternative scenarios must be considered.

Current models suggest that there was no single collision between the Gondwanan terranes and the Asian mainland. Many fragments separated from

Gondwana and amalgamated in Southeast Asia over a considerable period of time. For example, the Tanggula Block collided 200 million years ago and the Lhasa Block some 140 million years ago (Hall, 1998). Such repeated collisions would have permitted multiple introductions of faunas, fractionated any diverging populations on the Cimmerian terranes (see Figure 13), and initiated episodes of volcanism (from around 50 million years ago) as well as other barriers to later colonization (Xiao & Gao, 1984; Xu *et al.*, 1985). The result is to confound phylogeographies and to permit the introduction of pre-*Schistosoma* to mainland Asia at any time over the last 100 million years. In addition, if the less well-supported nodes are discounted, it appears that the phylogeny of Snyder and Loker (2000) reflects the definitive hosts (and to a lesser degree snails) involved in transmission of the schistosomes. In such instances it is important to be able to recognize, and discount, ecological factors from the effects of history and geography. In the case of *Schistosoma*, ecological considerations involve the nature of the host occupied, which is an aspect of habitat choice by the parasite. At present we lack sufficient data to enable clarification of the routes and times of the colonization events proposed by Snyder and Loker, which must agree well with both the implied palaeogeography and the radiation of the intermediate hosts. If a second colonization of Asia did occur it appears that it involved only members of the *S. indicum* group, as the biogeographical deployment of this group, alone, fails to reflect the evolution of river systems in the region and probably results from recent colonization events associated with human activity. It is now well accepted that the colonization of Southeast Asia by members of the *S. japonicum* group is linked with the opening of lotic habitats (Davis, 1982). Interestingly, several groups of cyprinid fish, which have ecological requirements close to those of triculine snails, show a similar distribution among the Mekong, Pahang and Ping river systems. This distribution is thought to reflect colonization via northern Burma in the Pliocene (Rainboth, 1991). No member of the *S. indicum* group was included in the above study; however, the importance of these taxa in resolving the origins of *Schistosoma* has been stated (Snyder *et al.*, 2001).

8.5. The *Schistosoma mekongi* Clade

Schistosoma sinensium of Sichuan Province, China, is crucial to our understanding of the origins of human schistosomiasis in Southeast Asia. Under either of the above scenarios, the ancestral form of *Schistosoma* that existed in northern Burma, Tibet and Yunnan during the Pliocene may well have resembled *S. sinensium* of Sichuan today. This ancestral schistosome could have entered China, off the Indian Plate, at the same time as ancestors of the Southeast Asian taxa or perhaps have dispersed much earlier off one of

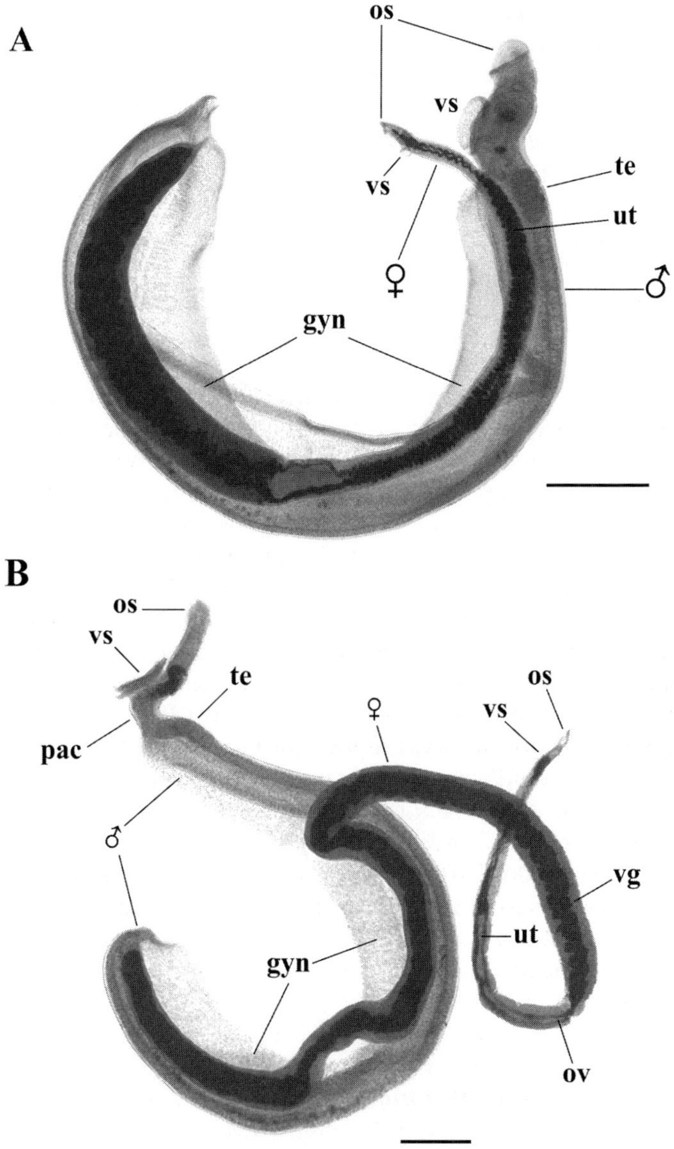

Figure 18 A. Adult *Schistosoma* n. sp. from Chiang Mai Province, Northwest Thailand; holotypes, male and female *in copula* (scale 200 μm). B. Adult *Schistosoma sinensium*, male and female *in copula*, from Mianzhu County, Sichuan Province, PR China (scale 500 μm). Abbreviations: gyn, gynaecophoric canal; os, oral sucker; ov, ovary; pac, postacetabular constriction; te, testes; ut, uterus; vg, vitelline gland; vs, ventral sucker.

the Gondwanan fragments accreted earlier (scenario two). The status of the *S. sinensium*-like taxa has become more important following the report of Snyder and Loker (2000) suggesting that *Schistosoma* originated in Asia. Bao (1958) noted that *S. sinensium* was of particular interest as it possessed characters seemingly intermediate between those of members of the *S. indicum* group (e.g., a subterminal-spined egg and single egg *in utero*) and the *S. japonicum* group (e.g., a triculine intermediate host and an atuberculate tegument). Members of the *S. indicum* group are widespread throughout India and those found in Southeast Asia (*S. incognitum* and *S. spindale*) are thought to have dispersed from India during the Holocene, probably as a result of human seafaring. As current hypotheses suggest an Indian origin for the *S. japonicum* group, with dispersal via the Brahmaputra and northern Burma, taxa such as *S. sinensium*, with characters of both groups, may best represent the ancestral form of *Schistosoma* that colonized southern China and Southeast Asia during the late Tertiary. The present host of *S. sinensium* is triculine, and this is the case for all but one member of the *S. japonicum* group. Indeed, *Schistosoma* may have colonized southern China and Southeast Asia in a snail of the Triculinae. The later colonization of the Yangtze Basin by Pomatiopsidae may have facilitated the divergence of *S. japonicum* from *S. sinensium*-like stock, with subsequent colonization of the mid-Yangtze plain by the former in oncomelanid snails. The extant Triculinae appear well adapted to mountain streams and minor rivers and, as such, represent a better vehicle than the Pomatiopsinae for the colonization of northern Burma, Laos and Thailand. The lack of involvement of pulmonate snails in the transmission of *S. japonicum*-group parasites (and their utilization in India and elsewhere) may be similarly explained. Once southern China had been colonized, the ecological situation would have been reversed and the amphibious *Oncomelania* (Pomatiopsinae) was clearly better adapted to the less fluviatile and more ephemeral habitats of the wetlands and canals of the middle Yangtze river system. Transmission of *S. sinensium* in Sichuan occurs in small streams draining the eastern margin of the Tibetan mountains and involves a species of *Tricula*; this would be expected given an origin for this clade in northern India and Burma. The definitive hosts of *S. sinensium* are bandicoots and other rodents. Humans would have become available to Asian *Schistosoma* once the lower rivers had been colonized. Human settlements are sparse in the highlands of Tibet and Sichuan but common around the habitats of *Oncomelania* and *N. aperta* in the south of China and Laos, respectively. Similarly, the invasion of human hosts by pre-*S. mekongi* may have led to its divergence from the highland taxon *Schistosoma* n. sp. found today in Northwest Thailand. In view of the above arguments we would expect *S. sinensium* to be basal to a clade leading to both *S. mekongi* and *S. japonicum*.

If *Schistosoma* originated or diverged extensively in India (Davis 1979) one would expect the *S. indicum* group to be polyphyletic, as either all ancestral forms in India are now extinct or some of these taxa are represented by members of the *S. indicum* group. *Schistosoma sinensium* of Sichuan would be expected to show an affinity with these Indian ('ancestral') taxa, whilst *Schistosoma* n. sp. of northern Thailand would show a closer relationship with taxa such as *S. mekongi*. It is hoped that study of these schistosomes will shed light on the factors involved in the evolution of human parasitism, and work on *S. sinensium* is currently underway in this laboratory. It is also expected that the findings will help decide between alternative hypotheses for the origin and dispersal of the Asian schistosomes. A number of interesting reports have been published which appear to support Snyder and Loker's view of an Asian origin for *Schistosoma*. For example, Southgate and Agrawal (1990) reported transmission of an *S. haematobium*-like schistosome by an ancylid (pulmonate) snail in India. More recently, Sherchand *et al.* (1999) reported the observation of *S. mansoni*-like eggs in the stools of villagers in southern Nepal. Subsequent ELISA tests for *S. mansoni* antibodies revealed a peak seroprevalence of nearly 43% in one of the villages sampled. However, the observation of a lateral-spined egg does not rule against an affinity with *S. sinensium*-like schistosomes and the eggs may have originated in infected rodents eaten by the villagers (V.R. Southgate, personal communication). The rodent schistosome *S. incognitum* also has an egg morphology similar to that of the eggs found by Sherchand and his co-workers.

9. CONCLUSIONS

We are now entering an exciting period in which population genetics, phylogeography and ecology are being combined in the study and control of Mekong schistosomiasis. Research over the past 20 years has been hampered by problems regarding access to field sites, and the patchy distributions of key taxa have made samples difficult to collect. Recent improvements in security and infrastructure in Cambodia and Laos will no doubt lead to a resurgence of interest in this problem. It is, however, unlikely that the culture of triculine snails in the laboratory will ever become a practical option. Much more data will soon become available for population genetic studies of both snails and schistosomes, and this will enable the evaluation of alternative hypotheses on the origin and Cenozoic dispersal of Southeast Asian *Schistosoma*. Unfortunately, past molecular systematic studies of the Asian schistosomes have involved samples from laboratory lines of various ages and degrees of reliability. It is hoped that many key populations, such as those of *S. mekongi* in southern Laos and *S. malayensis* in Malaysia, will be resampled and new DNA sequence data collected. A well-founded phylogeographical hypothesis is required for the group if we wish to predict the occurrence of *Schistosoma* in unsurveyed or inaccessible areas. In countries such as Thailand, where the problem is the exclusion (rather than control) of schistosomiasis, an ability to predict the distribution of *Schistosoma* in the rivers draining across border areas from Laos or Cambodia is vital.

The long-term control of human schistosomiasis in Laos and Cambodia will depend on combined chemotherapy, education and snail control. As it is now becoming apparent that conditions in the minor rivers of highland Laos (and possibly Vietnam) may better favour the growth of *N. aperta* populations than the Mekong river itself, any programme of snail control must include populations in these tributaries. Molecular ecological studies will be necessary to determine demographic parameters (including life cycles), migration rates and population stability wherever *N. aperta* is found. Such studies will enable the synchronization of molluscicide applications so as to prevent extensive recolonization of vacant habitats in endemic areas, and to limit the impact on non-target species.

Further work is required to elucidate fully the origin of Southeast Asian *Schistosoma* and to explain the present zoogeography of *S. mekongi*; the relative roles of history (vicariance) and ecology must be determined. The established view of a late Miocene divergence of the *S. japonicum* group (Davis, 1979, 1980) and an origin in Yunnan, China, must be tested against that of a Pliocene origin in the Irrawaddy drainage of Burma. The assessment of the two models will require a more refined palaeogeography and extensive sequence comparisons for various schistosome and snail taxa. Similarly, an understanding of the enigmatic *Schistosoma sinensium* in China will reveal important information regarding the characteristics of ancestral *Schistosoma*, useful in establishing polarity in the phylogeography of the group, and perhaps also the factors involved in the switch from animal to human hosts. The opportunities for investigation into Mekong schistosomiasis are diverse and the subject will benefit greatly from interdisciplinary research. Much progress will no doubt be made as advanced technologies become available in endemic countries and new approaches are adopted. It is hoped that the next 10 years will see the complete control of Mekong schistosomiasis in the human population and a solution to current biodiversity conservation problems in the region.

ACKNOWLEDGEMENTS

Dr L. Chitsulo, World Health Organization, and Dr P. Odermatt, Médecins Sans Frontières (Cambodia), for information on current schistosomiasis control activities. Dr D.A. Johnston, Natural History Museum, London, for suggestions regarding Figure 9. Dr W. Thammavit, Mahidol University, Bangkok, for loan of the photomicroscope. This work was supported by Wellcome Trust Project Grant number 058932.

REFERENCES

Allen, C.R., Gillespie, A.R., Yuan, H., Sieh, K.E., Buchun, Z. and Chengnan, Z. (1984). Red river and associated faults Yunnan Province, China: Quaternary geology, slip rates and seismic hazard. *Bulletin of the Geological Society of America* **95**, 686–700.

Attwood, S.W. (1994). Rates of recruitment among populations of the freshwater snail *Neotricula aperta* (Temcharoen) in North East Thailand. *Journal of Molluscan Studies* **60**, 197–200.

Attwood, S.W. (1995a). Uptake of acetate by *Neotricula aperta* (Gastropoda: Pomatiopsidae), the snail host of *Schistosoma mekongi* in the lower Mekong basin. *Journal of Molluscan Studies* **61**, 109–125.

Attwood, S.W. (1995b). A demographic analysis of *y-Neotricula aperta* (Gastropoda: Pomatiopsidae) populations in Thailand and southern Laos, in relation to the transmission of schistosomiasis. *Journal of Molluscan Studies* **61**, 29–42.

Attwood, S.W. (1996a). The impact of grazing by *Neotricula aperta* (Gastropoda: Pomatiopsidae) on post-spate recovery of the algal aufwuchs in the lower Mekong river: Changes in successional patterns and relative abundance of species. *Natural History Bulletin of the Siam Society* **44**, 61–74.

Attwood, S.W. (1996b). Changes in *Neotricula* β-*aperta* population density following construction of the Pak-Mul dam in Northeast Thailand, with implications for the transmission of schistosomiasis. *South East Asian Journal of Tropical Medicine and Public Health* **27**, 24–28.

Attwood, S.W. (1996c). The impact of grazing by *Neotricula aperta* (Gastropoda: Pomatiopsidae) on post-spate recovery of the algal aufwuchs in the lower Mekong river: Changes in standing crop and species diversity. *Natural History Bulletin of the Siam Society* **43**, 171–197.

Attwood, S.W. (1999). Genetic variation in *Neotricula aperta*, the snail intermediate host of *Schistosoma mekongi* in the lower Mekong basin. *Journal of Zoology* **249**, 153–164.

Attwood, S.W. (2001). The radular cusp formulae of *Neotricula aperta* (Gastropoda: Pomatiopsidae): taxonomic questions. *Journal of Natural History* **35**, 175–183.

Attwood, S.W. and Johnston, D.A. (2001). Nucleotide sequence differences reveal genetic variation in *Neotricula aperta* (Gastropoda: Pomatiopsidae), the snail host of schistosomiasis in the lower Mekong basin. *Bio. J. Linn. Soc* **73**, 23–41.

Attwood, S.W. and Upatham, E.S. (1999). A new strain of *Neotricula aperta* found in Khammouanne Province, central Laos, and its compatibility with *Schistosoma mekongi*. *Journal of Molluscan Studies* **65**, 371–374.

Attwood, S.W., Kitikoon, V. and Southgate, V.R. (1997). Infectivity of a Cambodian isolate of *Schistosoma mekongi* to *Neotricula aperta* from Northeast Thailand. *Journal of Helminthology* **71**, 183–187.

Attwood, S.W., Kitikoon, V. and Southgate, V.R. (1998). *Neotricula aperta* (Gastropoda: Pomatiopsidae) the intermediate hosts of human *Schistosoma mekongi*: Allozyme variation and relationships between Khmer, Lao and Thai populations. *Journal of Zoology* **246**, 309–324.

Attwood, S.W., Upatham, E.S. and Southgate, V.R. (2001). The detection of *Schistosoma mekongi* infections in a natural population of *Neotricula aperta* at Khong Island,

Laos, and the control of Mekong schistosomiasis. *Journal of Molluscan Studies* **67**, 404–409.

Audebaud, G., Tournier-Lasserve, C., Brumpt, V., Jolly, M., Mazaud, R., Imbert, X. and Bazillo, R. (1968). Première cas de bilharziose humaine observé au Cambodge (région de Kracheh). *Bulletin Société Pathologie Exotique* **5**, 778–784.

Baidikul, V., Upatham, E.S., Kruatrachue, M., Viyanant, V., Vichasri, S., Lee, P. and Chantanawat, R. (1984). Study on *Schistosoma sinensium* in Fang District, Chiangmai Province, Thailand. *South East Asian Journal of Tropical Medicine and Public Health* **15**, 141–147.

Banarescu, P. (1972). The zoogeographical position of the East Asian freshwater fish fauna. *Revue Roumaine de Biologie Série Zoologique* **17**, 315–323.

Bao, D.C. (1958). [Report on the discovery of a new species of schistosome in China (*Schistosoma sinensium sp. nov.* Schistosomatidae)]. *Chinese Medical Journal* **77**, 607–675 (in Chinese).

Barbier, M. (1966). Détermination d'un foyer de bilharziose artério-veineuse au Sud-Laos (Province de Sithandone). *Bulletin Société Pathologie Exotique* **6**, 974–981.

Barker, S.C. and Blair, D. (1996). Molecular phylogeny of *Schistosoma* species supports traditional groupings within the genus. *Journal of Parasitology* **82**, 292–298.

Biays, S., Stich, A.H.R., Odermatt, P., Long, C., Yersin, C., Men, C., Saem, C. and Lormand, J.-D. (1999). Foyer de bilharziose à *Schistosoma mekongi* redécouvert au Nord du Cambodge: I. Perception culturelle de la maladie; description et suivi de 20 cas cliniques graves. *Tropical Medicine and International Health* **4**, 662–673.

Blair, D., van Herwerden, L., Hirai, H., Taguchi, T., Habe, S., Hirata, M., Lai, K., Upatham, E.S. and Agatsuma, T. (1997). Relationships between *Schistosoma malayensis* and other Asian schistosomes deduced from DNA sequences. *Molecular and Biochemical Parasitology* **85**, 259–263.

Bøgh, H.O., Zhu, X.Q., Qian, B.Z. and Gasser, R.B. (1999). Scanning for nucleotide variations in mitochondrial DNA fragments of *Schistosoma japonicum* by single-strand conformation polymorphism. *Parasitology* **118**, 73–82.

Bowles, J., Hope, M., Tiu, W.U., Liu, X. and McManus, D.P. (1993). Nuclear and mitochondrial genetic markers highly conserved between Chinese and Philippine *Schistosoma japonicum*. *Acta Tropica* **55**, 217–229.

Brandt, R.A.M. (1968). Descriptions of new non-marine mollusks from Asia. *Archiv für Molluskenkunde* **98**, 213–289.

Brandt, R.A.M. (1970). New freshwater gastropods from the Mekong. *Archiv für Molluskenkunde* **100**, 183–205.

Brooks, D.R., O'Grady, R.T. and Glen, D.R. (1985). Phylogenetic analysis of the Digenea (Platyhelminthes: Cercomeria) with comments on their adaptive radiation. *Canadian Journal of Zoology* **63**, 411–443.

Bruce, J.I. and Schneider, C.R. (1976). Studies on schistosomiasis in the lower Mekong basin: the aquatic ecology and molluscicide sensitivity of *Lithoglyphopsis aperta*. In: *Final Report to the Committee for the Coordination of Investigations in the Lower Mekong Basin*, pp. 9–92. Bangkok: Mekong Secretariat.

Bruce, J.I., Sornmani, S., Asch, H.L. and Crawford, K.A. (eds) (1980). The Mekong schistosome. *Malacological Review*, supplement 2.

Bunopas, S. and Vella, P. (1983). Tectonic and geologic evolution of Thailand. In: *Proceedings of a Workshop on Stratigraphic Correlation of Thailand and Malaysia*. Vol. 1, pp. 307–322. Kuala Lumpur: Geological Society of Thailand, Bangkok/Geological Society of Malaysia.

Byram, J.E. and Von Lichtenberg, F. (1980). Experimental infection with *Schistosoma mekongi* in laboratory animals: parasitological and pathological findings. In: The

Mekong schistosome (J.I. Bruce, S. Sornmani, H.L. Asch and K.A. Crawford, eds), pp. 125–159. *Malacological Review*, supplement 2.

Chandler, A.C. (1926). A new schistosome infection in man, with notes on other human fluke infections in India. *Indian Journal of Medical Research* **14**, 179–183.

Chernin, E. and Antolics, V.M. (1975). Penetrative capacity of *Schistosoma mansoni* miracidia. *Journal of Parasitology* **63**, 560–561.

Chernin, E. and Dunavan, C.A. (1962). The influence of host–parasite dispersion upon the capacity of *Schistosoma mansoni* miracidia to infect *Australorbis glabratus*. *American Journal of Tropical Medicine and Hygiene* **11**, 455–471.

Cross, J.H. (1976). *Schistosomiasis japonica* in China: A brief review. *South East Asian Journal of Tropical Medicine and Public Health* **7**, 167–170.

Cuesta, R.A., Kaw, Y.T. and Duwaji, M.S. (1992). *Schistosoma mekongi* infection in a leiomyosarcoma of the small bowel: a case report. *Human Pathology* **23**, 471–473.

Davis, G.M. (1968). New *Tricula* from Thailand. *Archiv für Molluskenkunde* **98**, 291–317.

Davis, G.M. (1979). The origin and evolution of the gastropod family Pomatiopsidae, with emphasis on the Mekong river Triculinae. *Academy of Natural Sciences of Philadelphia, Monograph* **20**, 1–120.

Davis, G.M. (1980). Snail hosts of Asian *Schistosoma* infecting man: evolution and coevolution. In: The Mekong schistosome (J.I. Bruce, S. Sornmani, H.L. Asch and K.A. Crawford, eds), pp. 195–238. *Malacological Review*, supplement 2.

Davis, G.M. (1981). Different modes of evolution and adaptive radiation in the Pomatiopsidae (Prosobranchia: Mesogastropoda). *Malacologia* **21**, 209–262.

Davis, G.M. (1982). Historical and ecological factors in the evolution, adaptive radiation, and biogeography of freshwater molluscs. *American Zoology* **22**, 375–395.

Davis, G.M. (1992). Evolution of prosobranch snails transmitting Asian *Schistosoma*; coevolution with *Schistosoma*: a review. *Progress in Clinical Parasitology* **3**, 145–204.

Davis, G.M. and Greer, G.J. (1980). A new genus and two new species of Triculinae (Gastropoda: Prosobranchia) and the transmission of a Malaysian Mammalian *Schistosoma* sp. *Proceedings of the Academy of Natural Sciences of Philadelphia* **132**, 245–276.

Davis, G.M., Kitikoon, V. and Temcharoen, P. (1976). Monograph on '*Lithoglyphopsis*' *aperta*, the snail host of Mekong river schistosomiasis. *Malacologia* **15**, 241–287.

Davis, G.M., Kuo, Y.-H., Hoagland, K.E., Chen, P.-L., Yang, H.-M. and Chen, D.-J. (1985). *Erhaia*, a new genus and new species of Pomatiopsidae from China (Gastropoda: Rissoacea). *Proceedings of the Academy of Natural Sciences of Philadelphia* **137**, 48–78.

Davis, G.M., Subba Rao, N.V. and Hoagland, K.E. (1986). In search of *Tricula* (Gastropoda: Pomatiopsidae): *Tricula* defined, and a new genus described. *Proceedings of the Academy of Natural Sciences of Philadelphia* **138**, 426–442.

Davis, G.M., Chen, C.-E., Wu, C., Kuang, T.-F., Xing, X.-G., Li, L., Liu, W.-J. and Yan, Y.-L. (1992). The Pomatiopsidae of Hunan, China (Gastropoda: Rissoacea). *Malacologia* **34**, 143–342.

Davis, G.M., Chen, C.-E., Zeng, X.P., Yu, S.H. and Li, L. (1994). Molecular genetic and anatomical relationships among pomatiopsid (Gastropoda: Prosobranchia) genera from southern China. *Proceedings of the Academy of Natural Sciences of Philadelphia* **145**, 191–207.

Dupont, V.B.E., Soubrane, J., Halle, B. and Richir, C. (1957). Bilharziose à forme hépato-splénique révélée par une grande hématémèse. *Bulletin Mémoires de la Société Médicale.Hôpitaux Paris* **73**, 933–994.

Fletcher, M., Woodruff, D.S. and Lo Verde, P.T. (1980). Genetic differentiation between *Schistosoma mekongi* and *S. japonicum*: an electrophoretic study. In: The Mekong schistosome (J.I. Bruce, S. Sornmani, H.L. Asch and K.A. Crawford, eds), pp. 113–122. *Malacological Review*, supplement 2.

Fletcher, M., Lo Verde, P.T. and Woodruff, D.S. (1981). Genetic variation in *Schistosoma mansoni*: enzyme polymorphisms in populations from Africa, Southwest Asia, South America and the West Indies. *American Journal of Tropical Medicine and Hygiene* **30**, 406–421.

Gang, C.M. (1991). *Mission Report: Schistosomiasis Control Programme in Khong District*. Geneva: WHO/ICP/PDP/004.

Gibling, M. and Ratanasthien, B. (1980). Cenozoic basins of Thailand and their coal deposits: A preliminary report. *Bulletin of the Geological Society of Malaya* **13**, 27–42.

Gobert, G.N., Stenzel, D.J., Jones, M.K., Allen, D.E. and McManus, D.P. (1997). *Schistosoma japonicum*: paramyosin immunolocalisation during parasite development. *Parasitology* **114**, 45–52.

Gordon, R. (1882). The Irrawaddy and the Snapo. *Proceedings of the Royal Geographical Society* **9**, 559–563.

Goubert, L., Ly, C.S., Bunchan, K., Bitar, D., van der Velden, T., Lormand, J.-D., Biays, S. and Goemaere, E. (1994). Foyer de *Schistosoma mekongi* dans la Province de Kracheh, Cambodge du nord. *Médecins Sans Frontières Medical News* **3**, 15–19.

Gredler, P.V. (1881). Zur concylien-fauna von China. *Jahrbücher der Deutschen Malakozoologischen Gelleschaft* **8**, 119–132.

Greer, G.J., Ow-Yang, C.K. and Yong, H.S. (1988). *Schistosoma malayensis* n. sp.: a *Schistosoma japonicum*-complex schistosome from peninsular Malaysia. *Journal of Parasitology* **74**, 471–480.

Greer, G.J., Kitikoon, V. and Lohachit, C. (1989). Morphology and life cycle of *Schistosoma sinensium* Pao, 1959, from Northwest Thailand. *Journal of Parasitology* **75**, 98–101.

Gregory, J.W. (1925). The evolution of the river system of southeastern Asia. *Scottish Geographical Magazine* **41**, 129–141.

Guo, Y.H. and Gu, J.R. (1985). Studies on the intermediate host of *Schistosoma* and *Paragonimus*: 1. *Tricula jinhongensis*, a new species of *Tricula* from Yunnan Province (Gastropoda: Pomatiopsidae). *Acta Zootaxonomica Sinica* **10**, 250–252.

Hagan, P., Ndhlovu, P.D. and Dunne, D.W. (1998). Schistosome immunology: more questions than answers. *Parasitology Today* **14**, 407–412.

Hall, R. (1998). The plate tectonics of Cenozoic Asia and the distribution of land and sea. In: *Biogeography and Geological Evolution of SE Asia* (R. Hall and J.D. Holloway, eds), pp. 99–131. Leiden: Backbuys.

Hanski, I. (1994). A practical model of metapopulation dynamics. *Journal of Animal Ecology* **63**, 151–162.

Harinasuta, C. (1984). Epidemiology and control of schistosomiasis in Southeast Asia. *South East Asian Journal of Tropical Medicine and Public Health* **15**, 431–438.

Harinasuta, C. and Kruatrachue, M. (1962). The first recognised endemic area of bilharziasis in Thailand. *Annals of Tropical Medicine and Parasitology* **56**, 314–315.

Harinasuta, C., Sornmani, S., Kitikoon, V., Schneider, C.R. and Pathammavong, O. (1972). Infection of aquatic hydrobiid snails and animals with *Schistosoma japonicum*-like parasites from Khong Island, southern Laos. *Transactions of the Royal Society of Tropical Medicine and Hygiene* **66**, 184–185.

Harn, D.A., Mitsuyama, M., Huguenel, E.D., Oligino, L.D. and David, J.R. (1985). Identification by monoclonal antibody of a major (28 kDa) surface membrane antigen of *Schistosoma mansoni*. *Molecular Biochemistry and Parasitology* **16**, 345–354.

Hope, M. and McManus, D.P. (1994). Genetic variation in geographically isolated populations and subspecies of *Oncomelania hupensis* determined by a PCR-based RFLP method. *Acta Tropica* **57**, 75–82.

Huang, C.-Y., Liew, P.-M., Zhao, M., Chang, T.-C., Kuo, C.-M., Chen, M.-T., Wang, C.-H. and Zheng, L.-F. (1997). Deep sea and lake records of the Southeast Asian paleomonsoons for the last 25 thousand years. *Earth and Planetary Science Letters* **146**, 59–72.

Hutchinson, C.S. (1982). Southeast Asia. In: *The Ocean Basins and Margins: The Indian Ocean* (A.E.M. Nairn and F.G. Stehli, eds), Vol. 6, pp. 451–512. New York: Plenum Press.

Hutchinson, C.S. (1989). *Geological Evolution of South-east Asia*. Oxford: Clarendon Press.

Iijima, T. (1970). *Enquête sur la schistosomiase dans la bassin du Mékong: Cambodge. Rapport de Mission 13/11/68–08/05/69*. WPR/059/70. Genève: Organisation Mondiale de la Santé.

Iijima, T. and Garcia, E.G. (1967). *Preliminary Survey for Schistosomiasis in South Laos. WHO Assignment Report, WHO/BILH/67.64*. Geneva: World Health Organization.

Iijima, T., Lo, C.T. and Ito, Y. (1971). Studies on schistosomiasis in the Mekong basin. I. Morphological observation of the schistosomes and detection of their reservoir host. *Japanese Journal of Parasitology* **20**, 24–33.

Iijima, T., Garcia, E.G. and Lo, C.T. (1973). Studies on schistosomiasis in the Mekong Basin. III. Prevalence of *Schistosoma* infection among the inhabitants. *Japanese Journal of Parasitology* **22**, 338–341.

Jolly, M., Bazillo, R., Audebaud, G., Brumpt, V. and Sophinn, B. (1970a). Premières recherches épidémiologiques sur un foyer de bilharziose humaine au Cambodge, dans la région de Kratié. *Bulletin Société Pathologie Exotique* **63**, 476–479.

Jolly, M., Bazillo, R., Audebaud, G., Brumpt, V. and Sophinn, B. (1970b). Existence au Cambodge d'un foyer de bilharziose humaine, dans la région de Kratié II Enquête épidémiologique résultats préliminaires. *Medécin Tropicale* **30**, 462–471.

Jordan, P. and Webbe, G. (1969). *Human Schistosomiasis*. London: Heinemann.

Jourdane, J. and Théron, A. (1987). Larval development: eggs to cercariae. In: *The Biology of Schistosomes: From Genes to Latrines* (D. Rollinson and A.J.G. Simpson, eds), pp. 83–114. London: Academic Press.

Katsurada, F. (1904). *Schistosoma japonicum*, ein neuer menshlicher parasit durch welchen eine endemisch krankheit in verschiedenen genenden Japans verusacht wird. *Annotationes Zoologicae Japonenses* **5**, 147–160.

Katz, N., Chaves, A. and Pellegrino, J. (1972). A simple device for quantitative stool thick smears technique in schistosomiasis *mansoni*. *Revues do Instituto Medicale et Tropicale San Paulo* **14**, 397–400.

Kingman, J.F.C. (1982). On the genealogy of large populations. *Journal of Applied Probability* **19A**, 27–43.

Kitikoon, V. and Schneider, C.R. (1976). Notes on the aquatic ecology of *Lithoglyphopsis aperta*. *South East Asian Journal of Tropical Medicine and Public Health* **7**, 238–243.

Kitikoon, V., Schneider, C.R., Sornmani, S., Harinasuta, C. and Lanza, G.R. (1973). Mekong schistosomiasis: II. Evidence of the natural transmission of *Schistosoma japonicum*, Mekong strain at Khong Island, Laos. *South East Asian Journal of Tropical Medicine and Public Health* **4**, 350–358.

Lacassin, R., Replumaz, A. and Leloup, P.H. (1998). Hairpin river loops and slip-sense inversion on Southeast Asian strike-slip faults. *Geology* **26**, 703–706.

Le, T.H., Blair, D., Agatsuma, T., Humair, P.-F., Campbell, N.J.H., Iwagami, M., Littlewood, D.T.J., Peacock, B., Johnston, D.A., Bartley, J., Rollinson, D., Herniou, E.A., Zarlenga, D.S. and McManus, D.P. (2000a). Phylogenies inferred from mitochondrial gene orders – a cautionary tale from the parasitic flatworms. *Molecular Biology and Evolution* **17**, 1123–1125.

Le, T.H., Blair, D. and McManus, D.P. (2000b). Mitochondrial DNA sequences of human schistosomes: the current status. *International Journal for Parasitology* **30**, 283–290.

Le, T.H., Blair, D. and McManus, D.P. (2000c). Mitochondrial genomes of human helminths and their use as markers in population genetics and phylogeny. *Acta Tropica* **77**, 243–256.
Liang, Y.-S. and Kitikoon, V. (1980). Cultivation of *Lithoglyphopsis aperta* snail vector of *Schistosoma mekongi*. In: The Mekong schistosome (J.I. Bruce, S. Sornmani, H.L. Asch and K.A. Crawford, eds), pp. 35–45. *Malacological Review*, supplement 2.
Liu, S.X., Song, G.C., Xu, Y.X., Yang, W. and McManus, D.P. (1995). Anti-fecundity immunity induced in pigs vaccinated with recombinant *Schistosoma japonicum* 26 kDa glutathione *S*-transferase. *Parasite Immunology* **17**, 335–340.
Liu, S.X., He, Y., Song, G.C., Xu, Y.X., Yang, W. and McManus, D.P. (1997). Anti-fecundity immunity to *Schistosoma japonicum* induced in Chinese water buffaloes (*Bos buffelus*) after vaccination with recombinant 26 kDa glutathione-*S*-transferase (re-Sjc26GST). *Veterinary Parasitology* **69**, 39–47.
Lo, C.T., Berry, E.G. and Iijima, T. (1971). Studies on schistosomiasis in the Mekong Basin. II. Malacological investigations on human *Schistosoma* from Laos. *Chinese Journal of Microbiology* **4**, 168–181.
Lohachit, C., Sornmani, S. and Butrcham, P. (1980a). Development and maintenance of *Lithoglyphopsis aperta* in the laboratory. In: The Mekong schistosome (J.I. Bruce, S. Sornmani, H.L. Asch and K.A. Crawford, eds), pp. 19–34. *Malacological Review*, supplement 2.
Lohachit, C., Sritabutra, P. and Butrcham, P. (1980b). Pattern of emergence of *Schistosoma mekongi* cercariae from the beta race of *Lithoglyphopsis aperta*. In: The Mekong schistosome (J.I. Bruce, S. Sornmani, H.L. Asch and K.A. Crawford, eds), pp. 47–51. *Malacological Review*, supplement 2.
Maizels, R.M., Bundy, D.A.P., Selkirk, M.E., Smith, D.F. and Anderson, R.M. (1993). Immunological modulation and evasion by helminth parasites in human populations. *Nature* **365**, 797–805.
Manning, S.D., Woolhouse, M.E.J. and Ndamba, J. (1995). Geographic compatibility of the freshwater snail *Bulinus globosus* and schistosomes from the highveld. *International Journal for Parasitology* **25**, 37–42.
Maunoury, V., Guillemot, F., Mathieu-Chandelier, C., Dutoit, E., Gower-Rousseau, C., Cortot, A. and Paris, J.C. (1990). Bilharzioses à *Schistosoma mekongi* diagnostiquées par biopsie rectale et traitées par praziquantel: à propos de 5 cas. *Gastroenterology and Clinical Biology* **14**, 1032–1033.
McManus, D.P. (2000). A vaccine against Asian schistosomiasis: the story unfolds. *International Journal for Parasitology* **30**, 265–271.
McManus, D.P., Liu, S.X., Song, G., Xu, Y. and Wong, J.M. (1998). The vaccine efficacy of native paramyosin (Sj-97) against Chinese *Schistosoma japonicum*. *International Journal for Parasitology* **28**, 1739–1742.
Miao, Y.X., Liu, S.X. and McManus, D.P. (1998). Isolation of native, biochemically purified triosephosphate isomerase from a Chinese strain of *Schistosoma japonicum* and its protective efficacy in mice. *Parasitology International* **47**, 195–199.
Mitchell, A.H.G. (1981). Phanerozoic plate boundaries in mainland S.E. Asia, the Himalayas and Tibet. *Journal of the Geological Society of London* **138**, 109–122.
Morand, S., Manning, S.D. and Woolhouse, M.E.J. (1996). Parasite–host coevolution and geographic patterns of parasite infectivity and host susceptibility. *Proceedings of the Royal Society of London* **B263**, 119–128.
Nei, M. (1978). Estimation of average heterozygosity and genetic distance from a small number of individuals. *Genetics* **89**, 583–590.
Nei, M. and Li, W.-H. (1979). Mathematical model for studying genetic variation in terms of restriction endonucleases. *Proceedings of the National Academy of Sciences of the USA* **76**, 5269–5273.

Nei, M. and Miller, J.C. (1990). A simple method for estimating average number of nucleotide substitutions within and between populations from restriction data. *Genetics* **125**, 873–879.

Pantulu, V.R. (1998). Fish of the lower Mekong basin. In: *The Ecology of River Systems* (B.R. Davies and K.F. Walker, eds), pp. 721–741. Dordrecht, The Netherlands: Dr W. Junk.

Pao, T.-C. (1959). The description of a new schistosome *Schistosoma sinensium* sp. nov. (Trematoda: Schistosomatidae) from Szechuan Province. *Chinese Medical Journal* **78**, 278.

Pearce, E.J., James, S.L., Hieny, S., Lanar, D.E. and Sher, A. (1988). Induction of protective immunity against *Schistosoma mansoni* by vaccination with schistosome paramyosin (Sm97), a nonsurface parasite antigen. *Proceedings of the National Academy of Sciences of the USA* **85**, 5678–5682.

Pesigan, T.P., Hairston, N.G., Jauregui, J.J., Garcia, E.G., Santos, A.T., Santos, B.C. and Besa, A.A. (1958). Studies on *Schistosoma japonicum* infection in the Philippines. 2. The molluscan host. *Bulletin of the World Health Organization* **18**, 481–578.

Pholsena, K. (in press). *Schistosomiasis Control in Southern Laos. WHO Mission Report.* Geneva: World Health Organization.

Rainboth, W.J. (1991). Cyprinid fishes of Southeast Asia. In: *Cyprinid Fishes: Systematics, Biology and Exploitation* (I. Winfield and J.S. Nelson, eds), pp. 156–210. London: Chapman and Hall.

Rainboth, W.J. (1996). *The Taxonomy, Systematics, and Zoogeography of* Hypsibarbus, *a New Genus of Large Barbs (Pisces: Cyprinidae) from the Rivers of Southeastern Asia.* La Jolla: University of California Press.

Rollinson, D. and Southgate, V.R. (1987). The genus *Schistosoma*: a taxonomic appraisal. In: *The Biology of Schistosomes: From Genes to Latrines* (D. Rollinson and A.J.G. Simpson, eds), pp. 1–50. London: Academic Press.

Ross, A.G.P., Li, Y.S., Sleigh, A.C. and McManus, D.P. (1997). Schistosomiasis control in the People's Republic of China. *Parasitology Today* **13**, 152–155.

Schneider, C.R. (1976). Schistosomiasis in Cambodia: a review. *South East Asian Journal of Tropical Medicine and Public Health* **7**, 155–166.

Sen, A. (1973). *On Economic Inequality.* Oxford: Clarendon Press.

Shekhar, K.C. (1987). A comparative parasitological study of Malaysian schistosomes (Koyan and Baling strains) with *Schistosoma japonicum* (Philippine strain) and *S. mekongi* (Thai strain) in various laboratory animals. *Tropical Biomedicine* **4**, 132–144.

Sherchand, J.B., Ohara, H., Sherchand, S. and Matsuda, H. (1999). The suspected existence of *Schistosoma mansoni* in Dhanusha district, southern Nepal. *Annals of Tropical Medicine and Parasitology* **93**, 273–278.

Sleigh, A.C. (1989). *Community-based Praziquantel Therapy and National Schistosomiasis Control. WHO Document (WP) PDV/LAO/PDP/001.* Geneva: World Health Organization.

Smith, A.G., Hurley, A.M. and Briden, J.C. (1981). *Phanerozoic Paleocontinental World Maps.* Cambridge, UK: Cambridge University Press.

Snyder, S.D. and Loker, E.S. (2000). Evolutionary relationships among the Schistosomatidae (Platyhelminthes: Digenea) and an Asian origin for *Schistosoma. Journal of Parasitology* **86**, 283–288.

Snyder, S.D., Loker, E.S., Johnston, D.A. and Rollinson, D. (2001). The Schistosomatidae: Advances in phylogenetics and genomics. In: *Interrelationships of the Platyhelminthes* (D.T.J. Littlewood and R.A. Bray, eds), pp. 194–200. London: Taylor and Francis.

Sobhon, P. and Upatham, E.S. (1990). Introduction. In: *Snail Hosts, Life-cycle, and Tegumental Structure of Oriental Schistosomes* (P. Sobhon and E.S. Upatham, eds), pp. 1–17. Geneva: UNDP/World Bank/WHO.

Sørensen, E., Drew, A.C., Brindley, P., Bøgh, H.O., Gasser, R.B., Qian, B.Z., Chiping, Q. and McManus, D.P. (1998). Variation in the sequence of a mitochondrial NADH dehydrogenase I gene fragment among six natural populations of *Schistosoma japonicum* from China. *International Journal for Parasitology* **28**, 1931–1934.

Sørensen, E., Bøgh, H.O., Johansen, M.V. and McManus, D.P. (1999a). PCR-based identification of individuals of *Schistosoma japonicum* representing different subpopulations using a genetic marker in mitochondrial DNA. *International Journal for Parasitology* **29**, 1121–1128.

Sørensen, E., Johansen, M.V., Wilson, S. and Bøgh, H.O. (1999b). Elucidation of *Schistosoma japonicum* population dynamics in pigs using PCR-based identification of individuals representing distinct cohorts. *International Journal for Parasitology* **29**, 1907–1915.

Sornmani, S. (1969). Schistosomiasis in Thailand. In: *Proceedings of the Fourth Southeast Asian Seminar on Parasitology, Tropical Medicine, Schistosomiasis and Other Snail Transmitted Helminthiases. 22–27 February 1969* (C. Harinasuta, ed.), pp. 71–74. Manila: SEAMEO-TROPMED.

Sornmani, S. (1976). Current status of research on the biology of Mekong *Schistosoma*. *South East Asian Journal of Tropical Medicine and Public Health* **7**, 208–213.

Sornmani, S., Kitikoon, V., Harinasuta, C. and Pathammavong, O. (1971). Epidemiological study of schistosomiasis japonica on Khong Island, southern Laos. *South East Asian Journal of Tropical Medicine and Public Health* **2**, 365–374.

Sornmani, S., Kitikoon, V., Schneider, C.R., Harinasuta, C. and Pathammavong, O. (1973). Mekong schistosomiasis. I. Life cycle of *Schistosoma japonicum*, Mekong strain, in the laboratory. *South East Asian Journal of Tropical Medicine and Public Health* **4**, 218–225.

Sornmani, S., Kitikoon, V., Thirachantra, S. and Harinasuta, C. (1980). Epidemiology of Mekong schistosomiasis. In: The Mekong schistosome (J.I. Bruce, S. Sornmani, H.L. Asch and K.A. Crawford, eds), pp. 9–18. *Malacological Review*, supplement 2.

Southgate, V.R. and Agrawal, M.C. (1990). Human schistosomiasis in India? *Parasitology Today* **6**, 166–168.

Spolsky, C., Davis, G.M. and Yi, Z. (1996). Sequencing methodology and phylogenetic analysis: cytochrome *b* gene sequence reveals significant diversity in Chinese populations of *Oncomelania* (Gastropoda: Pomatiopsidae). *Malacologia* **38**, 213–221.

Staub, K.C., Woodruff, D.S., Upatham, E.S. and Viyanant, V. (1990). Genetic variation in *Neotricula aperta*, the intermediate host of *Schistosoma mekongi*: allozyme differences reveal a group of sibling species. *American Malacological Bulletin* **7**, 93–103.

Stich, A.H.R., Biays, S., Odermatt, P., Men, C., Saem, C., Sokha, K., Ly, C.S., Legros, P., Philips, M., Lormand, J.-D. and Tanner, M. (1999). Foci of schistosomiasis mekongi, northern Cambodia: II. The distribution of infection and morbidity. *Tropical Medicine and International Health* **4**, 674–685.

Stürchler, D. (1988). *Endemic Areas of Tropical Infections*. Basle: Roche.

Sun, W.Y., Liu, S.X., Brindley, P.J. and McManus, D.P. (1999). Bacterial expression and characterisation of functional recombinant triosephosphate isomerase from *Schistosoma japonicum*. *Protein Expression and Purification* **17**, 410–413.

Swan, L.W. (1981). The zoogeography of Tibet and its relation to the uplift of the Plateau. In: *Geological and Ecological Studies of the Qinghai-Xizang Plateau* (D.S. Liu, ed.), pp. 999–1004. Beijing: Science Press.

Tajima, F. (1983). Evolutionary relationship of DNA sequences in finite populations. *Genetics* **105**, 437–460.

Tapponier, P., Peltzer, G., Le Dain, A.Y., Armijo, R. and Cobbold, P. (1982). Propagating extrusion tectonics in Asia, new insights from simple experiments with plasticine. *Geology* **10**, 611–616.

Tapponier, P., Peltzer, G. and Armijo, R. (1986). On the mechanics of the collision between India and Asia. In: *Collision Tectonics* (M.P. Coward and A.C. Ries, eds), pp. 115–157. London: Geological Society of London.

Temcharoen, P. (1971). New aquatic molluscs from Laos. *Archiv für Molluskenkunde* **101**, 91–109.

Upatham, E.S., Sornmani, S., Thirachantra, S. and Sitaputra, P. (1980). Field studies on the bionomics of alpha and gamma races of *Tricula aperta* in the Mekong river of Khemmarat, Ubol Ratchathani Province, Thailand. In: The Mekong schistosome (J.I. Bruce, S. Sornmani, H.L. Asch and K.A. Crawford, eds), pp. 239–261. *Malacological Review*, supplement 2.

Vichasri-Grams, S., Grams, R., Korge, G., Viyanant, V. and Upatham, E.S. (1997). Cloning and sequence analysis of the 26 kDa glutathione-*S*-transferase gene of *Schistosoma mekongi. South East Asian Journal of Tropical Medicine and Public Health* **28**, 570–574.

Voge, M., Bruckner, D. and Bruce, J.I. (1978). *Schistosoma mekongi* sp. n. from man and animals, compared with four geographic strains of *Schistosoma japonicum. Journal of Parasitology* **64**, 577–584.

Wittes, R., MacLean, J.D., Law, C. and Lough, J.O. (1984). Three cases of schistosomiasis from northern Laos. *American Journal of Tropical Medicine and Hygiene* **33**, 1159–1165.

Woodruff, D.S. and Upatham, E.S. (1992). Snail-transmitted diseases of medical and veterinary importance in Thailand and the Mekong valley. *Journal of Medical and Applied Malacology* **4**, 1–12.

Woodruff, D.S., Merenlender, A.M., Upatham, E.S. and Viyanant, V. (1987). Genetic variation and differentiation of three *Schistosoma* species from the Philippines, Laos, and peninsular Malaysia. *American Journal of Tropical Medicine and Hygiene* **36**, 345–354.

Woodruff, D.S., Carpenter, M.P., Upatham, E.S. and Viyanant, V. (1999). Molecular phylogeography of *Oncomelania lindoensis* (Gastropoda: Pomatiopsidae), the intermediate host of *Schistosoma japonicum* in Sulawesi. *Journal of Molluscan Studies* **65**, 21–32.

Workman, D.R. (1972). *Geology of Laos, Cambodia, South Vietnam and the Eastern Part of Thailand: A Review*. London: Institute of Geological Science Overseas Division Report.

Workman, D.R. (1977). *Geology of Laos, Cambodia, South Vietnam and the Eastern Part of Thailand*. London: Institute of Geological Sciences.

Xiao, X. and Gao, Y. (1984). Tectonic evolution of the Tethys Himalayas of China. In: *Tectonics of Asia Colloquium 5*, pp. 181–189. Beijing: 27th International Geology Congress Reports.

Xu, R. (1981). Geological and ecological studies of Qinghai-Xizang Plateau. In: *Vegetational Changes in the Past and the Uplift of the Qinghai-Xizang Plateau* (D.S. Liu, ed.), pp. 139–144. Beijing: Science Press.

Xu, R.-H., Schärer, U. and Allègre, C.J. (1985). Magmatism and metamorphism in the Lhasa Block (Tibet): a geochronological study. *Journal of Geology* **93**, 41–57.

Yasuraoka, K. (1990). *Mission Report: Snail Control in Khong District*. Geneva: World Health Organization.

Yasuraoka, K. (1992). *Rapport de Mission: Lutte Contre les Mollusques dans le District de Khong*. Geneva: World Health Organization.

Yong, H.S., Greer, G.J. and Ow-Yang, C.K. (1985). Genetic diversity and differentiation of four taxa of Asiatic blood flukes (Trematoda: Schistosomatidae). *Tropical Biomedicine* **2**, 17–23.

Molecular Aspects of Sexual Development and Reproduction in Nematodes and Schistosomes

Peter R. Boag[1,2], Susan E. Newton[1] and Robin B. Gasser[2]

[1]*Victorian Institute of Animal Science, Attwood, Victoria 3049, Australia;*
[2]*Department of Veterinary Science, The University of Melbourne, Werribee, Victoria 3030, Australia*

ABSTRACT

In contrast to the free-living nematode *Caenorhabditis elegans*, surprisingly little is known about the molecular aspects of reproduction in parasitic helminths. Investigations into such aspects would provide an improved understanding of the fundamentals of sexual differentiation, development, maturation and behaviour, as well as sex-specific genes and their expression. Such knowledge could lead to new means of parasite control by interfering with or

ADVANCES IN PARASITOLOGY VOL 50
0065–308X $30.00

disrupting one or more of these processes, which is particularly important given the emerging problems with genetic resistance in parasitic nematodes against anthelmintic drugs. This chapter brings together some relevant information on the sexual biology of *C. elegans*, summarizes studies of gender-specific expression in selected parasitic helminths of socio-economic significance, describes advanced molecular techniques for the analysis of gender-specific genes, and indicates the prospects for genomic research on reproductive processes and the implications thereof for controlling parasitic helminths.

1. INTRODUCTION

Helminths represent one of the most diverse groups of organisms on the planet (Platt, 1994). They are found in both terrestrial and aquatic environments, existing as both free-living organisms and as parasites of plants and animals. Helminth infestations in livestock animals cause substantial production losses to growers due to poor productivity, failure to thrive or death (Smith, 1997). Current control strategies to overcome such problems have relied chiefly on the use of anthelmintic drugs. However, the effectiveness of two (benzimidazoles and imidothiazoles) of the three main drug classes is becoming compromised through the widespread development of drug resistance, particularly in sheep and goats (e.g., Roos, 1997; Sangster, 1999; Sangster and Gill, 1999). Therefore, other means of parasite control need to be investigated and developed. One potential approach is the disruption or suppression of reproductive processes by the identification of novel targets for prophylactic or therapeutic intervention.

Although the morphological differences between adult males and females of dioecious nematodes have been studied extensively (e.g., Skrjabin, 1952), comparatively little is known about sexual differentiation, maturation and reproductive processes in parasitic helminths. Nonetheless, some molecular aspects of reproduction have been investigated, for example in dioecious parasitic blood flukes (*Schistosoma* spp.) of major human health significance (Grevelding *et al.*, 1997; Schüssler *et al.*, 1997; Fantappie *et al.*, 1999). This has led to the isolation of a number of genes that are expressed in a gender-specific manner, the identification of potential regulatory elements for some genes, and a better understanding of the molecular biological interactions between the sexes.

In contrast to the paucity of information on reproductive processes in parasitic helminths, much is known about many different aspects of sexual biology in the free-living nematode *Caenorhabditis elegans*, which is considered a valuable 'model' for the study of parasitic nematodes (Blaxter, 1998). For over

35 years, *C. elegans* has been intensively investigated at various levels (e.g., morphology, physiology, biochemistry, neurology and genetics), culminating in the determination of its complete genome sequence (The *C. elegans* Sequencing Consortium, 1998). Hence, many of the pathways involved in its sexual determination as well as in the development and maturation of reproductive tissues have been identified, and genes involved in these processes characterized.

In a period of unparalleled growth of knowledge in genomics of helminths and *C. elegans*, including genome sequencing programs for several parasitic helminths of significance in humans, plants and animals (e.g., Opperman and Bird, 1998; Williams and Johnston, 1999; Blaxter, 2000; Maizels *et al.*, 2000), it is timely to take stock of current information on helminth genomics and reproductive biology. Therefore, the purpose of this chapter is to review relevant information on the sexual biology of *C. elegans* and other helminths, to summarize research on gender-specific genes and gene products for some parasitic helminths of socio-economic significance, to discuss novel molecular approaches for studying gender-specific genes of parasites, and to indicate the prospects and implications of investigating fundamental and applied aspects of their reproduction at the molecular level.

2. NEMATODES

2.1. The Free-living Nematode *Caenorhabditis elegans*

2.1.1. C. elegans *as a Model for Parasitic Helminths*

C. elegans is one of the best-characterized metazoan organisms (Riddle *et al.*, 1997). It is a free-living nematode consisting of 959 somatic cells in the hermaphrodite and 1031 somatic cells in the male. Its genome is ~97 Mb in size and contains five autosomal chromosomes and a single sex chromosome, producing a haploid number of $n = 12$ (10A : 2X) in the hermaphrodite and $2n = 11$ (10A : X) in the male. Although *C. elegans* has no medical or economic significance, it represents an invaluable research tool for investigating many biological processes. Some features that make *C. elegans* an attractive model species include its short life cycle (3 days at 25°C), ease of propagation using a simple bacterial food source (*Escherichia coli*), amenable characteristics for microscopy, relatively small genome size, the ability to produce clonal progeny from hermaphroditic worms and the ability to cross hermaphrodites with male worms. These attributes have allowed the acquisition of considerable knowledge and understanding of reproductive, developmental, physiological, neurological and genetic aspects of the nematode. For example, the complete cell lineage from zygote to adult has been determined for both hermaphroditic and male worms (Sulston and Horvitz, 1977; Sulston *et al.*, 1983). Also, the role of apoptosis in development (Hengartner, 1997) and many of the molecular events involved in sex determination have been investigated extensively (Meyer, 1997). Recently, *C. elegans* became the first metazoan to have its complete genome sequence determined (The *C. elegans* Sequencing Consortium, 1998). Of the ~20 000 predicted genes, ~58% appear to be nematode specific (Blaxter, 1998). Thus *C. elegans* can be considered a useful model organism for parasitic nematodes, particularly given that a number of key biological processes appear to be conserved between *C. elegans* and a range of parasitic nematodes (Blaxter, 1998; Favre *et al.*, 1998; Ashton *et al.*, 1999). The broad utility of *C. elegans* is also demonstrated by its applicability as a model for biomedical studies, such as in cancer biology (Chang and Sternberg, 1999) and human congenital disorders (Culetto and Sattelle, 2000).

2.1.2. *Sex Determination*

While the details of the sex determination pathway have been studied extensively in *C. elegans* (see Meyer, 1997), and increasingly in other closely related caenorhabdins (Kuwabara and Shah, 1994; Kuwabara, 1996a; Hansen and Pilgrim, 1998), using a combination of classical genetic and molecular biological techniques, a paucity of information is available for other nematodes. A number of excellent review articles summarize sex determination mechanisms in both somatic and germline tissues of *C. elegans* and related species (Cline and Meyer, 1996; Meyer, 1997, 2000). Hence, this section will be restricted to the general principles of somatic sex determination in *C. elegans*.

The number of X chromosomes determines the sex of *C. elegans*; XX worms develop as hermaphrodites and XO as males. In the young embryo, the number of X chromosomes in relation to autosomes is determined by several 'signal elements'. To date, two of these elements in the X chromosome, SEX-1 (Carmi *et al.*, 1998) and FOX-1 (Hodgkin *et al.*, 1994; Skipper *et al.*, 1999), have been cloned and characterized. Two additional regions in the X chromosome may contain other signal elements, but their precise location has not yet been determined (Akerib and Meyer, 1994). Both SEX-1 and FOX-1 act on the 'master switch' for sex determination, *xol-1*, but they operate via different mechanisms, and hence their effects are applied separately. SEX-1 is a member of the nuclear hormone receptor family of proteins and is a transcriptional regulator of *xol-1*, while FOX-1 is an RNA binding protein and regulates *xol-1* at the translational level. Both of these proteins, and potentially other signal elements, provide a tight regulation of sex determination throughout embryonic development (Skipper *et al.*, 1999). In wild-type hermaphrodite *C. elegans*, which possess only a single X chromosome, the *xol-1* master switch is expressed and initiates a cascade of suppression of alternate genes in the sex determination pathway, after which the terminal 'switching gene' of the cascade, *tra-1*, is either activated or repressed (reviewed by Meyer, 1997). The ability to produce mutants relating to the sex determination pathway of *C. elegans* has allowed genetic and epistasis studies to be conducted, and these have led to the discovery of the gene order in the pathway (reviewed in Meyer, 1997).

Several genes involved in this pathway have also been cloned from other caenorhabdin nematodes (deBono and Hodgkin, 1996; Kuwabara, 1996b; Streit *et al.*, 1999; Haag and Kimble, 2000) and from the parasitic nematode *Brugia malayi* (see Streit *et al.*, 1999). Compared with metabolic genes coding for essential functions, the genes involved in the initial steps of the sex determination pathway of *C. elegans* appear to have undergone elevated rates of evolutionary change (Civetta and Singh, 1998). Hence, the use of heterologous DNA probes to isolate orthologous genes from other nematodes has been of limited value. Nonetheless, comparative genome analyses between *C. elegans* and parasitic nematodes have revealed that some gene sequences are indeed related among species, and that there also appears to be some degree of conservation in the order and structure for some genes (reviewed in Blaxter, 1998). These findings have stimulated the use of synteny or positional cloning for the identification of orthologous genes (Kuwabara and Shah, 1994), where a highly conserved gene that is closely linked to a particular gene of interest in the characterized species is used as a probe to screen a genomic library of the target species. Streit *et al.* (1999) successfully cloned the *tra-2* orthologue from *Caenorhabditis briggsae* using this approach after the use of heterologous probes had failed.

Both *C. elegans* and *C. briggsae* are hermaphrodites, which raises questions as to how relevant their sex determination pathway is to that of dioecious nematodes. *B. malayi*, a dioecious nematode that causes lymphatic filariasis in humans, is currently the subject of a large expressed sequence tag (EST) sequencing initiative within the Filarial Genome Project (see Blaxter and Ivens, 1999). This project has identified a *her-1* homologue (*Bm-her-1*), which is predicted to encode a protein that shares 35% identity and 42% similarity with the *C. elegans* HER-1 protein, which is involved in the early events of sex determination. Despite the low level of sequence similarity between them, several features of the Bm-HER-1 predicted protein are characteristic of the *C. elegans* and *C. briggsae* HER-1 proteins. First, the Bm-HER-1 N-terminal secretion signal is predicted to be cleaved in almost the same relative position as in the *C. elegans* and *C. briggsae* proteins. Second, the Bm-HER-1 protein contains 14 cysteine residues, which are highly conserved spatially with the two caenorhabdin proteins. Third, 12 of 13 key amino acids (as defined by loss of function using mutational analysis) are highly conserved.

The relevance of sex determination genes in hermaphroditic nematodes is also being addressed in the gonochoristic *Caenorhabditis remanei*, a close relative of both *C. elegans* and *C. briggsae*. Haag and Kimble (2000) cloned the *tra-2* homologue from *C. remanei* using the synteny approach and determined that the *C. remanei* TRA-2 (Cr-TRA-2) protein had 43% and 49% sequence similarity with those from *C. elegans* and *C. briggsae*, respectively. Interestingly, despite the relatively low level of overall similarity, key regulatory elements were common between the *C. remanei* and *C. elegans* genes (Haag and Kimble, 2000). The predicted functional similarity suggested that the *Cr-tra-2* gene was indeed involved in sex determination, and indicated clearly that the sex determination pathway has similarities between the two nematodes, despite a distinct difference in sexual outcome. Moreover, suppression of *Cr-tra-2* gene function by double-stranded RNA-mediated interference (see Section 4.2) resulted in the masculinization of female worms, suggesting that the CR-TRA-2 protein is crucial for female development (Haag and Kimble, 2000).

Despite significant differences in reproductive modes of nematodes (i.e., gonochorism versus androdioecy), it appears that the general pathways of sex determination are relatively conserved but flexible enough to allow multiple variations in sex chromosome structure. The pathway appears to be similar for male/female and male/hermaphrodite systems, and also for XX/XO and XX/XY sex chromosome structures in nematodes. As more genomic and proteomic data become available for a wide range of parasitic nematodes, a comprehensive analysis of sex determination and subsequent growth and maturation will be possible. However, before this comparison can include parasitic nematodes, significant work needs to be carried out on the identification and characterization of genes involved in sex determination and gender-related gene expression for this group. From an academic viewpoint, this will provide a foundation for understanding nematode development and elucidating conserved biological pathways, and could aid in the identification of proteins of major functional relevance. From a practical perspective, this may also provide opportunities for identifying new targets for controlling parasitic nematodes through disruption of the reproductive cycle.

2.1.3. *Gametogenesis*

Gametogenesis is the process of producing sperm or oocytes in the germline tissues of a sexually reproducing organism. Early in the embryogenesis of the male and hermaphroditic *C. elegans*, reproductive tissues originate from four precursor cells, Z1, Z2, Z3 and Z4 (reviewed by Hubbard and Greenstein, 2000). The Z1 and Z4 cells differentiate to form the somatic structures of the mature adult gonad, and the Z2 and Z3 cells develop into the germline tissues.

The gonad begins to differentiate into the male or hermaphrodite form in the first larval stage, and the male gonad becomes functionally active during development of the fourth larval and adult stages (reviewed in Schedl, 1997). The gonad of the hermaphrodite also becomes active in the late fourth-stage larva, where it produces a limited amount of sperm. The first 40 cells undergoing meiosis in each lobe of the gonad develop into 160 spermatozoa, before the gonad switches to oocyte production in the adult. The anatomy of the reproductive tissues differs markedly in that the male gonad is asymmetrical (having a J-shape and connecting to the seminal vesicle and vas deferens) (Figure 1B), whereas the hermaphrodite possesses a symmetrical, bilobed gonad (with a U-shape, sharing a common uterus and vulva) (Figure 1A). The somatic gonad of the mature adult hermaphrodite forms the body of the reproductive organ and comprises the distal tip cells (DTCs), sheath cells, spermatheca and uterus. Oogenesis is initiated at the distal end of the gonad, where mitotically active stem cells proliferate under the control of somatic DTCs. Sheath cells, which are contractile myoepithelial cells required for correct meiotic maturation and ovulation, line the gonad (Rose *et al.*, 1997), although their precise function remains to be elucidated. As the oocytes move further proximal and continue their maturation, they undergo meiotic division, resulting in the production of oocytes with a haploid genome. The maturing oocytes undergo ovulation as they enter the spermatheca, are fertilized and then pass into the uterus, where they complete their maturation and where embryogenesis begins (Schedl, 1997). Recently, it has been shown that sperm-associated signals are implicated in the meiotic maturation of the oocyte, as mutant hermaphrodite adults incapable of sperm production are characterized by oocytes arrested in diakinesis (the last stage of meiotic prophase) (McCarter *et al.*, 1999). However, the most proximal oocytes in the gonad do mature and ovulate, but at a significantly decreased rate compared with normally developed hermaphrodites. Interestingly, mating of sperm-deficient hermaphrodites with male worms (even if the latter are incapable of spermatozoa formation and fertilization) reinvigorates their oocyte maturation and ovulation (McCarter *et al.*, 1999). This suggests that factors other than the presence of functional sperm are required for normal progression of oocyte maturation.

Sperm production in the male's single-lobed gonad is similar to that in the hermaphrodite and continues for the life of the adult worm (Kimble and Ward, 1988). DTCs at the distal end of the gonad control the activity of the stem cells, which develop as they move proximally, proceeding through mitotic and meiotic divisions. Spermatids are stored in the seminal vesicle until ejaculation, and they complete their differentiation into functional spermatozoa in the uterus (L'Hernault, 1997). From the uterus, the non-flagellated spermatozoa crawl into the spermatheca of the hermaphrodite and fertilize the maturing oocyte. The mode of locomotion of *C. elegans* sperm is similar to that of other nematodes, but unusual for the majority of metazoans (Bullock *et al.*, 1998)

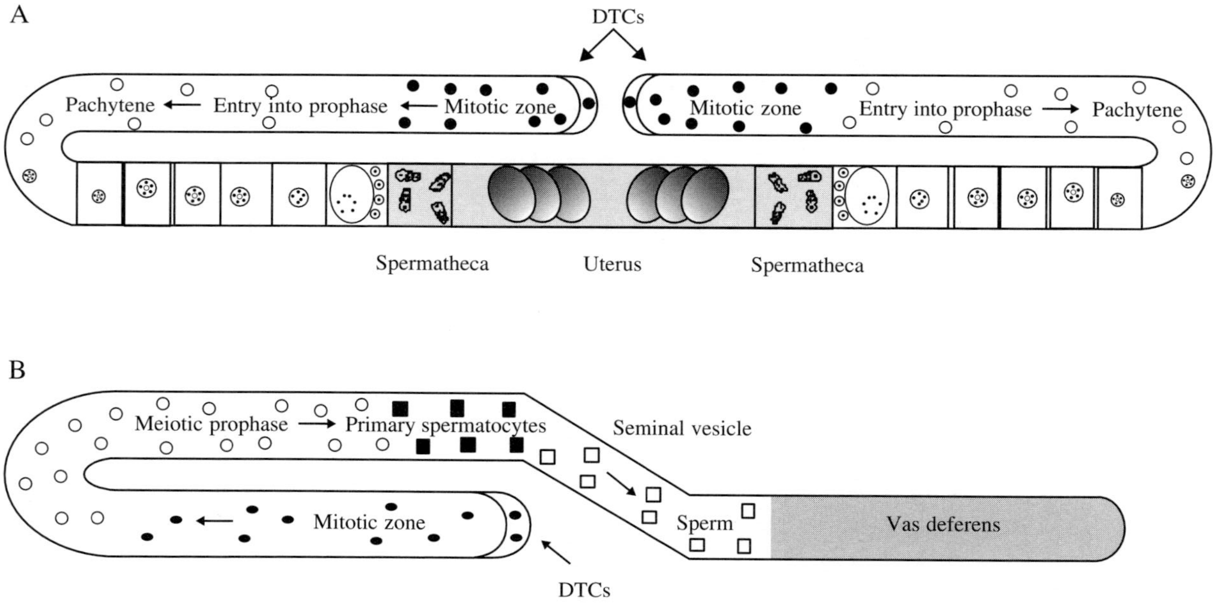

Figure 1 Schematic representation of gametogenesis in *C. elegans*. A. Hermaphrodite. B. Male. Gametogenesis begins at the distal end of both the hermaphrodite and male gonad, where the germ cells undergo mitotic proliferation under the control of the distal tip cells (DTCs). As they move further proximally, they enter into meiotic divisions. Hermaphrodite sperm is produced during the fourth larval stage and is stored in the spermatheca. Oocytes enter the spermatheca and are fertilized prior to passing into the uterus. In the male, spermatids are stored in the seminal vesicle, and differentiate into spermatozoa in the uterus of the hermaphrodite.

(see also Section 2.3). Sperm produced by male *C. elegans* is similar in morphology and motility to that produced by hermaphrodites, although spermatozoa of the male are larger (LaMunyon and Ward, 1998). It has been suggested that the increased size of male sperm provides a competitive advantage over hermaphrodite sperm during the fertilization process (LaMunyon and Ward, 1998, 1999), possibly providing an evolutionary advantage of out-crossing. At least five genes are required for the initiation of spermatogenesis in hermaphrodites, of which three, *fem-1*, *fem-2* and *fem-3*, are also involved in somatic and germline sex determination, while two other genes, *fog-1* and *fog-3*, are involved exclusively in germline cell fates (reviewed by Schedl, 1997). The *fog-3* gene is expressed in third and fourth stage larvae of *C. elegans*, but its expression diminishes in the young adult when the hermaphrodite ceases sperm production. This gene is believed to be transcriptionally regulated by several other genes, including the somatic sex determination master gene, *tra-1* (Chen and Ellis, 2000).

Apart from the genes associated with controlling the initiation of gametogenesis, ~60 different mutants affecting various stages of spermatogenesis in *C. elegans* have been identified, and a number thereof cloned (reviewed by L'Hernault, 1997). Some of the cloned genes have been shown to affect motility of sperm, while others affect chromosome segregation, maturation and/or fertilization (see L'Hernault, 1997). Characterization of these mutants will provide insights into the molecular events driving sperm production and fertilization in nematodes, and may provide a reference tool for the characterization of these processes in parasitic helminths.

2.2. Parasitic Nematodes

In contrast to *C. elegans*, there is limited information on fundamental aspects of reproduction (including sex determination and sexual maturation) for parasitic nematodes. Nonetheless, there have been studies of karyotypes (e.g., Post *et al.*, 1989; Mutafova, 1995), of pheromones and sexual attraction (reviewed by Green, 1980) and, more recently, of genes that are expressed in a gender-specific manner (e.g., Bessarab and Joshua, 1997; Llado *et al.*, 1998; Boag *et al.*, 2000).

2.2.1. *Karyotypes and Sex Determination*

For the majority of nematodes, sex determination is under genetic control, that is, the chromosomal complement of an individual worm defines the worm's sex. Cytogenetic investigations of nematodes have been carried out for over a century, with the first recorded microscopic analysis of meiosis being described for *Parascaris equorum* (see van Beneden in 1883, cited in Tobler, 1986). Predictions about the mechanisms of sex determination in parasitic nematodes may be drawn from numerous cytological studies (e.g., Walton, 1959; Triantaphyllou, 1983). The haploid chromosome number (n) in nematodes is usually small, with $n = 3$–6 being common, but ranging from 1 (*Diploscapter coronata*) to 19 (*Anguina tritici*) (see Triantaphyllou, 1983). Male nematodes are heterogametic, usually possessing either XO or XY sex chromosome complements, while females are homogametic, having an XX set of sex chromosomes. Interestingly, there is variation in the sex chromosome structures within certain groups, for example, spiruroids can possess both XX/XO and XX/XY chromosomes structures (Sakaguchi *et al.*, 1983; Hirai *et al.*, 1987; Mutafova, 1995; Post and Pinder, 1995; Spakulova *et al.*, 2000). The recent cloning of a chromosomal marker from *B. malayi* has confirmed, at the molecular level, the existence of a Y chromosome (Underwood and Bianco, 1999). A different sex chromosome structure is apparent for *Ascaris suum*, which has a single sex chromosome, but there are ten copies in the female and five in the male (i.e. $2n = 38$ autosomes + 10X and $2n = 38$ autosomes + 5X, respectively). In some species of nematodes, however, there are no detectable differences in the chromosomal complements of males and females (e.g., LeJambre, 1968; Goldstein and Triantaphyllou, 1979). This may reflect technical difficulties in producing reliable karyotypes for nematodes, as the chromosomes are often small and have relatively complex banding patterns that can be difficult to interpret. This may explain why there are conflicting descriptions of the haploid numbers and sex chromosome complements for several nematodes. For example, *Dirofilaria immitis* has been described as having XO (Taylor, 1960) and XY (Delves *et al.*, 1986) sex chromosomes. Also, the diploid number of *A. suum* has been determined as $2n = 24$ for males and 29 for females by Goldstein and Moens (1976), and as $2n = 43$ for males and 48 for females by Tobler (1986).

An interesting finding from karyotype analyses of some ascaridoids was that of chromatin diminution (Bennett and Ward, 1986; Müller and Tobler, 2000). This process relates to developmentally controlled chromosomal rearrangement and subsequent reduction in total DNA content in the somatic cells early in the development of the embryo. Chromatin diminution is well described for *Parascaris univalens* and *A. suum*, and consists of three distinct steps (Müller and Tobler, 2000). The first step involves chromosomal breakage, which occurs at particular sites throughout the genome. The second involves the addition of telomeric repeats $(TTAGGC)_n$, of 4–6 kb, to the ends of selected DNA fragments. The third step relates to the degradation of chromatin DNA. The result of this diminution process is to produce somatic cells that possess a significantly reduced DNA content compared with germline cells, estimated to be 80–95% for *P. univalens* and 25% for *A. suum* (see Tobler, 1986). In *P. univalens*, the chromosome number of somatic cells changes from $2n = 2$ to $2n = 60$. Chromatin diminution has been characterized for several other species of ascaridoid (Müller and Tobler, 2000), and it can also be found in other groups. For example, during mitotic parthenogenesis in *Strongyloides papillosus* chromatin diminution occurs, but the process appears to relate to sex determination rather than to a specific reduction of DNA content in somatic tissues (Albertson *et al.*, 1979). The precise mechanism by which this is achieved is currently unknown.

Although sex is determined chromosomally for the majority of nematodes studied to date, there are examples where environmental conditions can influence sex determination. For instance, an increase in the number of hermaphrodites relative to males has been demonstrated for *Heterorhabditis bacteriophora* when grown in culture *in vitro* under conditions of low nutrition, whereas the converse was observed when the worms were propagated in supplemented medium (Kahel-Raifer and Glazer, 2000). Another example is *Meloidodera floridensis*, which has been reported to produce an increased number of male worms when grown at high temperature (Triantaphyllou and Hirschmann, 1973). Hence, the precise mechanism(s) determining sexual development need to be characterized for these parasitic nematodes.

There is also a requirement to define molecular markers to allow detailed investigations into sex chromosome structures of nematodes, given the limitations of traditional karyotyping methods. Fluorescence *in situ* hybridization (FISH) experiments using such molecular markers (Drew and Brindley, 1995) should improve the accuracy of karyotyping and thus also enable investigations into the evolution of nematode sex chromosomes and mating systems. Such markers should become available through the EST sequencing programs currently underway (e.g., Blaxter and Ivens, 1999; Blaxter, 2000).

2.2.2. *Sexual Attraction and Pheromones*

Pheromones are chemical signalling molecules, produced by most metazoan organisms, which play a range of biological roles, from responding to environmental conditions to sex attraction (Renou and Guerrero, 2000). Sex pheromones are involved in the attraction of one sex by another, thus aiding in mate localization and achieving mating success. *Panagrolaimus rigidus* was the first nematode shown to produce sex pheromones, and currently more than 30 species of free-living and parasitic nematodes have been found to produce sex pheromones (reviewed by Green, 1980). Most studies of nematodes have identified substances produced by female worms that attract males, although there are examples of 'female' and 'homosexual' attractants (Green, 1980; Haseeb and Fried, 1988). Interestingly, the sex pheromones produced by the female of a particular species of nematode can sometimes attract males of a heterologous species (Green and Plumb, 1970; Riga *et al.*, 1996), suggesting that some level of conservation of both pheromones and their receptors exists between species. Also, individual species appear to produce more than one sex pheromone (Bone, 1982; Riga *et al.*, 1997).

The partial characterization of sex pheromones has been achieved mainly using *in vivo* and *in vitro* bioassays. For example, surgical transplantation of adult females of *Ancylostoma caninum* into the anterior of the small intestine of the dog and adult males into the posterior region results in the migration of males to females (Roche, 1966). This observation suggests that a pheromone is produced by the adult female nematode and diffuses down the lumen of the intestine to attract the male (Roche, 1966). Similar results were obtained with *Nippostrongylus brasiliensis* in the intestine of rodents (Glassburg *et al.*, 1981). However, the intrusive nature of experiments *in vivo* has led some investigators to use bioassays *in vitro* (such as agar plate methods and, more recently, electrophysiological responses to pheromone extracts (Riga *et al.*, 1996, 1997)) to determine the biochemical nature of sex pheromones. Despite the relatively large number of nematode species known to produce pheromones, only a few have received detailed study, with plant parasitic species of the genera *Globodera* and *Heterodera* and the animal parasite *N. brasiliensis* receiving most attention (Green and Plumb, 1970; Bone, 1982; Riga *et al.*, 1996, 1997). Bone and co-workers used multiple chromatography techniques to identify two fractions ($K_{av}0{\cdot}64$ and $K_{av}1{\cdot}0$) from adult female *N. brasiliensis* that attract male worms (Bone *et al.*, 1980; Bone, 1982; Ward and Bone, 1983). The extracts were chemically diverse; $K_{av}0{\cdot}64$ was soluble in water, while $K_{av}1{\cdot}0$ was soluble in both aqueous and organic solvents, but the precise nature of these extracts has not yet been determined. However, a sex pheromone identified by Jaffe *et al.* (1989) in extracts of female *Heterodera glycines* was shown to be vanillic acid, and was able to effectively attract male worms in a bioassay at concentrations of 10^{-5}–10^{-7} M.

Chemical signals from the environment are received by chemosensory receptors often found at the anterior end of a worm (Troemel, 1999), and it is likely that sex pheromones will be bound by such receptors. Again, *C. elegans* represents the best-studied nematode in term of chemosensation. In this species, there are 302 neurons, of which 32 appear to be chemotactic as they are associated with specialized structures on the surface of the worm, and thus are potentially exposed to hundreds of different chemicals (Ward *et al.*, 1975). The ability of a relatively small number of neurons to detect a broad range of different chemicals is thought to relate to the presence of multiple different chemosensory receptors in each neuron (Troemel, 1999).

Chemosensory receptors are usually proteins of the G protein-coupled receptor family and have been identified from a wide range of vertebrates and invertebrates (reviewed by Troemel, 1999). G proteins representing different receptors usually share a low level of sequence similarity but are characterized by the presence of seven transmembrane regions. The *C. elegans* genome is predicted to contain ~1000 genes encoding G protein-coupled receptors, which, based on protein sequence, can be divided into four families, namely *odr-10*-like, *sra*, *sro* and *srg* (Troemel, 1999). They are organized in clusters within the genome, with up to 15 genes per cluster. Interestingly, only ~50% of these genes are thought to be expressed, with the remainder appearing to be pseudogenes, because they contain stop codons and, if expressed, would produce truncated proteins. This raises questions as to the significance of the clustering and the presence of such pseudogenes. It is possible that the G protein-coupled receptor genes are located in regions of the chromosome susceptible to duplications and/or mutations, thus allowing novel genes to be produced, possibly with altered receptor specificity (Troemel, 1999).

The expression patterns of several G protein-coupled receptors have been investigated in transgenic *C. elegans*, with a reporter gene fused to the promoter region of the selected receptor genes (Troemel *et al.*, 1995). Three of the genes characterized to date, *sra-1*, *sra-6* and *srd-1*, are expressed in male-specific chemosensory neurons, suggesting that they could be involved in sensing hermaphrodite pheromones involved in mating (Troemel *et al.*, 1995). Knowledge of the G protein-coupled receptors and their genes in *C. elegans* may assist in the cloning of homologues from parasitic nematodes and may provide new avenues for investigating sex pheromones. Subsequent expression of these receptors from parasitic nematodes in transgenic *C. elegans* may allow the nature and roles of the chemical signals to be elucidated.

2.3. Gender-specific Genes of Free-living and Parasitic Nematodes

2.3.1. *Major Sperm Proteins*

Some of the first gender-specifically expressed proteins identified in nematodes were those of the major sperm protein (MSP) family, originally isolated from *C. elegans* (see Klass and Hirsh, 1981; Ward and Klass, 1982) and subsequently from *A. suum* (see Nelson and Ward, 1981). The MSPs are small (~14 kDa), nematode-specific, cytoskeletal proteins, and represent the most abundant protein in the spermatozoa, accounting for ~10–15% of the total cellular protein (Klass *et al.*, 1982).

MSPs are accumulated in the late primary spermatocyte, where they assemble into filamentous-fibrous bodies. These bodies are transient organelles that also contain other sperm-specific proteins, and which subsequently segregate with the nucleus and mitochondria into the developing spermatids (Figure 2) (Ward and Klass, 1982; Roberts *et al.*, 1986). In the developing spermatid, the filamentous-fibrous bodies disassemble, and the MSPs become distributed throughout the cytoplasm of the cell. It is at this stage that the spermatid's

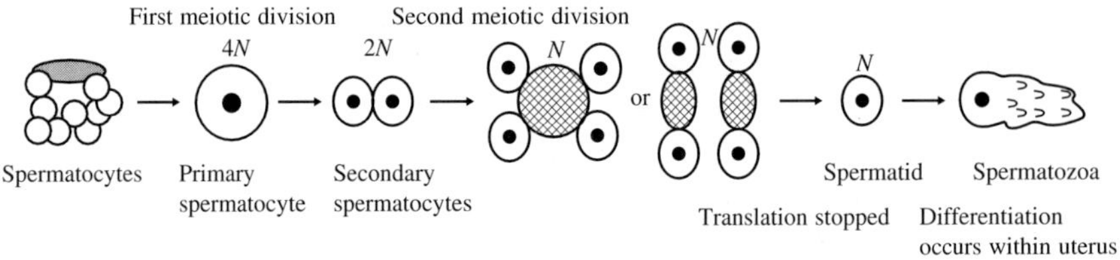

Figure 2 Sperm development in *C. elegans*. Spermatogenesis begins at the distal end of the male gonad where mitotic proliferation of spermatogonial cells produces the primary spermatocytes. These cells then mature as they move proximally, undergoing two meiotic divisions, after which the spermatids bud off from the parent cell, with the golgi apparatus, endoplasmic reticulum and ribosomes remaining in the residual body. Spermatids complete their development during copulation and become motile. Based on Roberts *et al.* (1986).

development arrests. Spermatogenesis is initiated during copulation, possibly by the release of secretions from the vas deferens. The MSPs reassemble, forming 2–3 nm filaments (Ward and Klass, 1982; Roberts *et al.*, 1986), which become located in the pseudopod of the motile spermatozoa. The reassociation of the MSPs into filaments can be stimulated *in vitro* by an increase in the pH through the addition of weak bases (Nelson and Ward, 1980) or of proteases (Ward *et al.*, 1983). Roberts and Stewart (2000) have suggested a mechanism whereby the extending pseudopod attaches to the underlying surface (over which the spermatozoon is crawling), and a series of polymerization reactions occurs at the extending end of the pseudopod, thereby pushing the pseudopod forward. The MSP filaments behind the attachment point undergo a depolymerization reaction, the MSPs are recycled and the cell body is pulled forward. The polymerization/depolymerization reactions are thought to be initiated, at least in part, by a small pH gradient between the leading edge of the pseudopod and the base of the cell body (King *et al.*, 1994).

Expression of *msp* genes is spatially and temporally regulated, being confined to the testis (in both *C. elegans* and *A. suum*) during the meiotic stages of spermatogenesis, a period of ~90 min in *C. elegans* (see Klass *et al.*, 1982; Ward and Klass, 1982). In *C. elegans*, the MSPs are encoded by a large family of ~60 genes located in six distinct clusters in three regions of chromosomes II and IV (Burke and Ward, 1983; Ward *et al.*, 1988). Most of these genes appear to be transcribed, with each gene contributing ~1–3% to the total cellular mRNA. This contrasts with the situation in *A. suum*, where only a single gene is transcribed (Nelson and Ward, 1981; Bennett and Ward, 1986).

The distribution of *msp* genes across a number of free-living and parasitic nematodes has been investigated by Southern blot analysis using *msp-3* from *C. elegans* and *msp* from *A. suum* as molecular probes (Scott *et al.*, 1989a).

This study revealed a difference in the distribution of *msp* genes among 16 species of nematodes representing a range of different orders, for example Spirurida, Rhabditida, Tylenchida and Ascaridida. Most of the parasitic nematodes investigated have 5–13 *msp* genes, while the free-living nematodes possess 15–50 *msp* genes. Interestingly, the distribution of *msp* genes contrasts with that of actin genes, which are usually more uniform across the nematodes studied, with 2–9 actin genes being present (except for *A. suum*, which has more than 20) (Scott *et al.*, 1989a). This raises the question as to why a gene essential for reproduction is present in significantly different numbers in different species. The high concentration of MSP in *C. elegans* sperm suggests that there is a large pool of *msp* mRNA available for translation, which may be achieved by the simultaneous expression of numerous *msp* genes. It has been proposed that MSP production is one of the rate-limiting steps in sperm production, and therefore a high copy number of *msp* genes is maintained (Scott *et al.*, 1989a). Parasitic nematodes, with life cycles of longer duration, or with larger testis, may not have the high rate of sperm production of *C. elegans*, and therefore only a few transcribed genes are needed to supply the required *msp* mRNA concentration. Alternatively, the rate of transcription of *msp* genes may be significantly greater in nematodes with fewer *msp* genes, possibly through a more efficient promoter structure, or they may have increased mRNA stability. However, these aspects have not yet been investigated for nematodes other than *C. elegans*.

The promoter structures of 10 *C. elegans msp* genes have been characterized by DNA sequence analysis (Klass *et al.*, 1988). Genomic DNA sequence similarity is restricted to a small region 100 bp 5′ to the translational start codon for all 10 genes, and analysis revealed various elements common to a range of eukaryotic promoter regions, including a TATA box as well as two other conserved regions (AGATCT and A/TGATAA), which conform to the binding motifs of the GATA family of transcription factors (Klass *et al.*, 1988; Shim, 1999). Shim (1999) demonstrated that the two putative GATA motifs are required for expression in a yeast reporter gene system, that the GATA transcription factor ELT-1 is capable of activating transcription of the reporter gene and that the *elt-1* gene is highly expressed in germline tissues of both males and hermaphrodites of *C. elegans*. Surprisingly, *Onchocera volvulus* is the only parasitic nematode for which the genomic organization of *msp* genes has been determined (Scott *et al.*, 1989b). Genomic clones for two *O. volvulus msp* genes, *Ovgs-1* and *Ovgs-2*, have been isolated, and these show ~80% identity to *A. suum msp* cDNA and 79% to the *C. elegans msp-3* cDNA sequence. Despite limited DNA sequence similarity between the promoters of the *O. volvulus msp* genes and those of *C. elegans*, two GATA binding motifs have been identified for *O. volvulus*, suggesting that these transcription factors may also be important for *msp* gene expression in this species. Hence, it would be of significant value to determine the DNA sequences adjacent to the *msp* transcriptional start site for a wide range of species, and to identify any regulatory elements involved in *msp* gene expression. Also, the relationship between the level of *msp* expression and gene copy number could be addressed by determining the efficiency of various promoters and identifying precisely which DNA sequence regions are associated with expression.

The number of *msp* gene sequences listed in nucleic acid and protein databases is increasing, mainly due to targetted gene cloning and EST sequencing programs for several important nematodes (e.g., Blaxter and Ivens, 1999). Usually the predicted MSP protein sequences share a high level of similarity among both closely and distantly related species of nematodes (Figure 3), although similarity is greatest between nematodes within an order. For example, MSPs from the filarioid nematodes, *B. malayi* and *O. volvulus*, are more similar in protein sequence to one another than to those of other nematodes. Interestingly, the putative MSP of *Dictyocaulus viviparus* (Strongylida) is distinct in sequence from other MSPs. The N-terminal half of the predicted protein shares significant similarity with other MSPs, but the similarity is significantly reduced at the C-terminus. While the *D. viviparus* MSP has been detected exclusively in adult worms (Schnieder, 1993), it is not yet known whether its expression is exclusive to the testes of the parasite. This warrants

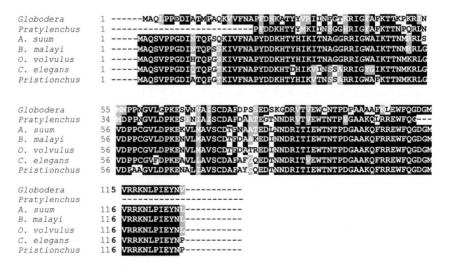

Figure 3 Alignment of major sperm proteins (MSPs) from selected nematodes. *Caenorhabditis elegans* MSP31 (AAB42253), *Pristionchus pacificus* (EST clone AW115172), *Globodera rostochiensis* MSP3 (P53023), *Pratylenchus penetrans* (AAB02251), *Ascaris suum* MSP1 (P27439), *Onchocerca volvulus* MSP2 (P13263), *Brugia malayi* (EST clone AI105502). Dark shading represents conserved residues; light shading represents similar amino acids.

further investigation. Also, given that there is a single base deletion in the published cDNA sequence of *D. viviparus msp* with respect to all other published sequences (Setterquist and Fox, 1995) resulting in a change in reading frame, the sequence data may need to be verified.

2.3.2. *Vitellogenins*

Vitellogenins are a ubiquitous family of large (170–700 kDa) phosphoglycolipoproteins found in a diverse range of vertebrate and invertebrate organisms, and are thought to function as a source of amino acids and lipids for the embryo to consume during its development within the egg (Chen *et al.*, 1997). Also, in some species, vitellogenins have the ability to non-covalently bind hormones, vitamins and metal ions (Chen *et al.*, 1997). In *C. elegans*, vitellogenins are expressed at high levels in the intestine of the late fourth-stage larval and adult hermaphrodites, and are secreted from the intestinal cells into the body cavity, where they are subsequently taken up by the gonad and absorbed into the oocyte by receptor-mediated endocytosis (Sharrock, 1983; Grant and Hirsh, 1999). They are processed into smaller molecules, either prior to uptake by the oocyte or after internalization. In *C. elegans*, there are six vitellogenin genes, *vit-1* to *vit-6*, of which *vit-6* encodes a protein that is proteolytically cleaved into two proteins (88 and 115 kDa) prior to uptake by the oocyte, whereas *vit-2*, *vit-3* and *vit-5* are absorbed without cleavage. Interestingly, *vit-1* and *vit-4* appear to be pseudogenes (Spieth *et al.*, 1991).

While there is relatively little published information regarding vitellogenin genes for parasitic nematodes, numerous vitellogenin ESTs have recently been identified for a range of nematodes, including *Haemonchus contortus*, *A. caninum*, *Oesophagostomum dentatum*, *Globodera rostochiensis* and *Pristionchus pacificus*. Additionally, an adult-female-specific cDNA clone from *H. contortus* with greatest similarity to *vit-6* from *C. elegans* has been isolated, and its expression in the intestine confirmed by hybridization *in situ* (Hartman *et al.*, 2001).

Although vitellogenins are present in a diverse range of taxa, database searches using *C. elegans vit-2*, *vit-5* and *vit-6* cDNA sequences do not identify any putative vitellogenin ESTs in the filarioid nematodes *B. malayi* and *O. volvulus*. This is in contrast to other nematodes groups, where there is sequence similarity between vitellogenins from insects and those of vertebrates. There are a number of possible explanations for the apparent lack of vitellogenin ESTs from filarioid nematodes. First, they may not be a major component of the oocyte in these two species. Second, their nucleic acid and protein sequences may have diverged substantially from other nematodes, as vitellogenin genes are believed to evolve rapidly (Winter *et al.*, 1996) and hence may not be detectable in EST database searches. Third, EST sequences are generally <500 bp in length, possibly preventing the identification of vitellogenins, which are usually encoded by mRNAs of several thousand nucleotides. Given that vitellogenin genes are usually expressed at high levels in the intestinal tract of most egg-laying metazoans, it may be possible to clone the vitellogenin genes of *B. malayi* and *O. volvulus*, should they exist, through a targetted approach, for example by polymerase chain reaction (PCR) using degenerate primers to conserved regions of the protein or by immunohistochemical screening of adult female expression libraries. If such genes were detected, this would indicate that caution is warranted in the sole use of EST databases as a resource for gene discovery.

In *C. elegans*, three of the vitellogenin genes are located on the X chromosome, and the most divergent gene, *vit-6*, is on chromosome IV. The vitellogenin promoter regions have been studied extensively in *C. elegans* using transgenic worms carrying reporter gene constructs (MacMorris *et al.*, 1994). This approach has allowed the identification of the minimal promoter region of 247 bp required for correct expression. This small region contains several elements common to all *C. elegans* vitellogenin genes, which have also been identified in the vitellogenin genes of *C. briggsae* (Zucker-Aprison and Blumenthal, 1989). The vitellogenin promoter element (VPE1) has a consensus sequence of TGTCAAT and is usually found at least three times within the 300 bases immediately adjacent to the transcriptional start site. An additional element (VPE2) has the consensus sequence of CTGATAA, which includes the binding site for the GATA family of transcription factors (MacMorris *et al.*, 1994). The functional requirement for the VPE1 and VPE2 elements was determined by MacMorris *et al.* (1994) using transgenic lines of *C. elegans* containing various modifications of the VPE elements, and it was concluded that both VPE elements are required for correct expression of vitellogenin in *C. elegans*. In the future, comparative analyses of the genomic organization and structure of vitellogenin genes across a range of parasitic nematodes would assist in identifying promoter regions critical for regulating sex-specific gene expression.

2.3.3. *Recently-identified Parasite Genes*

A number of workers (e.g., Bessarab and Joshua, 1997; Llado *et al.*, 1998; Michalski and Weil, 1999; Boag *et al.*, 2000) have recently isolated gender-specific genes from parasitic nematodes other than *msp* and vitellogenin, using the technique of differential display (DD). This technique relies on the PCR amplification of cDNAs from two or more sources (e.g., male and female) using random oligonucleotide primers. The products are resolved by denaturing gel electrophoresis, and bands which appear to be unique to a lane (e.g., male) can be excised, cloned and sequenced. Joshua and Hsieh (1995) used DD to isolate a female-specific gene fragment from adult *Angiostrongylus cantonensis*. The full-length cDNA (*Ac-fmp-1*) encodes a peptide of 417 amino acids, which is localized to the musculature adjacent to the pseudocoelomic space. However, no clear biological function has yet been ascribed to this protein (Bessarab and Joshua, 1997). More recently, several sex-specific transcripts of furin protease (an enzyme involved in the processing of a range of different proteins) have been isolated from the canine heartworm, *Dirofilaria immitis* (see Jin *et al.*, 1999). Three female-specific and five male-specific transcripts, resulting from differential splicing, were identified using reverse transcriptase-PCR and were proposed to encode proteins with distinct functions (Jin *et al.*, 1999). Interestingly, this is the first published report of gender-specific splicing of mRNA from any parasitic nematode.

Llado *et al.* (1998) identified by DD a novel, male-specific gene *(Hgm1)* from the soybean cyst nematode, *H. glycines*, while Michalski and Weil (1999) have characterized several gender-specific genes of *B. malayi* using DD combined with EST database analysis. Of the 12 adult sex-specific genes isolated from *B. malayi*, only five have similarity to nucleic acid or protein sequences contained within current databases. Some of the partial gene sequences encode proteins with similarity to protein families that could be expected to be expressed in a gender-specific manner based on their biological functions (e.g., the female-specific clone, MBAFCE2H11T3, encoding a putative eggshell protein), but for others no clear prediction could be made as to their gender-specific roles. For example, it is not clear what role a transmitter-gated ion channel may play in female reproductive development.

Recent reports have indicated that the porcine nodule worm, *O. dentatum* (Strongylida) provides a unique model system for studying fundamental aspects of reproductive biology in parasitic nematodes (Christensen *et al.*, 1995, 1997; Christensen, 1997). It has a direct, short life cycle (21 days) (Talvik *et al.*, 1997), produces large numbers of progeny and can be readily maintained as a laboratory line. Importantly, uni-sex or mixed-sex infections can be established by rectal transplantation to naive porcine hosts (Christensen *et al.*, 1996), thus allowing studies of mating behaviour and sexual maturation *in vivo*. Another feature is that the parasite can be maintained relatively effectively in cultures *in vitro* (Daugschies and Ruttkowski, 1998; Daugschies and Watzel, 1999). Recently, we identified gender-specific genes from *O. dentatum* by DD analysis of mRNAs from male or female adults (Boag *et al.*, 2000). Ten male-specific and two female-specific cDNAs were isolated which were confirmed to be expressed in a gender-specific manner. Of these, six cDNAs appeared to represent novel genes, while the others had varying levels of sequence similarity to either nucleic acid or protein sequences in the databases. One of the female-specific clones encoded a vitellogenin with significant similarity to *vit-6* of *C. elegans*, while one male-specific gene encoded the catalytic sub-unit of a serine/threonine protein phosphatase, sharing greatest

Table 1 Current EST sequencing initiatives and summary of EST data.

(a) Major EST initiatives

Project title	Species	Website
Parasitic Nematode Project	*Ancylostoma caninum* *Heterodera glycines* *Meloidogyne incognita* *Meloidogyne javanica* *Pristionchus pacificus* *Strongyloides stercoralis* *Zeldia punctata*	http://www.nematode.net/
Nematode Genomics	*Haemonchus contortus* *Trichuris muris* *Ascaris suum* *Necator americanus* *Loa loa* *Trichinella spiralis* *Litomosoides sigmodontis* *Globodera rostochiensis*	http://www.ed.ac.uk/ ~mbx/small_genomes
Filarial Genome Project	*Brugia malayi* *Wuchereria bancrofti* *Onchocerca volvulus*	http://nema.cap.ed.ac.uk/ fgn/filgen1.html
Schistosoma Genome Project	*Schistosoma japonicum* *Schistosoma mansoni*	http://www.nhm.ac.uk/ hosted_sites/schisto/

(b) EST summary by organism*

Species	Number of ESTs
Caenorhabditis elegans	109 215
Brugia malayi	22 392
Onchocerca volvulus	14 347
Schistosoma mansoni	14 039
Strongyloides stercoralis	10 979
Meloidogyne incognita	6 626
Ancylostoma caninum	5 546
Pristionchus pacificus	4 989
Haemonchus contortus	2 749
Caenorhabditis briggsae	2 424
Schistosoma japonicum	2 029
Heterodera glycines	1 421
Meloidogyne javanica	1 223
Globodera rostochiensis	894
Ascaris suum	588

* dbEST release 020901 – February 9, 2001.

similarity with a *C. elegans* protein implicated in sperm production (Reinke *et al.*, 2000). Characterization of these and other gender-specific genes should enable detailed investigations into the molecular aspects of reproduction in *O. dentatum* (both *in vitro* and *in vivo*).

Gender-specific genes can also be isolated by EST sequencing combined with electronic subtraction. Recently, consortia have been established for the analysis of gene expression in parasitic helminths (Blaxter and Ivens, 1999) (see Table 1). This involves 'single-pass' sequencing (<500 bp) of randomly selected clones from cDNA libraries, and has the advantage that sequence data can be obtained from libraries constructed from minute quantities of mRNA from different developmental stages, sexes or tissues of an organism. Also, EST sequencing is suited for automation and electronic data analysis. For instance, by comparing ESTs contained in male or female databases by 'electronic subtraction', gender-specific genes can be effectively identified (Michalski and Weil, 1999). Such an approach has enabled the identification of the *B. malayi* homologue of the *C. elegans her-1* gene, which is of comparative value in relation to sex determination (Streit *et al.*, 1999). However, the EST sequencing approach can have some limitations. Despite >100 000 ESTs having been generated from *C. elegans*, only 40% of the predicted genes have homologues in other nematodes (The *C. elegans* Sequencing Consortium, 1998), indicating that a large number of genes are expressed at low levels, are not present in the cDNA libraries sequenced or have not yet been sequenced (given the limited genome sequencing that has been done to date on parasitic nematodes). It is likely that many genes associated with sexual maturation and reproduction are expressed in a small number of tissues and/or at low levels, and as such may be difficult to identify by EST sequencing and analysis. Some of these limitations may be overcome by using subtractive suppressive hybridization (SSH) (Diatchenko *et al.*, 1996) because of its ability to isolate rare transcripts.

3. SCHISTOSOMES

Given the human health significance and unique biology of blood flukes (Trematoda: Schistosomatidae) (LoVerde and Chen, 1991; Ribeiro-Paes and Rodrigues, 1997; McManus, 1999), there has been considerable research on fundamental aspects of their biology, including reproduction. Early work involved karyotyping, studying sex ratios in schistosome populations and the pairing of male and female schistosomes. Recent work has focused on the isolation and characterization of gender-specific markers and genes, as well as molecules potentially involved in the transduction of molecular signals between the sexes.

3.1. Karyotypes and Sexual Biology

Schistosomes are unique trematodes in that they are dioecious. Like most nematodes, the sex of an individual is determined by the presence of sex chromosomes. Karyotype analysis of the Schistosomatidae demonstrated that the chromosome number is highly conserved among members, with a haploid number of $n = 8$, with seven pairs of autosomes and two sex chromosomes being most common (Short, 1957; Liberatos and Short, 1983). Female schistosomes are heterogametic, having a ZW sex chromosome composition, while the males are homogametic, having a ZZ composition. Studying karyotypes from a wide range of schistosomes has provided insights into the chromosomal mechanism of sex determination and the evolution of schistosomes (Grossman *et al.*, 1981) and, to a limited extent, has allowed the study of changes in sex ratios throughout the schistosome life cycle (e.g., Raghunathan and Bruckner, 1975; Liberatos and Short, 1983).

Investigations into the sexual biology of schistosomes has revealed two interesting observations. The first is a distinct bias in the sex ratio in chronic infections, in both intermediate and definitive hosts. As the sex of an individual schistosome is controlled by the sex chromosomes, an equal proportion of males and females would be expected. However, a male bias is common in chronic infections (both natural and experimental) with *Schistosoma* species (Liberatos, 1987; Mitchell *et al.*, 1990). Although Liberatos (1987) indicated that the male bias in *S. mansoni* was the result of greater infectivity and/or survival of males in both snails and the mammalian host, Mitchell *et al.* (1994) suggested that the bias observed in *S. japonicum* could be explained by a preferential immune response of the definitive host against female larvae, possibly through antigens encoded on the W chromosome. The biological explanation for this male bias in schistosome populations remains to be elucidated.

Another interesting observation is the requirement of the female worm to be paired with a male to complete and maintain sexual maturity (Clough, 1981; Popiel *et al.*, 1984). Pairing of male and female schistosomes occurs in the hepatic vein of the definitive vertebrate host, where the female lives encopula in the gynaecophoric canal of the significantly larger male worm (Figure 4). Early studies of schistosomes showed that *S. japonicum* females produced from experimental uni-sex infection failed to reach reproductive maturity and had a reduced body size compared with females from mixed-sex infection (Ribeiro-Paes and Rodrigues, 1997, and references therein). Similar results were obtained in studies of a range of other *Schistosoma* species, such as *S. mansoni* (see Moore *et al.*, 1954; Erasmus, 1973), although the dependence on pairing appears to be less pronounced for other species (e.g., *Schistosomatium douthitti*; see Short, 1957). In *S. mansoni*, female worms not only require pairing with the male to mature sexually, but also to maintain reproductive capacity (Clough, 1981; Popiel *et al.*, 1984). Clough (1981)

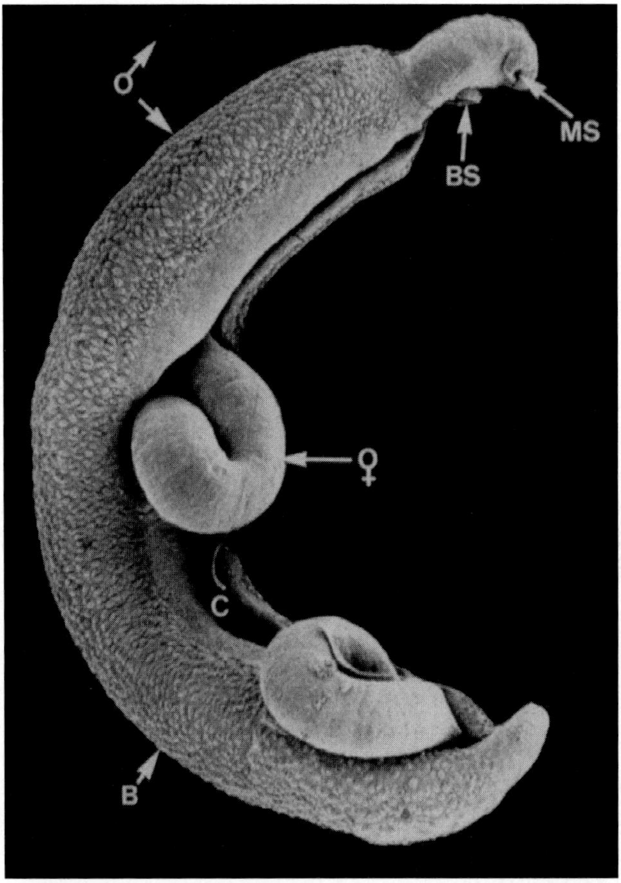

Figure 4 Paired *Schistosoma mansoni* male and female. The female resides within the gynaecophoric canal of the male. BS, ventral sucker; MS, oral sucker; B, bosses (protuberances) of the tegument; C, gynaecophoric canal. Reproduced with permission of H. Mehlhorn.

investigated the effect of separating the sexes of *S. mansoni* after transplantation into naive hamsters. The vitelline glands and ovaries of normally developed adult females degenerated 3 and 6 days after separation, respectively. This degeneration occurred despite the presence of residual sperm in the fertilization chamber of some females, suggesting that sperm is not the only male factor involved in stimulating female maturation and the maintenance of reproductive capacity. Clough (1981) also postulated that the termination of egg production following separation from males is the result of a decline in vitelline production.

Jungersen *et al.* (1997) demonstrated that transplantation of mature gravid *A. suum* females to establish a uni-sex infection results in the cessation of egg production 2 to 3 weeks after transplantation. Similar findings have been described for the canine hookworm *A. caninum* (see LeJambre and Georgi, 1970) and the porcine nodular worm *O. dentatum* (see Christensen, 1997), and there is also evidence that female *O. dentatum* need male *O. dentatum* worms to sexually mature (Christensen, 1997). These findings suggest that dependence by female worms on males for attainment and maintenance of sexual maturity may be a widespread phenomenon for helminths.

Re-pairing of female schistosomes with mature males reverses the degeneration of the reproductive system, whereby after 6 days the reproductive tissues are indistinguishable microscopically from females obtained from mixed-sex infections (Clough, 1981). Den Hollander and Erasmus (1985) used a biochemical assay to study sexual maturation of *S. mansoni in vitro* by measuring the uptake by female worms of [^{3}H] thymidine, which is a marker for DNA synthesis. Female worms cultured in an 'all female' environment showed little uptake of [^{3}H] thymidine compared with worms cultured in a mixed-sex environment, indicating that little DNA synthesis was occurring, which was in agreement with the histological observations of Popiel and Erasmus (1982) and Popiel *et al.* (1984). Interestingly, when uni-sex females of *S. mansoni* were paired with males from a uni-sex infection, the rate of [^{3}H] thymidine uptake after 24 h in culture was significantly lower than when uni-sex females were paired with males from a mixed-sex infection, although there was no difference between the two groups after 48 h. These results suggest that male worms from a uni-sex environment need to synthesize some factor(s) before they are fully stimulatory to the female, and thus the male also depends on the presence of the female for full sexual maturity. Indeed, there is some evidence that females influence the levels of lipase and glutathione in males (Siegel and Tracy, 1988; Haseeb *et al.*, 1989). Although there are no obvious morphological differences between adult males derived from a uni-sex versus a mixed-sex infection, the *in vitro* experiments clearly indicate that there are molecular differences, and that there is 'cross-talk' between the sexes (Den Hollander and Erasmus, 1985). Shaw *et al.* (1977) supported this by demonstrating that organic extracts of male *S. mansoni* could stimulate activity of vitelline cells in the female in a uni-sex environment. However, this result was restricted to a single line of *S. mansoni* (Popiel, 1986, cited in Ribeiro-Paes and Rodrigues, 1997).

Current evidence indicates that male schistosomes are required for females to complete their sexual maturation and to maintain reproductive capacity. However, there is still no consensus on how they achieve this. The steroid hormone ecdysone has been detected in *S. mansoni* and has been correlated to the sexual maturation of females (Nirde *et al.*, 1984, 1986). Moreover, glucose (Cornford and Huot, 1981; Cornford and Fitzpatrick, 1985), cholesterol

(Haseeb *et al.*, 1985), polypeptides and glycoproteins (Popiel and Basch, 1984; Gupta and Basch, 1987; Basch and Nicolas, 1989) have been identified as being transmissible from male to female worms. However, the relationship between these molecules and sexual development remains unclear, and there is a need to characterize their roles, as they may be a logical target for disease control by disrupting the life cycles of schistosomes.

3.2. Gender-specific Markers, and Genes Associated with Maturation and Reproduction

3.2.1. *Molecular Markers*

Molecular markers for identification of the sexes of *S. mansoni* have been reported by several groups (e.g., Spotila *et al.*, 1987; Walker *et al.*, 1989; Webster *et al.*, 1989; Gasser *et al.*, 1991; Drew and Brindley, 1995). Spotila *et al.* (1987) identified a 339 bp clone which generates a unique banding pattern when hybridized to genomic DNA on Southern blot, allowing the differentiation of male from female larvae. However, this method requires relatively large numbers (>200) of cercariae for hybridization, and thus is not applicable to determining the sex of individual larvae. Both Walker *et al.* (1989) and Webster *et al.* (1989) used a differential hybridization technique to screen genomic DNA libraries for female-specific markers and isolated clones with 600 bp and 476 bp (W1) inserts, respectively. Both clones contained repetitive DNA sequences predicted to represent some of the heterochromatin of the W chromosome of *S. mansoni*. With the advent of PCR, Gasser *et al.* (1991) used the W1 target to develop a rapid and simple method to determine the sex of individual miracidia and cercariae, providing an effective tool for sex ratio studies (cf. Liberatos, 1987; Mitchell *et al.*, 1990). Interestingly, Quack *et al.* (1998) showed that males of a Liberian line of *S. mansoni* contained the W1 marker, but the significance of this finding is unclear. Drew and Brindley (1995) isolated two novel female specific markers (W2 and SMαfem-1) from *S. mansoni* using the technique of representational difference analysis (RDA). Both of these appear to be associated with the W chromosome, with SMαfem-1 being related to the SM family of retrotransposons, found throughout the *S. mansoni* genome (Drew and Brindley, 1995).

3.2.2. *Differentially Expressed Genes and Their Regulation*

The unique reproductive biology of schistosomes and the pathological effects induced in the human host by immunological reactions to eggs have stimulated investigation into genes that are expressed in a stage- and gender-specific manner (see LoVerde and Chen, 1991). Understanding the molecular biological events associated with the sexual maturation process may lead to ways of disrupting reproduction, which, in turn, could result in a reduction in the severity of egg-induced granuloma formation in the liver (Bobek *et al.*, 1986; Kunz and Symmons, 1987). Initial experiments on the differences between male and female *S. mansoni* concentrated on the identification of differentially expressed proteins (Atkinson and Atkinson, 1982; Aronstein and Strand, 1983). However, reproducibility and interpretation of results was difficult because of the complexity of the protein profiles. The subsequent use of recombinant DNA techniques allowed the identification and cloning of stage- and gender-specific genes, and provided useful tools to study molecular events occurring during schistosome development. For instance, Aronstein and Strand (1985) identified an 80 kDa glycoprotein of *S. mansoni* expressed on the surface of adult females and, to a limited extent, on the surface of the gynaecophoric canal of adult males, which suggested that the protein played a significant role in the reproductive process. Male worms from a uni-sex infection express the 80 kDa protein at low levels compared with males from a mixed-sex infection, indicating that expression of this protein is increased in worms encopula. Subsequently, Bostic and Strand (1996) succeeded in cloning the *SmGCP* gene encoding the 80 kDa protein. The predicted amino acid sequence of SmGCP suggests that it is involved in cell adhesion, as it shares sequence and structural similarity with four proteins known to be involved in cell adhesion in *Drosophila*, sea urchin, mouse and human (Bostic and Strand, 1996). The observed increase in abundance of the protein in paired worms and the localization of the protein to the gynaecophoric canal suggest that it may be involved in female maturation.

Several genes involved in production of the eggshell have been isolated and cloned from *S. mansoni*, *S. japonicum* and *S. haematobium* (see Bobek *et al.*, 1986, 1989, 1991; Simpson and Knight, 1986; Johnson *et al.*, 1987; Koster *et al.*, 1988; Henkle *et al.*, 1990; Chen *et al.*, 1992). All of these genes share similar expression profiles, are exclusively expressed in the vitelline cells of mature females and are regulated indirectly by worm pairing. Eggshell protein genes are moderately represented (three to five copies) in the schistosome genome, and the eggshell protein genes of *S. mansoni*, *p14* and *p48*, have been estimated to contribute to 5–10% and to 0·3–0·5% respectively of the total mRNA in the mature female (Chen *et al.*, 1992). Each adult female of *S. mansoni* produces ~300 eggs per day, and thus requires a large amount of eggshell protein. A single egg is surrounded by 38 vitelline cells, all of which are thought to contribute to the formation of the eggshell, requiring ~11 000 vitelline cells to be produced per female per day (Erasmus and Davis, 1979).

The regulation of eggshell protein genes has received significant attention. For instance, promoter regions of several eggshell protein genes have been characterized for a range of species of schistosome (Bobek *et al.*, 1989, 1991; Henkle *et al.*, 1990; Chen *et al.*, 1992). Comparisons with promoter regions for chorion genes of silkmoth (*Bombyx mori*) and *Drosophila melanogaster* revealed a number of conserved elements (Mitsialis *et al.*, 1987). One of these, the hexamer TCACGT, has been identified in the promoter region of all eggshell proteins of *S. mansoni* as well as the *p14* gene of *S. japonicum* and *S. haematobium* (see LoVerde and Chen, 1991), and has been demonstrated to be essential for correct spatial and temporal expression of the gene in silkmoth and *Drosophila* (Mitsialis *et al.*, 1989). The TCACGT DNA sequence in *Drosophila* is the target of two transcription factors, one being a zinc finger protein and the other being a member of the steroid hormone receptor family (Shea *et al.*, 1990). Another conserved element, TRRAAT (where R is any pyrimidine), is found in the *p14*, *p48* and *Fs800* genes of *Schistosoma* spp., and in the chorion genes of *Drosophila* and *B. mori*. In *B. mori*, this element is bound by nuclear proteins and effects the qualitative and quantitative expression of reporter genes (Mitsialis *et al.*, 1989). An additional female-specific gene, *F-10*, has been identified and characterized for *S. mansoni* (see Rumjanek *et al.*, 1989; Giannini *et al.*, 1995; Fantappie *et al.*, 1999). The 3′-untranslated region of its mRNA contains a hexanucleotide and a pentanucleotide sequence identical to the hormone regulator elements found in genes regulated by steroids (Rumjanek *et al.*, 1989), suggesting that steroids may be involved in regulating the production of the F-10 protein, and potentially in female development.

Recently, mechanisms for regulating genes encoding proteins associated with eggshell production have been proposed (Fantappie *et al.*, 1999; Freebern *et al.*, 1999a,b). For instance, the promoter of the *p14* gene has been used as a model system to study the regulation of female-specific transcription in *S. mansoni* (see Freebern *et al.*, 1999a). A member of the retinoid X receptor (RXR) family has been implicated in regulation of the *s15* chorion gene of *Drosophila*, because of its binding to the conserved promoter elements (Freebern *et al.*, 1999b). This led Freebern *et al.* (1999b) to design PCR primers to conserved regions of previously characterized RXR proteins, which amplified a 170 bp product from *S. mansoni* adult (mixed-sex) cDNA. This PCR product was then used to screen an adult female *S. mansoni* cDNA library and several clones, which all encoded a 74 kDa retinoid X receptor (SmRXR), were isolated. Western blot analysis indicated that the SmRXR protein is constitutively expressed in adult males and females of *S. mansoni*, indicating that it may also be important in regulating other genes (Freebern *et al.*, 1999b). The ability of SmRXR to act as a transcriptional activator of the *p14* promoter was established using a yeast one-hybrid system and by demonstrating the binding of SmRXR to defined regions of the promoter using gel-shift assays. An additional RXR protein, SmRXR-2, which is also constitutively expressed, was isolated by Freebern *et al.* (1999a), but it was not determined whether it binds to the *p14* promoter. The identification of two steroid hormone receptors from *S. mansoni* may indicate that other steroid receptors with similar biological functions occur in other species of schistosome. The identification and characterization of additional RXR-type proteins from *S. mansoni* and related species, by both targeted cloning and searching EST databases, should provide an opportunity to further define the biological pathways mediated by this protein family and elucidate regulatory aspects of sexual maturation at the molecular level.

Several other female-specifc genes unrelated to eggshell proteins have also been identified in a range of species of schistosome. For example, Eshete and LoVerde (1993) characterized biochemically an abundant phenol oxidase of adult female *S. mansoni*. This enzyme is thought to be involved in cross-linking of eggshell precursors to form the mature eggshell through the conversion of tyrosine to dihydroxyphenylalanine, and subsequently quinones. Also, a yolk-ferritin gene *(fer-1)* of *S. mansoni*, encoding an iron-storage protein, has been characterized and shown to be expressed in the vitelline cells of mature females (Schüssler *et al.*, 1995), while the use of subtractive cDNA libraries enriched for female *S. mansoni* cDNAs allowed Menrath *et al.* (1995) and Schüssler *et al.* (1998) to identify additional female-specific genes. Menrath *et al.* (1995) identified a mucin-like protein (A11) expressed exclusively in the adult females of *S. mansoni*. *In situ* localization of the *A11* mRNA indicated that the gene is expressed in the epithelium surrounding the female reproductive tract adjacent to the entrance into the ootype. It was suggested that the function of the A11 protein may be to provide a protective layer in the reproductive tract and to inhibit premature eggshell formation by reducing the pH in the tract (Menrath *et al.*, 1995). More recently, Schüssler *et al.* (1998) identified a 2191 bp cDNA clone predicted to encode a 691 amino acid protein with sequence similarity to amidases from other organisms, including *C. elegans*, *Emericella nidulans*, *Aspergillus oryzae* and *Rattus norvegicus*. *In situ* hybridization experiments using anti-sense RNA localized the expression of this gene to the gastrodermis of *S. mansoni*, which was the first time that a female-specific gene had been detected external to the reproductive tissues. The predicted biochemical function of this putative amidase and its expression in the gastrodermis suggest that it may be associated with digestive processes in female *S. mansoni*.

Grevelding *et al.* (1997) used an *in vitro* culture system to analyse the expression profiles of three female-specific genes, namely *p14* (eggshell protein), *fer-1* (ferritin iron-storage protein) and *A11* (mucin-like protein) as well as two gender-independent genes, disulfide isomerase (*PDI*) and cathepsin L (*CapL*). In this system, mature females taken from mixed-sex infections were cultured and either paired with males or maintained separately. Expression of the three female-specific genes decreased rapidly when cultured in a uni-sex environment, and after 6 days of maintenance in culture no expression could be detected. Upon re-pairing of females with the males, expression of *p14* and *fer-1* could be detected, but not of *A11*. There was no evidence that the expression profiles for the two gender-independent genes (*PDI* and *CapL*) related to pairing.

The complex interplay between the sexes during pairing indicates that signal transduction mechanisms play an important role in regulating gene expression and hence development. Schüssler *et al.* (1997) characterized three highly conserved signal transduction proteins, Ras, MAP and GAP kinases, using Western blot analysis and showed that the abundance of the kinases varied according to sex and developmental stage. Ras is more abundant in mature than in immature females, GAP is more abundant in females paired with males than in unpaired females, and MAP is more abundant in females than males. Elucidation of the signalling pathways involved in the reception of the male signal and its propagation in the female, leading to sexual maturation, will be central to understanding schistosome biology and may also provide new opportunities for controlling these parasites (Schüssler *et al.*, 1997).

4. NEW TECHNIQUES FOR INVESTIGATING MOLECULAR REPRODUCTIVE PROCESSES

4.1. Expression Profiling

The completion of sequencing of the *C. elegans* genome has facilitated the development of DNA microarray analysis to study differential gene expression during key developmental and reproductive processes. Microarray analysis permits a 'global perspective' of gene expression (Gutierrez, 2000; Lockhart and Winzeler, 2000). The technique involves the automated 'spotting out' of oligonucleotides, cDNAs or genomic DNA (usually corresponding to previously characterized genes) onto glass slides in precise positions. mRNAs from two different stages or tissues are labelled with different fluorescent markers and hybridized to the array. The relative abundance of individual mRNA species in each population is then determined by comparing the relative signal intensity of each fluorescent marker.

Reinke *et al.* (2000) used a DNA microarray containing 11 917 (~63%) predicted genes of *C. elegans* to investigate gene expression during the development of germline tissues. A total of 1416 genes with enriched expression in the germline tissues were identified, which could be divided into three classes. The first class, termed 'germline intrinsic', comprises 508 genes, which are expressed in the germline of hermaphrodites producing either sperm or oocytes. These were proposed to have common functions in germline cells, such as meiosis and recombination, stem cell proliferation and germline development; this proposal was supported by the identification of several genes encoding proteins with sequence similarity to PIWI from *Drosophila melanogaster* and a related protein, ZWILLE, from the plant *Arabidopsis thaliana*, both of which are proteins required for the maintenance of germline stem cells (Cox *et al.*, 1998). The second class comprises 258 genes, which are expressed at elevated levels in hermaphrodites producing oocytes only. Of these, 49 genes are oocyte-specific in their expression while 209 have increased expression compared with that in other tissues. The third class contains 650 genes, which have elevated expression levels or are expressed exclusively in hermaphrodites producing sperm. The large number of genes identified using this microarray approach provided valuable insights into germline development and allowed the prediction of functions. The high incidence of sperm-specific genes suggests that germline cells are highly specialized and require a multitude of genes to function effectively.

Particular classes of proteins are abundantly expressed in spermatozoa. For instance, Reinke *et al.* (2000) found that almost half of the protein phosphatases in *C. elegans* are associated with spermatogenesis, and protein kinases are three times more abundant than random distribution would predict. This raises the question of the relevance of phosphatases and kinases in spermatozoa. Transcription and translation in spermatozoa is halted early in their development, which means that the subsequent maturing of the sperm occurs in an environment devoid of gene transcription and translation (see Figure 2). As kinases and phophatases are enzymes involved in regulation of the activity of other proteins, through the addition or removal of phosphate groups from specific residues, their abundance may reflect a requirement to regulate a range of different proteins involved in sperm maturation, ensuring that the proteins are active only when required.

Another example of the value of DNA microarray analysis is the work of Jiang *et al.* (2001), who investigated the developmental and sex-regulated gene expression profiles of 17 871 (~94%) predicted genes of *C. elegans*. Gene expression profiles of adult hermaphrodites (without eggs) and males were compared, as well as all developmental stages of hermaphrodites. A total of 2171 putative sex-regulated genes (1651 male-enriched and 520 hermaphrodite-enriched) were identified. Many of the genes identified are common to those identified by Reinke *et al.* (2000) and represent germline-expressed genes, while the remainder appeared to correspond to somatically expressed genes. The majority (75–80%) of the latter have sequence similarity to several well-characterized protein families, for example transcription factors, neuronal proteins or G-protein-coupled receptors. The identification of sex-regulated transcription factors should allow the characterization of pathways associated with the development of the different body plans and sex-specific gene expression.

In spite of its usefulness, DNA microarray technology can have some limitations. First, the production of arrays requires the availability of either large-scale genome sequencing or a large number of EST sequences to ensure that a significant proportion of gender-specifically expressed genes are represented.

Even with large EST data sets, it is possible that not all expressed genes will be present. Second, the current sensitivity of detection is not sufficient to identify genes expressed at low levels. Third, false positive results can occur as a consequence of non-specific hybridization of mRNA, although this problem can usually be overcome by using oligonucleotides in the arrays instead of cDNAs. As microarray technology is continuously improving, many of these methodological limitations are likely to be overcome in the very near future. Hence, together with our knowledge of the *C. elegans* genome, microarray approaches provide an exciting opportunity to rapidly improve our understanding of the molecular reproductive processes in parasitic helminths as the EST sequence data sets increase in size. Also, the characterization of *C. elegans* gene homologues in parasites, and the analysis of their functional roles using the *C. elegans* model (see Section 4.2), should provide insights into the reproductive biology of parasitic nematodes at the molecular level. The relatively large percentage of genes with high levels of expression in germline tissues, particularly those related to sperm development and maturation, suggests that they are highly specialized and may be suitable as targets for developing prophylactic or therapeutic interventions.

4.2. Double-stranded RNA-mediated Interference

RNA-mediated interference (RNAi) provides a valuable tool for the analysis of gene function in a number of organisms, including *C. elegans* (see Fire *et al.*, 1998; Tabara *et al.*, 1998), for several reasons. Only small amounts of double-stranded RNA (dsRNA) are required for the RNAi effect, which is thought to be due to an amplification of the dsRNA introduced into the nematode (Fire, 1999). The RNAi effect is systemic, with gene silencing occurring throughout the entire worm. Degradation of the target mRNA is highly specific and is also passed on to the F1 progeny in both *C. elegans* and *Drosophila*. Although the precise mechanism of RNAi is still relatively unclear, the current consensus (reviewed by Fire, 1999; Bass, 2000) is that introduction of dsRNA into an organism leads to a targeted degradation of the homologous mRNA, in many cases producing a null mutant phenotype.

In *C. elegans*, the dsRNA can be introduced into the worm in a variety of ways. The most common means is by microinjection into germline tissues, although injection into the intestine has also proven effective (Fire *et al.*, 1998). An alternative to microinjection is the soaking method, where the worm is bathed in dsRNA (Tabara *et al.*, 1998). However, the most practical, because of its applicability to large-scale screening, is the 'feeding' method (Fire *et al.*, 1998). In this method, *C. elegans* is cultured in the presence of *E. coli* expressing the specific dsRNAs. After ingestion of the *E. coli*, some dsRNA is absorbed by the worm, thus initiating RNAi-based gene silencing.

Although RNAi results are usually reliable in *C. elegans* because they produce phenotypes that resemble those of chromosomal gene knockouts (Kuwabara and Coulson, 2000), there are several potential limitations of the technique that need to be considered. For instance, gene redundancy and the existence of parallel pathways may mask RNAi effects, suppression of closely related non-target gene(s) may incorrectly attribute phenotype to particular genes, and there may be differential susceptibility of tissues to RNAi (Fire *et al.*, 1998; Fire, 1999). Also, there appears to be a limit to the number of different dsRNAs that can be injected simultaneously into a single worm of *C. elegans* before a reduction in the strength of each RNAi phenotype occurs (Gonczy *et al.*, 2000).

In spite of these limitations, the ability to rapidly assess the possible functional roles of EST sequences from helminths by RNAi is likely to improve our understanding of the reproductive biology of parasitic nematodes and may, in the long term, assist in designing effective therapeutic compounds or vaccines. RNAi has also been applied effectively to the protozoan parasite *Trypanosoma brucei* (see Ngo *et al.*, 1998; LaCount *et al.*, 2000; Shi *et al.*, 2000), but the challenge now is to adapt RNAi to helminth parasites. A major obstacle to be overcome is the inability to effectively propagate and maintain most parasitic helminths *in vitro* (Eckert, 1997). Nonetheless, RNAi feeding experiments could be conducted on the early developmental stages (e.g., first and second stage larvae of strongylid nematodes), which feed on bacteria. However, this is likely to identify only genes that are crucial during the early stages of development, and as such, may have limited value for characterizing sexual development and reproduction. Therefore, the development of an effective *in vitro* culture system for parasitic nematodes, which allows access to all life cycle stages, is required before RNAi can be fully exploited. However, where a high level of identity exists between a gene from a parasitic nematode and its *C. elegans* homologue, the putative function of the former can be deduced by RNAi experiments in *C. elegans*. For example, we have cloned a serine/threonine phosphatase from *O. dentatum* that is expressed exclusively in the male adult worm and that shares ~90% similarity with the *C. elegans* homologue (Boag *et al.*, 2000). RNAi experiments in *C. elegans* indicate that this homologue is indeed involved in reproduction, as a reduction in the number of offspring in the F1 generation was apparent in treated hermaphrodites (P.R. Boag, P. Ren, S.E. Newton and R.B. Gasser, personal observations).

4.3. Gene Transformation

Transformation of *C. elegans* has become a routine laboratory tool for assessing gene function since it was first reported (Stinchcomb *et al.*, 1985; Fire, 1986). It involves the microinjection of plasmid DNA into the syncytium (mitotically active) region of the adult hermaphrodite gonad. This DNA undergoes rearrangement to form extrachromosomal tandem arrays comprising hundreds of repeats of the plasmid DNA, which are inherited in a non-Mendelian fashion, whereby typically 5–30% of the progeny inherit the array (Stinchcomb *et al.*, 1985). To aid in the identification of transformed nematodes, a marker plasmid (e.g., the pRF4 plasmid, which contains the *rol-6* gene) is usually co-injected. *C. elegans* individuals containing this marker display a distinctive phenotype, which is readily identifiable.

Gene transformation in *C. elegans* has several potential applications. The expression profile of genes from parasitic nematodes can be determined using their promoter region to drive a reporter gene, such as the green fluorescent protein (GFP) or β-galactosidase. Promoters from several parasites have been shown to be functional in *C. elegans* (Qin *et al.*, 1998; Britton *et al.*, 1999; Page and Winter, 1999). For example, Qin *et al.* (1998) produced transgenic *C. elegans* containing 745 bp of the promoter region from the glyceraldehyde-3-phosphate-dehydrogenase gene from *G. rostochiensis* fused to GFP, and demonstrated GFP expression in muscle tissue. Similar work was carried out by Britton *et al.* (1999) using two promoters from *H. contortus* (*pep-1* and *AC-2*) and the cuticle collagen gene *colost-1* from *Teladorsagia circumcincta*. In these experiments, it was found that the spatial expression of the reporter genes correlated with the expression profiles in the parasite (see Figure 5). However, there were differences in timing of gene expression in *C. elegans* compared with that in the parasite.

A second valuable application of the transformation technology is 'genetic rescue' to demonstrate functional similarity among proteins (Fire and Waterston, 1989), although there is currently a limitation in that transgenes are usually not expressed in germline tissues (Kelly *et al.*, 1997). In such experiments, mutant phenotypes are 'rescued' by introducing the wild-type or a homologous gene into the worm by standard transformation techniques (Stinchcomb *et al.*, 1985; Fire, 1986). Restoration of the mutant to wild-type provides clear evidence that putative homologues are functionally similar. The availability of a large number of *C. elegans* lines carrying mutations for defined genes provides opportunities for carrying out such experiments using genes from parasites. For instance, Kwa *et al.* (1995) used the *C. elegans* line *ben-1*, which is resistant to the anthelmintic class of the benzimidazoles, to study the β-tubulin gene of benzimidazole-susceptible *H. contortus* and to assess the effect of a mutation in the protein at amino acid 200 (Phe → Tyr). *C. elegans* transformed with the wild-type *H. contortus* β-tubulin became sensitive to a benzimidazole, while those containing the altered β-tubulin remained resistant, indicating that resistance to benzimidazoles can be mediated through a single amino acid change as a consequence of a point mutation in the gene. Such an approach could be used to enhance our understanding of some molecular events relating to sexual differentiation, maturation and reproduction in parasitic helminths.

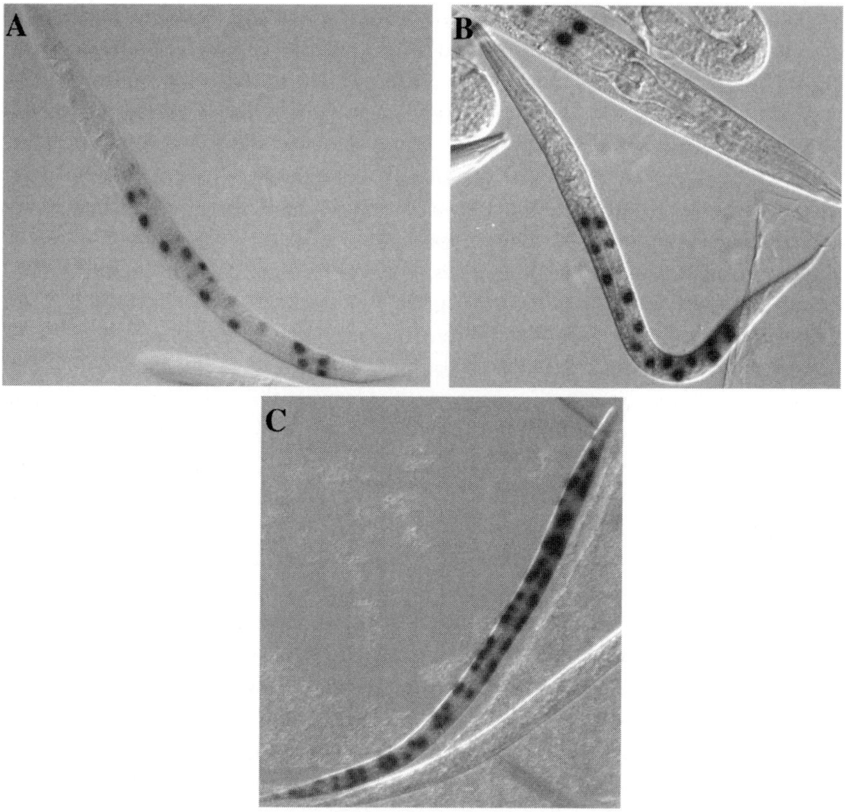

Figure 5 Expression of reporter genes in transgenic *Caenorhabditis elegans* under the control of promoters from parasitic nematodes. The *lac Z* reporter gene was cloned behind each promoter and transgenic *C. elegans* lines generated by microinjection. Expression was detected by staining with 5-bromo-4-chloro-3-indolyl β-D-galactopyranoside (X-gal) (Britton *et al.*, 1999). A and B. Expression of LAC Z in L3 *C. elegans* intestinal cells under control of the *Haemonchus contortus* cysteine protease AC2 promoter (A), and the *H. contortus* pepsinogen promoter (B). C. Expression of LAC Z in hypodermal cells of *C. elegans* L4 under control of the promoter for the *Teladorsagia circumcincta* collagen gene *colost-1*. These images were kindly provided by Dr C. Britton (Wellcome Centre for Molecular Parasitology, University of Glasgow).

5. CONCLUSIONS AND PROSPECTS

Many helminths (e.g., trematodes, cestodes and nematodes) that parasitize plants, animals and humans are of socio-economic importance because of the diseases and production losses they cause. Their sexual reproduction within the host results in the production of developmental stages that are infective to the next host. Therefore, understanding reproductive processes in dioecious parasitic helminths is of fundamental scientific relevance, and may also have major implications for control by interfering with parasite development or maturation. Central to studying reproductive biology is the identification and characterization of genes that exhibit sex-specific expression patterns. However, to date, only a small number of such genes have been isolated from parasitic helminths of animal and human health importance. This is surprising, given that molecules that are involved in sexual development may be expressed for short periods of time and hence may provide unique candidates amenable to intervention.

Recent technological advances now pave the way for rapid progress in discovering and characterizing the functions of genes associated with reproductive processes. Large-scale EST-sequencing programs for parasitic helminths (e.g., Blaxter and Ivens, 1999; Blaxter, 2000) will allow catalogues of genes to be established, which should assist in the identification of genes related to sexual differentiation, maturation, development, and attraction and behaviour. Such EST data sets will also provide a foundation for functional genomics using a range of new techniques currently being pioneered in the free-living nematode *C. elegans*. These include large-scale protein–protein interaction studies with the yeast two-hybrid system, gene expression studies using DNA microarrays, gene deletion studies and/or gene silencing in *C. elegans* by double-stranded RNA-mediated interference. Importantly, the availability of the *C. elegans* model, knowledge of its complete genome and information emerging on gene function provide unique opportunities for assessing the putative functions of gene orthologues from parasitic helminths, given that most of the latter are difficult or impossible to propagate or maintain in culture *in vitro*. However, since *C. elegans* is a free-living nematode, it is reasonable to expect that some genes and pathways will be unique to parasites, including some aspects involved in reproduction, as the reproductive stages occur within their host. Moreover, differences in the niches occupied by different parasites in their hosts and the characteristics of their interactions with the host are likely to be reflected in differences in genes and biological pathways between different species, possibly including reproduction. Understanding reproductive processes at the molecular level by employing these advanced techniques, or adaptations thereof, to the study of parasitic helminths in an integrated way should provide insights into sex determination and subsequent development of reproductive tissues and sexual behaviour, and even into components of signal transduction and transcription pathways, including sex attractants, their receptors, and secondary messages and downstream transcription factors. These insights will provide a molecular basis for understanding the fundamentals of reproductive biology in parasitic helminths. This will be of particular relevance if there is only a limited number of pathways controlling sexual differentiation and development, because being able to disrupt or block such pathways in parasitic helminths could to lead to novel and innovative approaches for their control.

ACKNOWLEDGEMENTS

Project support through the Australian Research Council, Novartis Animal Health Australia, the Department of Natural Resources and Environment Victoria, and the Danish Centre for Experimental Parasitology is gratefully acknowledged. P.R.B. is the recipient of a scholarship from The University of Melbourne and Novartis Australia. We are grateful to Dr Collette Britton for kindly providing the images for Figure 5.

REFERENCES

Akerib, C.C. and Meyer, B.J. (1994). Identification of X chromosome regions in *Caenorhabditis elegans* that contain sex-determination signal elements. *Genetics* **138**, 1105–1125.

Albertson, D.G., Nwaorgu, O.C. and Sulston, J.E. (1979). Chromatin diminution and a chromosomal mechanism of sexual differentiation in *Strongyloides papillosus*. *Chromosoma* **75**, 75–87.

Aronstein, W.S. and Strand, M. (1983). Identification of species-specific and gender-specific proteins and glycoproteins of three human schistosomes. *Journal of Parasitology* **96**, 1006–1017.

Aronstein, W.S. and Strand, M. (1985). A glycoprotein antigen of *Schistosoma mansoni* expressed on the gynecophoral canal of mature male worms. *American Journal of Tropical Medicine and Hygiene* **34**, 508–512.

Ashton, F.T., Li, J. and Schad, G.A. (1999). Chemo- and thermosensory neurons: structure and function in animal parasitic nematodes. *Veterinary Parasitology* **84**, 297–316.

Atkinson, G.G. and Atkinson, K.H. (1982). *Schistosoma mansoni*: One-two dimensional electrophoresis of proteins synthesized *in vitro* by male, female, and juveniles. *Experimental Parasitology* **53**, 26–38.

Basch, P.F. and Nicolas, C. (1989). *Schistosoma mansoni*: pairing of male worms with artificial surrogate females. *Experimental Parasitology* **68**, 202–207.

Bass, B.L. (2000). Double-stranded RNA as a template for gene silencing. *Cell* **101**, 235–238.

Bennett, G. and Ward, S. (1986). Neither a germ line-specific nor several somatically expressed genes are lost or rearranged during embryonic chromatin diminution in the nematode *Ascaris lumbricoides* var. *suum*. *Developmental Biology* **118**, 141–147.

Bessarab, I.N. and Joshua, G.W. (1997). Stage-specific gene expression in *Angiostrongylus cantonensis*: characterisation and expression of an adult-specific gene. *Molecular and Biochemical Parasitology* **88**, 73–84.

Blaxter, M. (1998). *Caenorhabditis elegans* is a nematode. *Science* **282**, 2041–2046.

Blaxter, M. (2000). Genes and genomes of *Necator americanus* and related hookworms. *International Journal for Parasitology* **30**, 347–355.

Blaxter, M. and Ivens, A. (1999). Reports from the cutting edge of parasitic genome analysis. *Parasitology Today* **15**, 430–431.

Boag, P.R., Newton, S.E., Hansen, N.-P., Christensen, C.M., Nansen, P. and Gasser, R.B. (2000). Isolation and characterisation of sex-specific transcripts from *Oesophagostomum dentatum* by RNA arbitrarily-primed PCR. *Molecular and Biochemical Parasitology* **108**, 217–224.

Bobek, L., Rekosh, D.M., van Keulen, H. and LoVerde, P.T. (1986). Characterization of a female-specific cDNA derived from a developmentally regulated mRNA in the human blood fluke *Schistosoma mansoni*. *Proceedings of the National Academy of Sciences of the USA* **83**, 5544–5548.

Bobek, L.A., LoVerde, P.T. and Rekosh, D.M. (1989). *Schistosoma haematobium*: analysis of eggshell protein genes and their expression. *Experimental Parasitology* **68**, 17–30.

Bobek, L.A., Rekosh, D.M. and LoVerde, P.T. (1991). *Schistosoma japonicum*: analysis of eggshell protein genes, their expression, and comparison with similar genes from other schistosomes. *Experimental Parasitology* **72**, 381–390.

Bone, L.W. (1982). *Nippostrongylus brasiliensis*: female incubation, release of pheromone, fractionation of incubates. *Experimental Parasitology* **54**, 12–20.

Bone, L.W., Gaston, L.K. and Reed, S.K. (1980). Production and activity of the Kav 0.64 pheromone fraction of *Nippostrongylus brasiliensis*. *Journal of Parasitology* **66**, 268–273.

Bostic, J.R. and Strand, M. (1996). Molecular cloning of a *Schistosoma mansoni* protein expressed in the gynecophoral canal of male worms. *Molecular and Biochemical Parasitology* **79**, 79–89.

Britton, C., Redmond, D.L., Knox, D.P., McKerrow, J.H. and Barry, J.D. (1999). Identification of promoter elements of parasite nematode genes in transgenic *Caenorhabditis elegans*. *Molecular and Biochemical Parasitology* **103**, 171–181.

Bullock, T.L., McCoy, A.J., Kent, H.M., Roberts, T.M. and Stewart, M. (1998). Structural basis for amoeboid motility in nematode sperm. *Nature Structural Biology* **5**, 184–189.

Burke, D.J. and Ward, S. (1983). Identification of a large multigene family encoding the major sperm protein of *Caenorhabditis elegans*. *Journal of Molecular Biology* **171**, 1–29.

Carmi, I., Kopczynski, J.B. and Meyer, B.J. (1998). The nuclear hormone receptor SEX-1 is an X-chromosome signal that determines nematode sex. *Nature* **396**, 168–173.

Chang, C. and Sternberg, P.W. (1999). *C. elegans* vulval development as a model system to study the cancer biology of EGFR signaling. *Cancer and Metastasis Reviews* **18**, 203–213.

Chen, P. and Ellis, R.E. (2000). TRA-1A regulates transcription of *fog-3*, which controls germ cell fate in *C. elegans*. *Development* **127**, 3119–3129.

Chen, L.L., Rekosh, D.M. and LoVerde, P.T. (1992). *Schistosoma mansoni p48* eggshell protein gene: characterization, developmentally regulated expression and comparison to the *p14* eggshell protein gene. *Molecular and Biochemical Parasitology* **52**, 39–52.

Chen, J.S., Sappington, T.W. and Raikhel, A.S. (1997). Extensive sequence conservation among insect, nematode, and vertebrate vitellogenins reveals ancient common ancestry. *Journal of Molecular Evolution* **44**, 440–451.

Christensen, C.M. (1997). The effect of three distinct sex ratios at two *Oesophagostomum dentatum* worm population densities. *Journal of Parasitology* **83**, 636–640.

Christensen, C.M., Barnes, E.H., Nansen, P., Roepstorff, A. and Slotved, H.C. (1995). Experimental *Oesophagostomum dentatum* infection in the pig: worm populations resulting from single infections with three doses of larvae. *International Journal for Parasitology* **25**, 1491–1498.

Christensen, C.M., Grøndahl-Nielsen, C. and Nansen, P. (1996). Non-surgical transplantation of *Oesophagostomum dentatum* to recipient pigs via rectal intubation. *Veterinary Parasitology* **65**, 139–145.

Christensen, C.M., Nansen, P. and Barnes, E.H. (1997). The effect of concurrent or sequential *Oesophagostomum dentatum* and *O. quadrispinulatum* infections on the worm burdens of the two species in pigs. *Parasitology* **114**, 273–278.
Civetta, A. and Singh, R.S. (1998). Sex-related genes, directional sexual selection, and speciation. *Molecular Biology and Evolution* **15**, 901–909.
Cline, T.W. and Meyer, B.J. (1996). Vive la difference: males vs females in flies vs worms. *Annual Review of Genetics* **30**, 637–702.
Clough, E.R. (1981). Morphology and reproductive organs and oogenesis in bisexual and unisexual transplants of mature *Schistosoma mansoni* females. *Journal of Parasitology* **67**, 535–539.
Cornford, E.M. and Fitzpatrick, A.M. (1985). The mechanism and rate of glucose transfer from male to female schistosomes. *Molecular and Biochemical Parasitology* **17**, 131–141.
Cornford, E.M. and Huot, M.E. (1981). Glucose transfer from male to female schistosomes. *Science* **213**, 1269–1271.
Cox, D.N., Chao, A., Baker, J., Chang, L., Qiao, D. and Lin, H. (1998). A novel class of evolutionarily conserved genes defined by piwi are essential for stem cell self-renewal. *Genes and Development* **12**, 3715–3727.
Culetto, E. and Sattelle, D.B. (2000). A role for *Caenorhabditis elegans* in understanding the function and interactions of human disease genes. *Human Molecular Genetics* **9**, 869–877.
Daugschies, A. and Ruttkowski, B. (1998). Modulation of migration of *Oesophagostomum dentatum* larvae by inhibitors and products of eicosanoid metabolism. *International Journal for Parasitology* **28**, 355–362.
Daugschies, A. and Watzel, C. (1999). *In vitro* development of histotropic larvae of *Oesophagostomum dentatum* under various conditions of cultivation. *Parasitology Research* **85**, 158–161.
deBono, M. and Hodgkin, J. (1996). Evolution of sex determination in *Caenorhabditis*: unusually high divergence of *tra-1* and its functional consequences. *Genetics* **144**, 587–595.
Delves, C.J., Howells, R.E. and Post, R.J. (1986). Gametogenesis and fertilization in *Dirofilaria immitis* (Nematoda: Filarioidea). *Parasitology* **92**, 181–197.
Den Hollander, J.E. and Erasmus, D.A. (1985). *Schistosoma mansoni*: male stimulation and DNA synthesis by the female. *Parasitology* **91**, 449–457.
Diatchenko, L., Lau, Y.F., Campbell, A.P., Chenchik, A., Moqadam, F., Huang, B., Lukyanov, S., Lukyanov, K., Gurskaya, N., Sverdlov, E.D. and Siebert, P.D. (1996). Suppression subtractive hybridization: a method for generating differentially regulated or tissue-specific cDNA probes and libraries. *Proceedings of the National Academy of Sciences of the USA* **93**, 6025–6030.
Drew, A.C. and Brindley, P.J. (1995). Female-specific sequences isolated from *Schistosoma mansoni* by representational difference analysis. *Molecular and Biochemical Parasitology* **71**, 173–181.
Eckert, J. (1997). Alternatives to animal experimentation in parasitology. *Veterinary Parasitology* **71**, 99–120.
Erasmus, D.A. (1973). A comparative study of the reproductive system of mature, immature and 'unisexual' female *Schistosoma mansoni*. *Parasitology* **67**, 165–183.
Erasmus, D.A. and Davis, T.W. (1979). *Schistosoma mansoni* and *S. haematobium*: calcium metabolism of the vitelline cell. *Experimental Parasitology* **47**, 91–106.
Eshete, F. and LoVerde, P.T. (1993). Characteristics of phenol oxidase of *Schistosoma mansoni* and its functional implications in eggshell synthesis. *Journal of Parasitology* **79**, 309–317.
Fantappie, M.R., Correa-Oliveira, R., Caride, E.C., Geraldo, E.A., Agnew, A. and Rumjanek, F.D. (1999). Comparison between site-specific DNA binding proteins of

male and female *Schistosoma mansoni*. *Comparative Biochemistry and Physiology. B: Comparative Biochemistry* **124**, 33–40.
Favre, R., Cermola, M., Nunes, C.P., Hermann, R., Muller, M. and Bazzicalupo, P. (1998). Immuno-cross-reactivity of CUT-1 and cuticlin epitopes between *Ascaris lumbricoides*, *Caenorhabditis elegans* and *Heterorhabditis*. *Journal of Structural Biology* **123**, 1–7.
Fire, A. (1986). Integrative transformation of *Caenorhabditis elegans*. *EMBO Journal* **5**, 2673–2680.
Fire, A. (1999). RNA-triggered gene silencing. *Trends in Genetics* **15**, 358–363.
Fire, A. and Waterston, R.H. (1989). Proper expression of myosin genes in transgenic nematodes. *EMBO Journal* **8**, 3419–3428.
Fire, A., Xu, S., Montgomery, M.K., Kostas, S.A., Driver, S.E. and Mello, C.C. (1998). Potent and specific genetic interference by double-stranded RNA in *Caenorhabditis elegans*. *Nature* **391**, 806–811.
Freebern, W.J., Niles, E.G. and LoVerde, P.T. (1999a). RXR-2, a member of the retinoid X receptor family in *Schistosoma mansoni*. *Gene* **233**, 33–38.
Freebern, W.J., Osman, A., Niles, E.G., Christen, L. and LoVerde, P.T. (1999b). Identification of a cDNA encoding a retinoid X receptor homologue from *Schistosoma mansoni*. Evidence for a role in female-specific gene expression. *Journal of Biological Chemistry* **274**, 4577–4585.
Gasser, R.B., Morahan, G. and Mitchell, G.F. (1991). Sexing single larval stages of *Schistosoma mansoni* by polymerase chain reaction. *Molecular and Biochemical Parasitology* **47**, 255–258.
Giannini, A.L., Caride, E.C., Braga, V.M. and Rumjanek, F.D. (1995). *F-10* nuclear binding proteins of *Schistosoma mansoni*: structural and functional features. *Parasitology* **110**, 155–161.
Glassburg, G.H., Zalisko, E. and Bone, L.W. (1981). *In vivo* pheromone activity in *Nippostrongylus brasiliensis* (Nematoda). *Journal of Parasitology* **67**, 898–905.
Goldstein, P. and Moens, P.B. (1976). Karyotype analysis of *Ascaris lumbricoides* var. *suum*. Male and female pachytene nuclei by 3-D reconstruction from electron microscopy of serial sections. *Chromosoma* **58**, 101–111.
Goldstein, P. and Triantaphyllou, A.C. (1979). Karyotype analysis of the plant-parasitic nematode *Heterodera glycines* by electron microscopy. 1. The diploid. *Journal of Cell Science* **40**, 171–179.
Gonczy, P., Echeverri, G., Oegema, K., Coulson, A., Jones, S.J., Copley, R.R., Duperon, J., Oegema, J., Brehm, M., Cassin, E., Hannak, E., Kirkham, M., Pichler, S., Flohrs, K., Goessen, A., Leidel, S., Alleaume, A.M., Martin, C., Ozlu, N., Bork, P. and Hyman, A.A. (2000). Functional genomic analysis of cell division in *C. elegans* using RNAi of genes on chromosome III. *Nature* **408**, 331–336.
Grant, B. and Hirsh, D. (1999). Receptor-mediated endocytosis in the *Caenorhabditis elegans* oocyte. *Molecular Biology of the Cell* **10**, 4311–4326.
Green, C.D. (1980). Nematode sex attractants. *Helminthological Abstracts Series B* **49**, 81–93.
Green, C.D. and Plumb, S.C. (1970). The interrelationships of some *Heterodera* spp. indicated by the specificity of the male attractants by their females. *Nematologica* **16**, 39–46.
Grevelding, C.G., Sommer, G. and Kunz, W. (1997). Female-specific gene expression in *Schistosoma mansoni* is regulated by pairing. *Parasitology* **115**, 635–640.
Grossman, A.I., Short, R.B. and Cain, G.D. (1981). Karyotype evolution and sex chromosome differentiation in schistosomes (Trematoda, Schistosomatidae). *Chromosoma* **84**, 413–430.
Gupta, B.C. and Basch, P.F. (1987). Evidence for transfer of a glycoprotein from male to female *Schistosoma mansoni* during pairing. *Journal of Parasitology* **73**, 674–675.

Gutierrez, J.A. (2000). Genomics: from novel genes to new therapeutics in parasitology. *International Journal for Parasitology* **30**, 247–252.

Haag, E.S. and Kimble, J. (2000). Regulatory elements required for development of *Caenorhabditis elegans* hermaphrodites are conserved in the *tra-2* homologue of *C. remanei*, a male/female sister species. *Genetics* **155**, 105–116.

Hansen, D. and Pilgrim, D. (1998). Molecular evolution of a sex determination protein FEM-2 (pp2c) in *Caenorhabditis*. *Genetics* **149**, 1353–1362.

Hartman, D., Donald, D.R., Nikolaou, S., Savin, K.W., Hasse, D., Presidente, P.J.A. and Newton, S.E. (2001). Analysis of developmentally regulated genes of the parasite *Haemonchus contortus*. *International Journal for Parasitology* **31**, 1236–1245.

Haseeb, M.A. and Fried, B. (1988). Chemical communication in helminths. *Advances in Parasitology* **27**, 169–207.

Haseeb, M.A., Eveland, L.K. and Fried, B. (1985). The uptake, localization and transfer of [4-^{14}C]cholesterol in *Schistosoma mansoni* males and females maintained *in vitro*. *Comparative Biochemistry and Physiology. A: Comparative Physiology* **82**, 421–423.

Haseeb, M.A., Fried, B. and Eveland, L.K. (1989). *Schistosoma mansoni*: female-dependent lipid secretion in males and corresponding changes in lipase activity. *International Journal for Parasitology* **19**, 705–709.

Hengartner, M.O. (1997). Cell death. In: *C. elegans II* (D.L. Riddle, T. Blumenthal, B.J. Meyer and J.R. Priess, eds), pp. 383–415. Cold Spring Harbor: Cold Spring Harbor Laboratory Press.

Henkle, K.J., Cook, G.A., Foster, L.A., Engman, D.M., Bobek, L.A., Cain, G.D. and Donelson, J.E. (1990). The gene family encoding eggshell proteins of *Schistosoma japonicum*. *Molecular and Biochemical Parasitology* **42**, 69–82.

Hirai, H., Tada, I., Takahashi, H., Nwoke, B.E. and Ufomadu, G.O. (1987). Chromosomes of *Onchocerca volvulus* (Spirurida: Onchocercidae): a comparative study between Nigeria and Guatemala. *Journal of Helminthology* **61**, 43–46.

Hodgkin, J., Zellan, J.D. and Albertson, D.G. (1994). Identification of a candidate primary sex determination locus, *fox-1*, on the X chromosome of *Caenorhabditis elegans*. *Development* **120**, 3681–3689.

Hubbard, E.J. and Greenstein, D. (2000). The *Caenorhabditis elegans* gonad: a test tube for cell and developmental biology. *Developmental Dynamics* **218**, 2–22.

Jaffe, H., Huettel, R.N., Demilo, A.B., Hayes, D.K. and Rebois, R.V. (1989). Isolation and identification of a compound from soybean cyst nematode, *Heterodera glycines*, with sex pheromone activity. *Journal of Chemical Ecology* **15**, 2031–2043.

Jiang, M., Ryu, J., Kiraly, M., Duke, K., Reinke, V. and Kim, S.K. (2001). Genome-wide analysis of developmental and sex-regulated gene expression profiles in *Caenorhabditis elegans*. *Proceedings of the National Academy of Sciences of the USA* **98**, 218–223.

Jin, J., Poole, C.B., Slatko, B.E. and McReynolds, L.A. (1999). Alternative splicing creates sex-specific transcripts and truncated forms of the furin protease in the parasite *Dirofilaria immitis*. *Gene* **237**, 161–175.

Johnson, K.S., Taylor, D.W. and Cordingley, J.S. (1987). Possible eggshell protein gene from *Schistosoma mansoni*. *Molecular and Biochemical Parasitology* **22**, 89–100.

Joshua, G.W. and Hsieh, C.Y. (1995). Stage-specifically expressed genes of *Angiostrongylus cantonensis*: identification by differential display. *Molecular and Biochemical Parasitology* **71**, 285–289.

Jungersen, G., Eriksen, L., Nansen, P. and Fagerholm, H.P. (1997). Sex-manipulated *Ascaris suum* infections in pigs: implications for reproduction. *Parasitology* **115**, 439–442.

Kahel-Raifer, H. and Glazer, I. (2000). Environmental factors affecting sexual differentiation in the entomopathogenic nematode *Heterorhabditis bacteriophora*. *Journal of Experimental Zoology* **287**, 158–166.

Kelly, W.G., Xu, S., Montgomery, M.K. and Fire, A. (1997). Distinct requirements for somatic and germline expression of a generally expressed *Caernorhabditis elegans* gene. *Genetics* **146**, 227–238.

Kimble, K. and Ward, S. (1988). Germ-line development and fertilization. In: *The Nematode* Caenorhabditis elegans. (B. Wood, ed.), pp. 191–213. Cold Spring Harbor: Cold Spring Harbor Laboratory Press.

King, K.L., Essig, J., Roberts, T.M. and Moerland, T.S. (1994). Regulation of the *Ascaris* major sperm protein (MSP) cytoskeleton by intracellular pH. *Cell Motility and the Cytoskeleton* **27**, 193–205.

Klass, M.R. and Hirsh, D. (1981). Sperm isolation and biochemical analysis of the major sperm protein from *Caenorhabditis elegans*. *Developmental Biology* **84**, 299–312.

Klass, M., Dow, B. and Herndon, M. (1982). Cell-specific transcriptional regulation of the major sperm protein in *Caenorhabditis elegans*. *Developmental Biology* **93**, 152–164.

Klass, M., Ammons, D. and Ward, S. (1988). Conservation in the 5′ flanking sequences of transcribed members of the *Caenorhabditis elegans* major sperm protein gene family. *Journal of Molecular Biology* **199**, 15–22.

Koster, B., Dargatz, H., Schroder, J., Hirzmann, J., Haarmann, C., Symmons, P. and Kunz, W. (1988). Identification and localisation of the products of a putative eggshell precursor gene in the vitellarium of *Schistosoma mansoni*. *Molecular and Biochemical Parasitology* **31**, 183–198.

Kunz, W. and Symmons, P. (1987). Gender-specifically expressed genes in *Schistosoma mansoni*. *Acta Tropica Supplement* **12**, 90–93.

Kuwabara, P.E. (1996a). Interspecies comparison reveals evolution of control regions in the nematode sex-determining gene *tra-2*. *Genetics* **144**, 597–607.

Kuwabara, P.E. (1996b). A novel regulatory mutation in the *C. elegans* sex determination gene *tra-2* defines a candidate ligand/receptor interaction site. *Development* **122**, 2089–2098.

Kuwabara, P.E. and Coulson, A. (2000). RNAi – prospects for a general technique for determining gene function. *Parasitology Today* **16**, 347–349.

Kuwabara, P.E. and Shah, S. (1994). Cloning by synteny: identifying *C. briggsae* homologues of *C. elegans* genes. *Nucleic Acids Research* **22**, 4414–4418.

Kwa, M.S., Veenstra, J.G., Van Dijk, M. and Roos, M.H. (1995). Beta-tubulin genes from the parasitic nematode *Haemonchus contortus* modulate drug resistance in *Caenorhabditis elegans*. *Journal of Molecular Biology* **246**, 500–510.

LaCount, D.J., Bruse, S., Hill, K.L. and Donelson, J.E. (2000). Double-stranded RNA interference in *Trypanosoma brucei* using head-to-head promoters. *Molecular and Biochemical Parasitology* **111**, 67–76.

LaMunyon, C.W. and Ward, S. (1998). Larger sperm outcompete smaller sperm in the nematode *Caenorhabditis elegans*. *Proceedings of the Royal Society of London. Series B: Biological Sciences* **265**, 1997–2002.

LaMunyon, C.W. and Ward, S. (1999). Evolution of sperm size in nematodes: sperm competition favours larger sperm. *Proceedings of the Royal Society of London. Series B: Biological Sciences* **266**, 263–267.

LeJambre, L.F. (1968). The chromosome numbers of *Oesophagostomum columbianum* curtice and *Chabertia ovina* fabricius (Nematoda, Strongylata). *Transactions of the American Microscopical Society* **87**, 105–106.

LeJambre, L.F. and Georgi, J.R. (1970). Influence of fertilization on ovogenesis in *Ancylostoma caninum*. *Journal of Parasitology* **56**, 131–137.

L'Hernault, S.W. (1997). Spermatogenesis. In: *C. elegans II* (D.L. Riddle, T. Blumenthal, B.J. Meyer and J.R. Priess, eds), pp. 271–294. Cold Spring Harbor: Cold Spring Harbor Laboratory Press.

Liberatos, J.D. (1987). *Schistosoma mansoni*: male-biased sex ratios in snails and mice. *Experimental Parasitology* **64**, 165–177.

Liberatos, J.D. and Short, R.B. (1983). Identification of sex of schistosome larval stages. *Journal of Parasitology* **69**, 1084–1089.

Llado, R.R., Urwin, P., Atkinson, H. and Gilmartin, P.M. (1998). *Hgm1*, a novel male-specific gene from *Heterodera glycines* identified by differential mRNA display. *Molecular and Biochemical Parasitology* **95**, 45–52.

Lockhart, D.J. and Winzeler, E.A. (2000). Genomics, gene expression and DNA arrays. *Nature* **405**, 827–836.

LoVerde, P.T. and Chen, L. (1991). Schistosome female reproductive development. *Parasitology Today* **7**, 303–308.

MacMorris, M., Spieth, J., Madej, C., Lea, K. and Blumenthal, T. (1994). Analysis of the VPE sequences in the *Caenorhabditis elegans vit-2* promoter with extrachromosomal tandem array-containing transgenic strains. *Molecular and Cell Biology* **14**, 484–491.

Maizels, R.M., Tetteh, K.K. and Loukas, A. (2000). *Toxocara canis*: genes expressed by the arrested infective larval stage of a parasitic nematode. *International Journal for Parasitology* **30**, 495–508.

McCarter, J., Bartlett, B., Dang, T. and Schedl, T. (1999). On the control of oocyte meiotic maturation and ovulation in *Caenorhabditis elegans*. *Developmental Biology* **205**, 111–128.

McManus, D.P. (1999). The search for a vaccine against schistosomiasis – a difficult path but an achievable goal. *Immunology Reviews* **171**, 149–161.

Menrath, M., Michel, A. and Kunz, W. (1995). A female-specific cDNA sequence of *Schistosoma mansoni* encoding a mucin-like protein that is expressed in the epithelial cells of the reproductive duct. *Parasitology* **111**, 477–483.

Meyer, B.J. (1997). Sex determination and X chromosome dosage compensation. In: *C. elegans II*. (D.L. Riddle, T. Blumenthal, B.J. Meyer and J.R. Priess, eds), pp. 209–240. Cold Spring Harbor: Cold Spring Harbor Laboratory Press.

Meyer, B.J. (2000). Sex in the worm: counting and compensating X-chromosome dose. *Trends in Genetics* **16**, 247–253.

Michalski, M.L. and Weil, G.J. (1999). Gender-specific gene expression in *Brugia malayi*. *Molecular and Biochemical Parasitology* **104**, 247–257.

Mitchell, G.F., Garcia, E.G., Wood, S.M., Diasanta, R., Almonte, R., Calica, E., Davern, K.M. and Tiu, W.U. (1990). Studies on the sex ratio of worms in schistosome infections. *Parasitology* **101**, 27–34.

Mitchell, G.F., Garcia, E.G., Rivera, P.T., Tiu, W.U. and Davern, K.M. (1994). Evidence for and implications of anti-embryonation immunity in schistosomiasis. *Experimental Parasitology* **79**, 546–549.

Mitsialis, S.A., Spoerel, N., Leviten, M. and Kafatos, F.C. (1987). A short 5′-flanking DNA region is sufficient for developmentally correct expression of moth chorion genes in *Drosophila*. *Proceedings of the National Academy of Sciences of the USA* **84**, 7987–7991.

Mitsialis, S.A., Veletza, S. and Kafatos, F.C. (1989). Transgenic regulation of moth chorion gene promoters in *Drosophila*: tissue, temporal, and quantitative control of four bidirectional promoters. *Journal of Molecular Evolution* **29**, 486–495.

Moore, D.V., Yolles, T.K. and Meleney, H.E. (1954). The relationship of male worms to the sexual development of female *Schistosoma mansoni*. *Journal of Parasitology* **40**, 166–185.

Müller, F. and Tobler, H. (2000). Chromatin diminution in the parasitic nematodes *Ascaris suum* and *Parascaris univalens*. *International Journal for Parasitology* **30**, 391–399.

Mutafova, T. (1995). Meiosis and some aspects of cytological mechanisms of chromosomal sex determination in nematode species. *International Journal for Parasitology* **25**, 453–462.

Nelson, G.A. and Ward, S. (1980). Vesicle fusion, pseudopod extension and amoeboid motility are induced in nematode spermatids by the ionophore monensin. *Cell* **19**, 457–464.

Nelson, G.A. and Ward, S. (1981). Amoeboid motility and actin in *Ascaris lumbricoides* sperm. *Experimental Cell Research* **131**, 149–160.

Ngo, H., Tschudi, C., Gull, K. and Ullu, E. (1998). Double-stranded RNA induces mRNA degradation in *Trypanosoma brucei. Proceedings of the National Academy of Sciences of the USA* **95**, 14687–14692.

Nirde, P., De Reggi, M.L., Tsoupras, G., Torpier, G., Fressancourt, P. and Capron, A. (1984). Excretion of ecdysteroids by schistosomes as a marker of parasite infection. *FEBS Letters* **168**, 235–240.

Nirde, O., De Reggi, M.L. and Capron, A. (1986). Fundamental aspects and potential roles of ecdysteroids in schistosomiasis. An update overview. *Journal of Chemical Ecology* **12**, 1863–1884.

Opperman, C.H. and Bird, D.M. (1998). The soybean cyst nematode, *Heterodera glycines*: a genetic model system for the study of plant-parasitic nematodes. *Current Opinion in Plant Biology* **1**, 342–346.

Page, A.P. and Winter, A.D. (1999). Expression pattern and functional significance of a divergent nematode cyclophilin in *Caenorhabditis elegans. Molecular and Biochemical Parasitology* **99**, 301–306.

Platt, H.M. (1994). Foreword. In: *The Phylogenetic Systematics of Free-living Nematodes* (S. Lorenzen, ed.), pp. i–ii. London: The Ray Society.

Popiel, I. and Basch, P.F. (1984). Putative polypeptide transfer from male to female *Schistosoma mansoni. Molecular and Biochemical Parasitology* **11**, 179–188.

Popiel, I. and Erasmus, D. (1982). *Schistosoma mansoni*: The survival and reproductive status of mature infections in mice treated with oxamniquine. *Journal of Helminthology* **56**, 257–262.

Popiel, I., Cioli, D. and Erasmus, D.A. (1984). The morphology and reproductive status of female *Schistosoma mansoni* following separation from male worms. *International Journal for Parasitology* **14**, 183–190.

Post, R.J. and Pinder, M. (1995). Oogenesis and embryogenesis in *Loa loa. Journal of Helminthology* **69**, 351–356.

Post, R.J., McCall, P.J., Trees, A.J., Delves, C.J. and Kouyate, B. (1989). Chromosomes of six species of *Onchocerca* (Nematoda: Filarioidea). *Tropical Medicine and Parasitology* **40**, 292–294.

Qin, L., Smant, G., Stokkermans, J., Bakker, J., Schots, A. and Helder, J. (1998). Cloning of a trans-spliced glyceraldehyde-3-phosphate-dehydrogenase gene from the potato cyst nematode *Globodera rostochiensis* and expression of its putative promoter region in *Caenorhabditis elegans. Molecular and Biochemical Parasitology* **96**, 59–67.

Quack, T., Doenhoff, M., Kunz, W. and Grevelding, C.G. (1998). *Schistosoma mansoni*: the varying occurrence of repetitive elements in different strains shows sex-specific polymorphisms. *Experimental Parasitology* **89**, 222–227.

Raghunathan, L. and Bruckner, D. (1975). Identification of sex in *Schistosoma mansoni* cercariae. *Journal of Parasitology* **61**, 66–68.

Reinke, V., Smith, H.E., Nance, J., Wang, J., Van Doren, C., Begley, R., Jones, S.J., Davis, E.B., Scherer, S., Ward, S. and Kim, S.K. (2000). A global profile of germline gene expression in *C. elegans. Molecular Cell* **6**, 605–616.

Renou, M. and Guerrero, A. (2000). Insect parapheromones in olfaction research and semiochemical-based pest control strategies. *Annual Review of Entomology* **45**, 605–630.

Ribeiro-Paes, J.T. and Rodrigues, V. (1997). Sex determination and female reproductive development in the genus *Schistosoma*: a review. *Revista do Instituto de Medicina Tropical de Sao Paulo* **39**, 337–344.

Riddle, D.L., Blumenthal, T., Meyer, B.J. and Priess, J.R. (eds) (1997). *C. elegans II*. Cold Spring Harbor: Cold Spring Harbor Laboratory Press.

Riga, E., Perry, R.N., Barrett, J. and Johnston, M.R.L. (1996). Electrophysiological response of males of the potato cyst nematodes, *Globodera rostochiensis* and *G. pallida*, to their sex pheromones. *Parasitology* **112**, 239–246.

Riga, E., Holdsworth, D.R., Perry, R.N., Barrett, J. and Johnston, M.R. (1997). Electrophysiological analysis of the response of males of the potato cyst nematode, *Globodera rostochiensis*, to fractions of their homospecific sex pheromone. *Parasitology* **115**, 311–316.

Roberts, T.M. and Stewart, M. (2000). Acting like actin. The dynamics of the nematode major sperm protein (msp) cytoskeleton indicate a push–pull mechanism for amoeboid cell motility. *Journal of Cell Biology* **149**, 7–12.

Roberts, T.M., Pavalko, F.M. and Ward, S. (1986). Membrane and cytoplasmic proteins are transported in the same organelle complex during nematode spermatogenesis. *Journal of Cell Biology* **102**, 1787–1796.

Roche, M. (1966). Influence of male and female *Ancylostoma caninum* on each other's distribution in the intestine of the dog. *Experimental Parasitology* **19**, 327–331.

Roos, M.H. (1997). The role of drugs in the control of parasitic nematode infections: must we do without? *Parasitology* **114**, S137–S144.

Rose, K.L., Winfrey, V.P., Hoffman, L.H., Hall, D.H., Furuta, T. and Greenstein, D. (1997). The POU gene *ceh-18* promotes gonadal sheath cell differentiation and function required for meiotic maturation and ovulation in *Caenorhabditis elegans*. *Developmental Biology* **192**, 59–77.

Rumjanek, F.D., Braga, V.M. and Kelly, C. (1989). DNA binding proteins of *Schistosoma mansoni* recognizing a hexanucleotide motif occurring in genes regulated by steroids. *Comparative Biochemistry and Physiology. B: Comparative Biochemistry* **94**, 807–812.

Sakaguchi, Y., Tada, I., Ash, L.R. and Aoki, Y. (1983). Karyotypes of *Brugia pahangi* and *Brugia malayi* (Nematoda: Filarioidea). *Journal of Parasitology* **69**, 1090–1093.

Sangster, N.C. (1999). Anthelmintic resistance: past, present and future. *International Journal for Parasitology* **29**, 115–124.

Sangster, N.C. and Gill, J. (1999). Pharmacology of anthelmintic resistance. *Parasitology Today* **15**, 141–146.

Schedl, T. (1997). Developmental genetics of the germ line. In: *C. elegans II* (D.L. Riddle, T. Blumenthal, B.J. Meyer and J.R. Priess, eds), pp. 241–269. Cold Spring Harbor: Cold Spring Harbor Laboratory Press.

Schnieder, T. (1993). The diagnostic antigen encoded by gene fragment Dv3–14: a major sperm protein of *Dictyocaulus viviparus*. *International Journal for Parasitology* **23**, 383–389.

Schüssler, P., Potters, E., Winnen, R., Bottke, W. and Kunz, W. (1995). An isoform of ferritin as a component of protein yolk platelets in *Schistosoma mansoni*. *Molecular Reproduction and Development* **41**, 325–330.

Schüssler, P., Grevelding, C.G. and Kunz, W. (1997). Identification of Ras, MAP kinases, and a GAP protein in *Schistosoma mansoni* by immunoblotting and their putative involvement in male–female interaction. *Parasitology* **115**, 629–634.

Schüssler, P., Kohrer, K., Finken-Eigen, M., Michel, A., Grevelding, C.G. and Kunz, W. (1998). A female-specific cDNA sequence of *Schistosoma mansoni* encoding an amidase that is expressed in the gastrodermis. *Parasitology* **116**, 131–137.

Scott, A.L., Dinman, J., Sussman, D.J. and Ward, S. (1989a). Major sperm protein and actin genes in free-living and parasitic nematodes. *Parasitology* **98**, 471–478.

Scott, A.L., Dinman, J., Sussman, D.J., Yenbutr, P. and Ward, S. (1989b). Major sperm protein genes from *Onchocerca volvulus*. *Molecular and Biochemical Parasitology* **36**, 119–126.

Setterquist, R.A. and Fox, G.E. (1995). *Dictyocaulus viviparus*: nucleotide sequence of Dv3-14. *International Journal for Parasitology* **25**, 137–138.
Sharrock, W.J. (1983). Yolk proteins of *Caenorhabditis elegans*. *Developmental Biology* **96**, 182–188.
Shaw, J.R., Marshall, I. and Erasmus, D.A. (1977). *Schistosoma mansoni*: *in vitro* stimulation of vitelline cell development by extracts of male worms. *Experimental Parasitology* **42**, 14–20.
Shea, M.J., King, D.L., Conboy, M.J., Mariani, B.D. and Kafatos, F.C. (1990). Proteins that bind to *Drosophila* chorion cis-regulatory elements: a new C2H2 zinc finger protein and a C2C2 steroid receptor-like component. *Genes and Development* **4**, 1128–1140.
Shi, H., Djikeng, A., Mark, T., Wirtz, E., Tschudi, C. and Ullu, E. (2000). Genetic interference in *Trypanosoma brucei* by heritable and inducible double-stranded RNA. *RNA* **6**, 1069–1076.
Shim, Y.H. (1999). *elt-1*, a gene encoding a *Caenorhabditis elegans* GATA transcription factor, is highly expressed in the germ lines with *msp* genes as the potential targets. *Molecules and Cells* **9**, 535–541.
Short, R.B. (1957). Chromosome and sex in *Schistomatium douthitti*. *Journal of Heredity* **48**, 2–6.
Siegel, D.A. and Tracy, J.W. (1988). Effect of pairing in vitro on the glutathione level of male *Schistosoma mansoni*. *Journal of Parasitology* **74**, 524–531.
Simpson, A.J. and Knight, M. (1986). Cloning of a major developmentally regulated gene expressed in mature females of *Schistosoma mansoni*. *Molecular and Biochemical Parasitology* **18**, 25–35.
Skipper, M., Milne, C.A. and Hodgkin, J. (1999). Genetic and molecular analysis of *fox-1*, a numerator element involved in *Caenorhabditis elegans* primary sex determination. *Genetics* **151**, 617–631.
Skrjabin, K.I. (ed.) (1952). *Keys to Parasitic Nematodes*, vol. 3. New York: E.J. Brill. (English translation; Israel program for scientific translation, 1961).
Smith, G. (1997). The economics of parasite control: obstacles to creating reliable models. *Veterinary Parasitology* **72**, 437–444.
Spakulova, M., Casanova, J.C., Laplana Guillen, N. and Kral'Ova, I. (2000). A karyological study of the spirurid nematode *Mastophorus muris* (Nematoda: Spirocercidae). *Parasite* **7**, 173–177.
Spieth, J., Nettleton, M., Zucker-Aprison, E., Lea, K. and Blumenthal, T. (1991). Vitellogenin motifs conserved in nematodes and vertebrates. *Journal of Molecular Evolution* **32**, 429–438.
Spotila, L.D., Rekosh, D.M., Boucher, J.M. and LoVerde, P.T. (1987). A cloned DNA probe identifies the sex of *Schistosoma mansoni* cercariae. *Molecular and Biochemical Parasitology* **26**, 17–20.
Stinchcomb, D.T., Shaw, J.E., Carr, S.H. and Hirsh, D. (1985). Extrachromosomal DNA transformation of *Caenorhabditis elegans*. *Molecular and Cell Biology* **5**, 3484–3496.
Streit, A., Li, W., Robertson, B., Schein, J., Kamal, I.H., Marra, M. and Wood, W.B. (1999). Homologs of the *Caenorhabditis elegans* masculinizing gene *her-1* in *C. briggsae* and the filarial parasite *Brugia malayi*. *Genetics* **152**, 1573–1584.
Sulston, J.E. and Horvitz, H.R. (1977). Post-embryonic cell lineages of the nematode, *Caenorhabditis elegans*. *Developmental Biology* **56**, 110–156.
Sulston, J.E., Schierenberg, E., White, J.G. and Thomson, J.N. (1983). The embryonic cell lineage of the nematode *Caenorhabditis elegans*. *Developmental Biology* **100**, 64–119.
Tabara, H., Grishok, A. and Mello, C.C. (1998). RNAi in *C. elegans*: soaking in the genome sequence. *Science* **282**, 430–431.

Talvik, H., Christensen, C.M., Joachim, A., Roepstorff, A., Bjørn, H. and Nansen, P. (1997). Prepatent periods of different *Oesophagostomum* spp. isolates in experimentally infected pigs. *Parasitology Research* **83**, 563–568.

Taylor, A.E.R. (1960). Spermatogenesis and embryology of *Litomosoides carinii* and *Dirofilaria immitis*. *Journal of Helminthology* **34**, 3–12.

The *C. elegans* Sequencing Consortium (1998). Genome sequence of the nematode *C. elegans*: a platform for investigating biology. *Science* **282**, 2012–2018.

Tobler, H. (1986). The differentiation of germ and somatic cell lines in nematodes. In: *Results and Problems in Cell Differentiation* (W. Hennig, ed.), vol. 13, pp. 1–69. Berlin: Springer-Verlag.

Triantaphyllou, A.C. (1983). Cytogenetic aspects of nematode evolution. In: *Concepts in Nematode Systematics* (A.R. Stone, H.M. Platt and L.F. Khalil, eds), vol. 22, pp. 55–71. New York: Academic Press.

Triantaphyllou, A.C. and Hirschmann, H. (1973). Environmentally controlled sex determination in *Meloidodera floridensis*. *Journal of Nematology* **5**, 181–185.

Troemel, E.R. (1999). Chemosensory signaling in *C. elegans*. *Bioessays* **21**, 1011–1020.

Troemel, E.R., Chou, J.H., Dwyer, N.D., Colbert, H.A. and Bargmann, C.I. (1995). Divergent seven transmembrane receptors are candidate chemosensory receptors in *C. elegans*. *Cell* **83**, 207–218.

Underwood, A.P. and Bianco, A.E. (1999). Identification of a molecular marker for the Y chromosome of *Brugia malayi*. *Molecular and Biochemical Parasitology* **99**, 1–10.

Walker, T.K., Rollinson, D. and Simpson, A.J. (1989). A DNA probe from *Schistosoma mansoni* allows rapid determination of the sex of larval parasites. *Molecular and Biochemical Parasitology* **33**, 93–100.

Walton, A.C. (1959). Some parasites and their chromosomes. *Journal of Parasitology* **45**, 1–20.

Ward, J.B. and Bone, L.W. (1983). Chromatography and isolation of the Kav 1.0 pheromone of female *Nippostrongylus brasiliensis* (Nematoda). *Journal of Parasitology* **69**, 302–306

Ward, S. and Klass, M. (1982). The location of the major protein in *Caenorhabditis elegans* sperm and spermatocytes. *Developmental Biology* **92**, 203–208.

Ward, S., Thomson, N., White, J.G. and Brenner, S. (1975). Electron microscopical reconstruction of the anterior sensory anatomy of the nematode *Caenorhabditis elegans*. *Journal of Comparative Neurology* **160**, 313–337.

Ward, S., Hogan, E. and Nelson, G.A. (1983). The initiation of spermatogenesis in the nematode *Caenorhabditis elegans*. *Developmental Biology* **98**, 70–79.

Ward, S., Burke, D.J., Sulston, J.E., Coulson, A.R., Albertson, D.G., Ammons, D., Klass, M. and Hogan, E. (1988). Genomic organization of major sperm protein genes and pseudogenes in the nematode *Caenorhabditis elegans*. *Journal of Molecular Biology* **199**, 1–13.

Webster, P., Mansour, T.E. and Bieber, D. (1989). Isolation of a female-specific, highly repeated *Schistosoma mansoni* DNA probe and its use in an assay of cercarial sex. *Molecular and Biochemical Parasitology* **36**, 217–222.

Williams, S.A. and Johnston, D.A. (1999). Helminth genome analysis: the current status of the filarial and schistosome genome projects. Filarial Genome Project. Schistosome Genome Project. *Parasitology* **118**, S19–S38.

Winter, C.E., Penha, C. and Blumenthal, T. (1996). Comparison of a vitellogenin gene between two distantly related rhabditid nematode species. *Molecular Biology and Evolution* **13**, 674–684.

Zucker-Aprison, E. and Blumenthal, T. (1989). Potential regulatory elements of nematode vitellogenin genes revealed by interspecies sequence comparison. *Journal of Molecular Evolution* **28**, 487–496.

Antiparasitic Properties of Medicinal Plants and Other Naturally Occurring Products

Senyo Tagboto and Simon Townson

Tropical Parasitic Diseases Unit, Northwick Park Institute for Medical Research, Harrow, Middlesex, HA1 3UJ, UK

ADVANCES IN PARASITOLOGY VOL 50
0065–308X $30.00

ABSTRACT

Parasitic diseases remain a major public health problem affecting hundreds of millions of people, particularly in tropical developing countries. The limited availability and affordability of pharmaceutical medicines means that the majority of the world's population depends on traditional medical remedies, and it is estimated that some 20 000 species of higher plant are used medicinally throughout the world. Many well-known drugs listed in the modern pharmacopoeia have their origins in nature, including, for example, quinine from the bark of the *Cinchona* tree for the treatment of malaria, which has been followed by the subsequent development of the synthetic derivatives chloroquine, amodiaquine, primaquine and mefloquine. More recently, the wider recognition of the antimalarial activity of artemisinin from the herb *Artemisia annua* has led current research to focus on the development of a large number of synthetic and semisynthetic compounds, which are more active than artemisinin.

There is an increasing awareness of the potential of natural products, which may lead to the development of much-needed new antiparasitic drugs. In this chapter, we have drawn together a comprehensive list of medicinal plants and other natural products that have been shown to have activity against human and, to a lesser extent, animal parasites. In addition, some of the opportunities and difficulties in working with natural products have been reviewed and discussed, including the problems involved with evaluating complex mixtures of compounds which may occur in extracts, problems associated with differentiating between general cytotoxicity and genuine antiparasitic activity, and the hope that new technologies will rapidly accelerate new drug discovery and development in this field. Nevertheless, the way forward for natural product medicines, including the conservation of recognized natural products and protection of general biodiversity, the discovery and development process, and the promotion and usage of existing remedies, presents some difficult challenges. Following an initiative by the World Health Organization in August 2000, there is now the opportunity to evaluate scientifically many more traditional medicines and other natural products in validated antiparasite and toxicity screens, which will help establish which substances have potential for new pharmaceutical products. The use of 'untested' traditional medicines will no doubt continue, and there is an urgent need to distinguish between the efficacious and safe products and the ineffective and/or unsafe products, particularly since many remedies are being more widely promoted in developing countries.

1. INTRODUCTION

Parasitic diseases remain a major public health problem affecting hundreds of millions of people and in many parts of the world. Economic and social conditions such as inadequate sanitation, ignorance and poverty may encourage their spread. The immense suffering caused by these illnesses and the consequent loss of productivity is a major drain on the limited resources of the communities in which they occur.

There are rather limited numbers of safe and effective antiparasitic drugs licensed for human use (WHO, 1990). Furthermore, increasing drug resistance has limited the usefulness of some existing compounds. Parasitic diseases occur mostly in poorer countries, where the technical expertise and financial resources necessary for new drug development are scarce. Despite efforts made by organizations like the World Health Organization to help find new treatments, there have been few new drugs in recent times.

Traditional medical remedies for several diseases abound in most endemic regions and it is estimated that some 20 000 species of higher plant are used medicinally throughout the world (Phillipson, 1994). Many of these preparations have been used extensively and knowledge about them has been accrued by several generations of practitioners from experience, trial and error. Although formal toxicology studies are limited, most of the extensively used local remedies are unlikely to be severe toxins and are worthy of further evaluation for novel antiparasitic compounds. It has been estimated that almost two-thirds of the earth's 6·1 billion people rely on these preparations because of limited availability or affordability of pharmaceutical medicines. In industrialized countries, where scientifically formulated drugs are readily available, there is increasing confidence in and growing use of non-prescription drugs from plant sources. In the USA, it has been estimated that $5 billion was spent on such preparations in 1997 (Swerdlow, 2000).

Ethnomedicine and ethnobotany have long been of interest to medical researchers, physicians, the pharmaceutical industry, anthropologists and botanists. The value of ethnomedical and ethnobotanical information in drug development is highly variable. There are many splendid texts (Dalziel, 1937; Ayensu, 1978; Oliver-Bever, 1986; Xiao and Fu, 1986) cataloguing the ethnobotanical uses of plant species by traditional peoples, and publications on this subject in specialist journals, including the *Journal of Ethnopharmacology*. A number of databases are referred to in the literature including NAPRALERT, which includes over 150 genera with folklore reputations as antimalarials (see Phillipson and O'Neill, 1986; Phillipson and Wright, 1991). There are, however, relatively few publications of the ethnomedical uses of other natural products. Large numbers of plants are rapidly becoming extinct and need to be investigated for their medicinal properties with some urgency.

Various well-known drugs listed in modern pharmacopoeia have their origins in nature. These include digitalis and related cardiac glycosides isolated from the leaves of the foxglove plant (*Digitalis lantana* and *Dig. purpurea*). These drugs are presently used to treat certain abnormal heart rhythms and chronic heart failure. William Withering, who trained as a physician in Edinburgh, first described digitalis in 1785. The foxglove plant had been used as a topical preparation for treating heart problems since the Middle Ages (Groves and Bisset, 1991). Ephedrine, a component of many treatments for respiratory disorders, is derived from the ephedra plant (*Ephedra sinica*, *Eph. equisetina*, *Eph. gerardiana*, *Eph. intermedia*, *Eph. nebrodensis*) and morphine is a widely used potent analgesic derived from the opium poppy (*Papaver somniferum*). These drugs were first used as traditional herbal remedies. Salicin, a natural product of the willow (*Salix* sp.), was discovered accidentally during attempts to use its bitter bark to treat malaria following the success of *Cinchona* bark. Salicylates were later developed as semisynthetic derivatives of salicin (Greenwood, 1992). The drugs vincristine and vinblastine from the rosy periwinkle, *Vinca rosea* (*Catharanthus roseus*), are used to treat a number of haematological and other malignancies. Periwinkle extracts have been used traditionally to treat diabetes in many parts of the world (Noble, 1990). Tubocurarine, used as a muscle relaxant during general anaesthesia, is one of the ingredients in the famous South American arrow poisons and is a bisbenzylisoquinolone alkaloid from *Chondrodendron tomentosum*. Paclitaxel (taxol) is a new drug derived from the Pacific yew tree, *Taxus brevifolia*. The use of this drug has been a major advance in the treatment of breast, ovarian and other cancers (Gotaskie and Andreassi, 1994). These anticancer agents were the result of scientific research into the bioactive molecules from these plants. While most traditional remedies originate from plant sources, it is becoming increasingly evident that natural products from fungi, or animal toxins and venoms may have therapeutic applications. With regard to parasites, natural product research has contributed to outstanding new drugs for treating some infections. These drugs include quinine and artemisinin for treating malaria and ivermectin for onchocerciasis and lymphatic filariasis. These are described in greater detail elsewhere in this chapter. There continue to be increasing numbers of reports of antiparasitic activities of natural products which will undoubtedly be a major source of new medicines yet to be identified and developed.

There has been a growing awareness by governments and the scientific and medical communities of the importance of medicinal plants in health-care systems in many developing countries. Greater importance is now being attached to the use of locally available medicines as a means of reducing reliance on expensive imported drugs. Recently, there have been some initiatives to promote research into the utilization of traditional plant-based medicines (Bodeker and Willcox, 2000).

2. AIMS AND LIMITATIONS

There has been a rapid increase in new reports of the antiparasitic activity of natural products, both from scientific studies and from studies into the traditional uses of these products for treating diseases. The principal aim of this contribution has been to draw together, in the form of a series of tables, a comprehensive list of medicinal plants and other natural products that have been shown to have activity against human, and to a lesser extent, animal parasites. Information has been gleaned from a wide range of databases and other sources, and we hope that this will provide an invaluable and timely reference for all those interested in natural products medicine. In addition, we discuss promising new areas of research, trends, problems and what we see as the way forward for natural product drug discovery, development and usage. However, the scale of our task means that it is beyond the scope of this chapter to cover all the approaches currently being taken, for example the ethnobotanical surveys, which have a large literature all of their own. Our main focus has been to include the studies that present scientific evidence for natural product activity against parasites, although it is fair to say that we have had some difficulty in defining the limits of this review. Nevertheless, we do believe that there are no major omissions at the time of writing, bearing in mind that new discoveries are being made on a daily basis in this fast-evolving and exciting field.

The generic and family names of plants used in this text were checked against the nomenclature in a standard taxonomic reference source (Mabberley, 1997). Generic names used by authors have all been listed in the tables but where these names have been superseded, they have been cross-referenced to the modern name, where relevant information relating to that plant product is recorded.

We believe that this text will be useful for researchers with an interest in natural products as chemotherapeutic agents, the pharmaceutical industry and persons with an interest in ethnobotany, ethnomedicine or ethnopharmacology. It may guide clinicians and healthworkers in remote areas or in times of civil uprising or other disturbance where commercially manufactured drugs are not available.

3. NATURAL PRODUCTS WITH ANTIPROTOZOAL PROPERTIES

Diseases caused by protozoa are responsible for considerable mortality and morbidity throughout the world. There are an estimated 20 million people infected with *Leishmania* species (Goto *et al.*, 1998) and nearly the same number infected with *Trypanosoma cruzi* (Buckner *et al.*, 1998). There are 50 million cases of amoebiasis with up to 100 000 deaths each year (Huston and Petri, 1998). Current estimates indicate that 60 million people are at risk of infection with African trypanosomiasis, with about 300 000 new cases each year (WHO, 1998). There are 2·8 billion people living in malaria endemic areas, and every year there are 300–500 million clinical cases of malaria with over 1 million deaths due to the disease (Trigg and Wernsdorfer, 1999). It has been predicted that global warming will cause the spread of many tropical diseases and could be responsible for a major malaria epidemic in the second half of this century (Sharp, 1996). In 1994, it was estimated that chloroquine was the second or third most widely consumed drug in the world, and that the global market for antimalarial drugs was worth $100–$120 million per annum (Foster, 1994). The globalization and improvement in the economies of many tropical countries presents an opportunity for the economic development of new antimalarial and other antiprotozoal agents.

There are many problems with the currently available drugs for treating protozoal diseases. Many of these drugs are poorly tolerated because of side effects. There is inadequate drug therapy for the treatment of some of these illnesses such as the chronic stages of Chagas disease. Other problems include limited availability, prohibitive cost and increasing drug resistance. As a consequence of this, new, cheap, safe and effective drugs are urgently needed. Plant products that have undergone scientific evaluation for antiprotozoal activity are listed in Tables 1–8. In addition, Table 9 lists plant products evaluated against *Pneumocystis carinii* (this organism is no longer classified as a protozoan, but as a yeast).

Established human antiprotozoal drugs from natural sources include quinine from *Cinchona* species, artemisinin from *Artemisia annua* (used in treating malaria) and emetine from *Psychotria* (*Cephaelis*) *ipecacuanha* (used in treating amoebiasis).

The red bark of various *Cinchona* species was used by the Incas of South America to treat tropical fevers and was introduced into Europe from Peru in 1630. Further evaluation established this as a valuable treatment for malaria in the 17th century (Greenwood, 1992). It is thought that the French chemists Pierre Pelletier and Joseph Caventou first isolated quinine in 1820. *Cinchona* (*calisaya*) *ledgeriana*, a Bolivian species, was found to have the highest quinine content. At the beginning of the 21st century, this drug remains a first-line drug for the treatment of this illness. Following further research and development, the semisynthetic derivatives of quinine, chloroquine, amodiaquine, primaquine and mefloquine were developed as useful antimalarials. Due to its efficacy and ease of administration, chloroquine rapidly became the second or third most widely consumed drug in the world, although its use has declined owing to the development of drug resistance (Foster, 1994).

Quinine and three other alkaloids with significant antimalarial activity, quinidine, cinchonine and cinchonidine (found in roughly equal proportions), have been isolated from *Cinchona* trees. In the past, the antimalarial totaquine, containing all four alkaloids, was available as a cheap alternative to quinine sulphate (Dobson, 1998). There are growing reports of malaria parasites resistant to quinine. Experimental studies have shown synergy between the various *Cinchona* alkaloids with improved activity over quinine against resistant

Plasmodium falciparum in vitro, particularly when quinine is combined with cinchonine (Druilhe *et al.*, 1988). Clinical studies have shown that the quinine–quinidine–cinchonine combination has similar clinical efficacy to quinine alone when used in uncomplicated malaria (Sowunmi *et al.*, 1990).

The use of the herb *Artemisia annua* for treating febrile illnesses has been mentioned in an ancient Chinese publication thought to date from the year AD 341 by Ge Heng (Hien and White, 1993). Despite this, its potential for treating malaria was only recently recognized when Chinese scientists discovered its antimalarial activity in 1971. The active principle was shown to be a novel sesquiterpene lactone called quinghaosu or artemisinin in the Western World (Qinghaosu Antimalarial Coordinating Research Group, 1979). It has a complex tetracyclic 1,2,4-trioxane structure containing a peroxide moiety. A water-soluble derivative sodium artesunate, suitable for oral use, and an oil-soluble derivative artemether, suitable for intramuscular injection, showed improved antimalarial activity over artemisinin (Hien and White, 1993).

Since the realization that the essential part of the molecule is centred on the endoperoxide bridge, simple structures called trioxanes and tetroxanes have been synthesized (over 1000 molecules belonging to several classes). The mode of action involves the cleavage of this bridge by intraparasitic iron and haem, generating unstable free radicals that lead to the alkylation of specific malaria proteins (Meshnick *et al.*, 1996). These compounds show great promise, with some preparations showing activity *in vitro* several thousand times greater than artemisinin. They are collectively called 'Malperox', and are generally easy and inexpensive to prepare and may offer more stable and safer drugs than the original naturally occurring compound.

Arteflene, a synthetic antimalarial peroxide, has already been shown to be safe and effective in clinical trials. This compound is derived from yingzhaosu, a naturally occurring antimalarial peroxide from *Artabotrys* species. Unfortunately, treatment of malaria with arteflene is characterized by recrudescences. Nevertheless, there is great hope that further research on these compounds may eventually yield new replacement antimalarials (Meshnick *et al.*, 1996).

Species of Simaroubaceae are widely used throughout the tropics as traditional herbal antimalarial agents. They contain bitter pentacyclic terpenoids known as quassinoids with antineoplastic, antiamoebic and antiplasmodial activity (Trager and Polonsky, 1981; Gillin *et al.*, 1982; Wright *et al.*, 1988). Several of these are potent inhibitors of protein synthesis in malaria parasites (Kirby *et al.*, 1989). Amongst the most active are simalikalactone and bruceantin, which have IC_{50} values of 0·0009 and 0·0008 $\mu g\ ml^{-1}$ respectively against *P. falciparum in vitro* (Phillipson and O'Neill, 1986). These compounds also possess antiamoebic activity (Van Assendelft *et al.*, 1956, Wright *et al.*, 1988). The quassinoid bruceantin is 10 times more potent against *Entamoeba histolytica in vitro* than metronidazole. In general, the activity of quassinoids against *P. falciparum* and *E. histolytica in vitro* tend to parallel each other (Wright *et al.*, 1988). These compounds are, unfortunately, generally toxic to mammalian cells including tumour cell lines (Trager and Polonsky, 1981). However, a small number of quassinoids possess selective activity against *P. falciparum*. The use of modern combinatorial chemistry to produce semi-synthetic derivatives for further screening will be a useful next step.

Other pure compounds with antimalarial activity include corialstonine and corialstonidine, indole alkaloids isolated from *Alstonia coriaceae* (Wright *et al.*, 1993b), cryptolepine from *Cryptolepis sanguinolenta* (Kirby *et al.*, 1995; Grellier *et al.*, 1996), ancistrocladine, ancistrobrevine, dioncopeltine A and dioncophylline C from species of Ancistrocladaceae and Dioncophyllaceae (Francois *et al.*, 1994, 1995, 1997a). A bisbenzylisoquinoline alkaloid isolated from *Triclisia patens* was shown to have an antimalarial to mammalian cell cytotoxicity ratio equivalent to that of chloroquine (Phillipson, 1994).

Other leads include isoquinoline alkaloids such as berberine that have antimalarial (Vennerstrom and Klayman, 1988) and anti-amoebic (Subbaiah and Amin, 1967) activity. The indole alkaloids harmaline and vinblastine have effects against *Leishmania amazonensis in vitro* and in a mouse model (Evans and Croft, 1987), and against *Trypanosoma cruzi in vitro* (Cavin *et al.*, 1987) respectively. Ataphillinine is an acridone alkaloid from the Rutaceae family with activity against *Plasmodium berghei* in mice (Fujioka *et al.*, 1989) and a number of limonoids with antiplasmodial activity have been isolated from the neem tree and other members of the Meliaceae family. Disopyrin is a quinone active against *Leishmania donovani* promastigotes *in vitro* (Hazra *et al.*, 1987). Other compounds including gossypol, a polyphenolic compound from cottonseed oil, have been shown to be active against *Plasmodium falciparum*, *Trypanosoma cruzi* and *Entamoeba histolytica* (Gonzalez-Garza and Said-Fernandez, 1988), and allicin isolated from garlic clove has been shown to have effects against *E. histolytica in vitro* (Mirelman *et al.*, 1987).

To date, several plants have been identified from ethnobotanical information as having useful antiprotozoal activity. Some of them have been tested as crude extracts and a proportion of these have had active compounds isolated from them. There is a great opportunity and an urgent need for synthetic chemistry programmes to generate chemical analogues for further testing as potential new drugs.

4. NATURAL PRODUCTS WITH ANTHELMINTIC PROPERTIES

There are several natural products reported to have anthelmintic activity in scientific studies, although these predominantly relate to gut helminths. These products and their published activity are recorded in Tables 10–14.

Nevertheless, helminth parasites are ubiquitous and responsible for a tremendous degree of morbidity and mortality in tropical countries.

River blindness caused by the filarial worm *Onchocerca volvulus* affects 17·7 million people of whom 270 000 are blind and a further 500 000 severely visually disabled (WHO, 1995). In certain parts of Africa, blindness in up to 15% of the population of badly affected villages has been reported (Lindley, 1987). Lymphatic filariasis is thought to affect 2% of the world's population (approximately 119 million cases) (Michael *et al.*, 1996). However, in badly affected areas, up to 66% prevalence of microfilaraemia has been reported (Kazura *et al.*, 1997). The world prevalence of *Ascaris lumbricoides* is estimated at 1400 million (Albonico *et al.*, 1998). A Chinese survey in 30 provinces with a population of nearly 1·5 million showed overall prevalences of 47%, 18·8% and 17·2% for *Ascaris lumbricoides*, *Trichuris trichiura* and hookworm infections (Xu *et al.*, 1995). The World Health Organization (WHO, 1993) estimates that 200 million people are infected with schistosomiasis despite major international control efforts, with 600 million at risk of acquiring the disease. Although helminth infections are more prevalent in the poorer sections of society, the sheer numbers of people infected presents an opportunity for the economic development of new drugs by pharmaceutical companies and in addition could be hugely important in developing public relations by drug companies.

There are some effective pharmaceutical drugs with good safety margins for treating helminth infections (Grove, 1990). These include the antitrematode agent praziquantel; antinematode drugs such as the benzimidazole carbamates mebendazole and albendazole; the imidazothiazole levamisole; the macrocyclic lactone ivermectin; and the anticestode drugs niclosamide and praziquantel. However, the spectrum of chemotherapeutic coverage is incomplete. There are still no potent safe macrofilaricides or drugs that reliably kill or cause the physical extrusion of *Dracunculus medinensis*. Although there are presently no major problems with resistance to anthelmintic drugs used to treat human infections, this is a major problem in the veterinary field where intensive drug use has led to resistance to each major group of compounds. There is clearly the risk of developing resistance to the limited numbers of drugs available for treating human helminthic infections, which makes the need for new therapies a continuous one.

Despite the lack of pharmaceutical plant-based anthelmintics, there are nevertheless anthelmintics from natural sources, including ivermectin from the actinomycete *Streptomyces avermitilis* and moxidectin from *Streptomyces cyanogriseus*. These types of drugs are classified as avermectins and milbemycins respectively.

The drug company Merck & Co. Inc. developed ivermectin in 1975 as a veterinary anthelmintic. The manufacturers, through the Mectizan Donation Programme, provide this drug free of charge for the treatment of onchocerciasis.

It has now replaced diethylcarbamazine and suramin (both with serious side effects) as the drug of choice for treating onchocerciasis. However, it needs to be administered every 6–12 months to control the disease by reducing the numbers of microfilariae in the skin and eyes for the life span of the adult worms (a mean of 11 but up to 18 years). Although moxidectin is not yet licensed for human use, trials *in vitro* and *in vivo* have demonstrated its activity against *Onchocerca* microfilariae, also showing that its superior activity *in vivo* may be due to its persistence in host tissues (Tagboto and Townson, 1996). Clinical trials have confirmed the efficacy of ivermectin in eliminating the microfilariae of other filarial parasites including *Loa loa* (Richard-Lenoble *et al.*, 1988), *Wuchereria bancrofti* (Nguyen *et al.*, 1996) and *Brugia malayi* (Mak *et al.*, 1993). The drug is also effective in eliminating certain human gut helminths (*Strongyloides stercoralis* and *Ascaris lumbricoides*) (Marti *et al.*, 1996), and in treating visceral larva migrans caused by *A. suum* (Maruyama *et al.*, 1996).

Although there is considerable published ethnobotanical information regarding treatments, especially for gut helminths, there are few published reports of active components in the scientific literature. There are reasons for this. There are a limited number of good screens for drug activity against helminths. These screens are often fairly complex, expensive and laborious to operate. They may be difficult to set up properly and to interpret. Bioassays such as the *Onchocerca*/monkey kidney cell assay (Townson *et al.*, 1987; Townson, 1988) that provide a means for the simultaneous determination of filaricidal activity and primate cell toxicity are more useful than assays *in vitro* employing no measure of mammalian toxicity.

Although there are a number of highly effective antiprotozoal agents from plant sources, there is still no clinically useful anthelmintic of plant origin. The difficulty in finding a plant-based product with selective anthelmintic toxicity may be because of the greater phylogenetic similarity between humans and helminths. Our review of the literature suggests that there have probably been fewer samples of plant products screened for anthelmintic activity than for antiprotozoal activity. The lack of clear ethnomedical correlation between symptoms and the presence/removal of certain parasites may have hindered the development of traditional drugs for controlling them.

There are several well-known plant species whose parts are used in traditional medicine as anthelmintic agents. These include the seeds, leaves and roots of the pawpaw plant (*Carica papaya*) (Kumar *et al.*, 1991) and an extract of the root of the pomegranate plant (*Punica granatum*) (Hukkeri *et al.*, 1993), which are reputed to have activity against some gastrointestinal helminths. The active constituents of many of these products are poorly understood. There is a dearth of good quality clinical trials and of documentation of selective toxicity. Despite this, there is good evidence of activity in some preliminary scientific studies.

A number of compounds from plant sources have been shown to have definite anthelmintic activity in laboratory trials. These include benzylthiocyanate from *Carica papaya* seeds active against *Ascaris lumbricoides* (Dar *et al.*, 1965), and diospyrol from *Diospyros mollis* fruit active against *Necator americanus* (Sen *et al.*, 1974). Atanine from *Evodia rutecarpa* fruit, artemether from *Artemisia annua* and embelin from *Embelia schimperi* have also been shown to be active against *Schistosoma mansoni* larvae (Perrett and Whitfield, 1995a,b), *S. japonicum* (You *et al.*, 1992) and *Hymenolepis diminuta* (Bogh *et al.*, 1996) respectively. It is not entirely clear why some of these initial leads have not been further researched, although it is generally well known that pharmaceutical companies have carried out unpublished research on antiparasite natural products for many years. There is an urgent need for imaginative funding to allow the full evaluation of medicinal plant products as potential anthelmintics as an initial step in developing new drugs.

5. LEADS FROM OTHER NATURAL PRODUCT AREAS AND PROMISING NEW TECHNOLOGIES

There has been considerable recent research activity identifying and evaluating candidate molecules from non-plant sources as potential new antiparasitic drugs. These products and their published activity are recorded in Tables 15 and 16.

There has been growing research interest in venomous animals and their toxins, with a surprising number of toxic substances in nature demonstrating pharmacological and therapeutic applications, ranging from immunosuppressants from scorpion venoms, analgesics and neuroprotectants from marine snails, to analgesics from frog skin (Harvey, 1999).

Of particular interest are some of the substances obtained from the skin of amphibians; over the past 30 years, over 400 alkaloids have been detected from the poison glands of amphibian skins. These substances help to protect them from predators and also from microbial infection through their soft moist skins. It is unclear if these are synthesized *de novo* from precursors by amphibians or are accumulated from dietary sources. Available evidence suggests that they probably originate from arthropods, including beetles, ants, mites and flies, eaten by these creatures. The arthropods probably accumulate them from plant sources although it is not entirely clear if they can synthesize some molecules themselves (Daly, 1998). There has recently been considerable interest in peptides with antibacterial properties isolated from the skin of the African clawed frog (*Xenopus laevis*). These so-called magainins, together with other peptide molecules including cecropins from insects, mellitin from honeybees and alamethicin from the fungus *Trichoderma viride*, may form the basis of new pharmacologically active compounds (Bechinger, 1997) with broad antibacterial and antiparasitic activity (Morvan *et al.*, 1994). A number of these peptides and their semisynthetic derivatives have recently been shown to be active against the trophozoites of *Acanthamoeba castellanii*, *A. polyphaga* and *Cryptosporidium parvum* (Arrowood *et al.*, 1991; Feldman *et al.*, 1991; Schuster and Jacobs, 1992). In general, there has been little scientific evaluation of these sources of products as antiparasite drugs.

Insects produce specialized inducible antimicrobial proteins in response to infection. The development of their immune system is perhaps important in determining their abundance and success. A large number of such proteins have been described and classified as abaecins, apidaecins, attacins, cecropins, defencins, dipterins and lysozymes (Kimbrell, 1991). Cecropins were initially isolated from the giant silk moth (*Hyalophora cecropia*) but have now been identified in several other insects. The three principal cecropins, A, B and D, are highly homologous. This class of compounds has been shown to be active against a number of protozoan and helminth parasites (Chalk *et al.*, 1995). Following experimental research, Gwadz *et al.* (1989) demonstrated the disruption of sporogonic development of *Plasmodium* parasites by magainins and cecropins. They have suggested that an attempt to introduce and express genes coding for these peptides into mosquitoes may be an effective transmission-blocking strategy. If successful, this strategy may have profound implications for disease control in a number of other insect-transmitted illnesses. There may, however, be practical problems in administering proteinaceous drugs, since these are typically rapidly metabolized. Nevertheless, they may prove useful as a microbial agent which may be applied topically to treat parasitic infections and this warrants further study.

Some plants produce chemical substances in response to infection with fungi, bacteria, viruses and parasites. These responses are thought to be fairly specific to particular infections (Rich *et al.*, 1977). The compounds have been shown to have antimicrobial properties and are called phytoalexins, a term derived from the Greek meaning 'warding-off agent in plants'. They are usually produced within 4–5 days of infection and may induce death, inhibit development or prevent the spread of microbial agents in plants. The first phytoalexin isolated in response to nematode infection was phaseolin from the red kidney bean (*Phaseolus vulgaris*) in response to *Pratylenchus penetrans* infection. However, studies *in vitro* could show no effect of phaseolin on this nematode (Veech, 1982). Subsequently, phytoalexins have been isolated with demonstrable *in vitro* efficacy against plant nematodes. These include glyceollin from *Glycine max* (soy bean) (Kaplan *et al.*, 1980a,b) and gossypol from *Gossypium hirsutum* (cotton plant) (Veech, 1982) against *Meloidogyne incognita* and coumestrol from *Phaseolus lunatus* (lima bean) against *Pratylenchus scribneri* (Rich *et al.*, 1977). Phytoalexins have a number of chemical structures including diterpenes, pterocarpan, isoflavonoids, flavonoids, sesquiterpenes, steroidglycoalkaloids and polyacetylenes (O'Neill,

1986). Basic laboratory studies have demonstrated that gossypol inhibits the growth of *Trypanosoma cruzi in vitro* (Turrens, 1986). These studies raise several questions and present potentially exciting opportunities for further research. Very recently, it has become possible to engineer some common plants to produce many different chemical compounds and it has been shown that plants engineered to produce specific proteins may excrete them into morning dewdrops. This may potentially be applied to obtain and purify antiparasitic natural products from plants (Boyce, 2000).

Naturally occurring antibiotics could also play a role in the control of some parasitic diseases. The presence of intracellular bacteria in the Onchocercidae was recorded over 25 years ago (McLaren *et al.*, 1975; Vincent *et al.*, 1975; Kozek and Marroquin, 1977), but the significance of these organisms as antifilarial drug targets was not fully recognized until very recently. It appears that these endobacteria (genus *Wolbachia*) might play some essential role in the well-being and survival of the parasite (Taylor and Hoerauf, 1999). Several studies have demonstrated that these endobacteria are susceptible to antirickettsial antibiotics, which in turn may lead to deleterious effects on the host filarial worms (Bandi *et al.*, 1999; Hoerauf *et al.*, 1999; McCall *et al.*, 1999; Townson *et al.*, 2000). There are several antibiotic substances occurring in nature, including penicillin from the fungus *Penicillium notatum*. It remains a possibility that this approach of attacking the filarial worm's endobacteria could open up new methods of control using naturally occurring antibiotics in endemic areas.

At present, the control of gastrointestinal nematode parasites of man entirely involves case treatment with anthelmintic drugs. However, the greatest biomass of certain parasites resides in the external environment as free-living stages (*Necator americanus* and *Ancylostoma duodenale*) in moist, shady soils or as eggs (*Ascaris lumbricoides*). These stages may be vulnerable to destruction by a range of abiotic factors (extremes in temperature and desiccation) or biotic factors (macro- and micro-organisms) (Waller and Faedo, 1996). Arthropods, protozoa, viruses, bacteria and fungi could potentially act as control agents but this possibility has not been studied in man. Several fungi (*Arthobotrys* sp., *Duddingtonia flagrans*, *Dactylaria* sp., *Monacrosporium eudermatum* and *M. candidum*, *Nemactoctonus* sp. and *Harposporium leptospira*) have been shown to be nematophagous for animal nematodes (Waller and Larsen, 1993; Faedo *et al.*, 1997; Hay *et al.*, 1997; Flores Crespo *et al.*, 1999). Furthermore, oral treatment with *Duddingtonia flagrans* showed a substantial ($>80\%$) reduction in infective larvae derived from eggs in sheep faeces (Larsen *et al.*, 1998), and in a separate study, a reduction of *Ostertagia ostertagi* infective larvae on pasture (Fernandez *et al.*, 1999). After deposition, it has been shown that nematophagous fungi in the local environment rapidly infest sheep faeces within a few days (Hay *et al.*, 1997). These studies raise the prospect of the control of human gastrointestinal nematodes by oral administration or by treating infected soils with these fungi or other organisms. It will be useful to study the natural predators of these helminth stages and identify fungi that are found in and survive passage through the human gut as a first step.

6. SOME PROBLEMS IN ANTIPARASITIC NATURAL PRODUCT RESEARCH

There are a considerable number of practical problems involved with natural product research and many of these are immediately evident from reading on this subject. These include the reliability of ethnobotanical information, the supply of sufficient quantities of the product, and the possibility of overcollection and depletion. The quality and uniformity of the chemical constituents and their concentrations in natural products may be affected by factors such as subspecies or age of plant, geographical and seasonal variations, time and method of collection and storage, and other environmental variables (Chung and Staba, 1986; Makinde *et al.*, 1993; Laughlin, 1994). There may be major difficulties in isolating pure compounds from complex mixtures of substances often found in extracts submitted for screening.

Local medicinal plant usage may provide valuable information about lesser-known plants. Unfortunately, local uses can be very numerous and may differ completely from one tribe to another for the same plant (Oliver-Bever, 1986). According to a recent report (Derbyshire, 2000), traditional uses may vary wildly. For example, *Aloe vera* is used to induce abortion in Argentina, to treat constipation in Bolivia, for diabetes in the Canary Islands, as an aphrodisiac in India, for stomach ulcers in Panama, for asthma in Peru, for piles in Saudi Arabia, as a contraceptive in South Korea, for hepatitis in Taiwan and to prevent syphilis in the West Indies. Also, it should not be forgotten that superstition and the placebo effect might play a role in folk medicine. For this reason, purgatives, emetics, diuretics and vesicants are often used in the belief that they may eliminate or oppose evil influences or disease.

The very nature of the disease being studied may play a significant role in whether or not effective natural products have been identified for its treatment. For example, the filarial disease onchocerciasis, caused by the tissue-dwelling nematode *Onchocerca volvulus*, results in immunopathological lesions in the skin and eyes. For this chronic disease, it is particularly difficult to find reliable leads from ethnobotanical surveys since there is no clear link between taking a preparation and the treatment of diseases or symptoms. Indeed a substance that causes the destruction of *Onchocerca* microfilariae may even exacerbate symptoms, discomfort and pathology in the short term (WHO, 1995), while a substance that provides temporary relief from the common symptom of itching is unlikely to have any significant effect on the course of the disease. This is in contrast, for example, to treating gut helminths, where taking a preparation will result in the expulsion of clearly visible intestinal worms, or to the correlation between the treatment of fever and the elimination of malaria parasites.

The reliability of 'scientific' information may be a major problem. There are too many examples of poorly conducted trials that have been inadequately controlled, often involving no measure of general toxicity to mammalian cells and no positive control compound, resulting in research of only limited value. As far as possible, new compound samples should be evaluated in defined, controlled and validated assays as an essential first step to determine if real intrinsic activity exists. Such a defined system is also essential for comparing like with like, preferably on an equi-molar or at least weight basis, with comparisons against known active compounds, thus enabling rational decisions to be made on the potential of a new compound for further development. One of the fundamental concepts of 'activity' is about a selective toxicity against the target parasite, but with little or tolerable toxicity to the host. Unfortunately, there is a high probability that many of the products that have been classified as 'active' against a particular organism *in vitro* are likely to be general toxins, and quite unsuitable for development as an antiparasitic product. A perceived problem is the sometimes-observed lack of correlation between tests *in vitro* and *in vivo* (Kirby, 1996), where we often see good activity *in vitro* but poor or no activity *in vivo*. However, this phenomenon is seen in all areas of drug research and is essentially due to the limitations of *in vitro* assays, which may be excellent for measuring the intrinsic activity of a substance, but cannot possibly emulate the complex situation *in vivo*, including the absorption, distribution, metabolism and excretion of the substance. Indeed, a compound may be unstable *in vivo* and be rapidly broken down to inactive constituents, or, more unusually, a substance may be inactive *in vitro* and require metabolism by the host to produce an active compound (for example, *Berberis* alkaloids against *E. histolytica* (see Subbaiah and Amin, 1967, and Phillipson *et al.*, 1995)). Some compounds may act in concert with the immune response, which may be very difficult to replicate *in vitro*; one of the best examples of this is diethylcarbamazine (DEC), used as the standard treatment of onchocerciasis before the advent of ivermectin (WHO, 1995), which invokes a massive allergic-type response in its mode of action (Mazzotti reaction) against microfilariae in the skin and eyes, but is virtually inactive *in vitro* (Rivas-Alcala *et al.*, 1984) or less active in immunocompromized (T-cell deprived) mice (Bianco *et al.*, 1986). Nevertheless, no screening system is perfect and a properly controlled screen *in vitro*, to measure the intrinsic activity of the substance, is generally considered to be the first step in drug discovery. Alternatively, where sophisticated incubation, tissue-culture facilities and reliable power supply are not available, it may be more practical to evaluate products/compounds directly in small-animal models.

Even where some clear antiparasitic activity has been established, natural products used in traditional medicine for humans or domestic animals may produce serious side effects, and may be of a chemical nature with characteristics that would be unacceptable in pharmaceutical medicine. A good example of this problem is discussed by Whitfield (1996) and concerns the Chinese medicinal plant *Acorus gramineus*, which is used widely in the Chinese and Ayurvedic traditional medical systems for a variety of indications ranging from sedative, analgesic and anticonvulsant properties (Morelli *et al.*, 1983), to treatment for insomnia, memory loss and remittent fevers (Vohora *et al.*, 1990), to activity against the ascarid nematodes of pigs *in vitro* (Chang and But, 1986). Perrett and Whitfield (1995b) investigated the effects of a hexane extract of the rhizomes of this plant against a range of helminths and arthropods *in vitro* and reported good levels of activity. However, they also demonstrated that activity was essentially due to two phenylpropanoids, alpha and beta asarone. Unfortunately, these compounds are known cytotoxins and carcinogens and are capable of inducing chromosome aberrations (Taylor *et al.*, 1967; Moralez-Ramirez *et al.*, 1992). Overall, these studies indicate that products from the plant *Aco. gramineus* undoubtedly possess a wide range of interesting biological effects, including activity against some parasites. However, it is also probably the case that there is only a small therapeutic index and that these extracts may be unsafe to use at any concentration, with the possibility of acute or long-term deleterious effects on the patient. Another widely used plant extract with proven anthelmintic activity but potentially serious side effects is the latex of *Ficus* species (Amorin *et al.*, 1999), which, on scientific evaluation, produced high acute toxicity, with haemorrhagic enteritis in mice. A recent study (Navarette and Hong, 1996) on the decoction of the stem bark of *Zanthoxylum liebmannianum* demonstrated that it decreased the egg counts of intestinal nematodes from naturally infected sheep, and α-sanshool was identified as the active ingredient; however, it was also demonstrated that when this component was administered to mice at doses higher than 10 mg kg^{-1} it induced convulsions, and the LD_{50} was found to be only 54·77 mg kg^{-1}. Many studies suggest that significant numbers of natural product traditional medicines are likely to be substantially toxic to the patient. It is probable that some preparations used against gastrointestinal helminths are equally toxic to the host but show selective activity against the parasite because of poor absorption from the host gut. There appears to be a general misconception in the developed world that natural product medicines are 'more natural' and therefore intrinsically safer than medicines from a synthetic chemistry laboratory. We feel it is essential that each compound or treatment, whether found occurring naturally or manufactured, be evaluated on its merits. In the absence of affordable pharmaceutical medicines in much of the developing world, natural product medicines are being widely promoted. However, there is an urgent need to examine carefully the use of such products and carry out scientific safety and efficacy studies, and essential follow-up studies on treated patients. A recent report (Derbyshire, 2000) has indicated that statisticians would need to monitor many thousands of natural product patients in order to observe a low incidence of serious side effects. Indeed, the herbal formula sho-sako-to was used in Japanese kampo medicine for 2000 years without reported side effects until recent evidence emerged associating it with liver damage. With regard to the search for new antiparasitic natural product compounds or extracts, it is necessary to include at least a basic acute toxicity test during the initial evaluation *in vitro*. Kirby (1996) has drawn attention to the possible problem of antagonism between established drugs and natural products used in traditional medicine. Studies by Chawira and Warhurst (1987) and Chawira *et al.* (1987) have demonstrated that both *in vitro* and in malaria-infected mice, there is antagonism between artemisinin and standard antifolates used in the treatment of malaria. Further studies *in vitro* (Al-Khayat *et al.*, 1991; Ekong *et al.*, 1991; Kirby *et al.*, 1995) have reported antagonism when testing the antiplasmodial effects of combinations of chloroquine with a number of plant-derived antiplasmodial extracts or compounds. There may be a risk that treament will fail if patients take chloroquine and simultaneously use traditional plant-derived remedies (Kirby *et al.*, 1995). Al-Khayat *et al.* (1991) demonstrated that at least two highly active antimalarial quassinoids, glaucarubinone and bruceantin, potentiate one another when tested in combination *in vitro*.

In our experience, the receipt of natural product extracts for antiparasite screening has presented us with a number of real practical difficulties in how to proceed (Townson, 2000). For example, one typical sample was an extract with the consistency of toffee, probably containing a complex mixture of compounds at unknown concentrations, which may even interact in a synergistic or antagonistic manner. This type of sample does not easily fit into our well-defined and validated test system, since at this stage none of the constituent compounds can be tested on an equi-molar or weight basis. At the very least, this sample will require considerable effort and resources to determine its toxicity to mammalian cells *in vitro* or the maximum tolerated dose *in vivo*, followed by trials with parasites to determine whether activity is present. If sufficient activity is found, this will justify purification and further research, possibly including a synthetic chemistry programme in order to attempt to improve on nature. However, if no activity is found up to a level that is toxic to mammalian cells or host, then it is quite possible that the activity of potentially interesting compounds may be masked by the presence of other general cytotoxins, and the sample will be discarded. This presents the researcher with a chicken and egg situation, in that many investigators will want to see activity before purification. Another problem is that a number of crude plant extracts show biological activity, which cannot always be confirmed on fractionation (Dhar *et al.*, 1968). This may be explained by the loss of synergistic activity from compounds selectively concentrated in different fractions, loss of labile constituents or elimination of inorganic constituents by the process of fractionation.

From a biological point of view, testing complex mixtures at unknown concentrations is probably not a good strategy for discovering new active compounds against a particular disease, unless there is good prior prima facie evidence of active components. For many drug discovery programmes, particularly in tropical parasitic diseases where there are very limited resources and little prospect of profits, the evaluation of unpurified natural products would have to be weighed carefully against the very much larger number of purified (usually synthesized) compounds that could be evaluated for the equivalent effort.

7. THE WAY FORWARD

The way forward for natural product medicines, including the conservation of the natural products themselves, the discovery and development process, and the promotion and usage of existing remedies, presents some difficult challenges. Natural forests are being rapidly destroyed for timber, agricultural use and human habitation, fuelled by rapid population growth and economic need, particularly in tropical developing countries where the greatest wealth of biodiversity is found. The disappearance of valuable flora and fauna from these habitats has increased the urgency for evaluating this potential source of new medically useful chemical compounds before they are lost. Perhaps the fact that at least a quarter of all prescription drugs are derived from plant sources (Anonymous, 1994) may emphasize the scale of the problem. The sustainable use of these threatened habitats must be the highest priority for the conservation of these resources; if there is political will, it should be possible to manage tropical forests in such a way as to preserve the ecosystem and biodiversity, while taking sustainable 'economic' crops of flora and fauna. The collection of wild plant species for medicinal purposes is thought to be one reason for their depletion, but effective management of reserves or even the 'farming' of some species should be promoted. New leads for human medicine may emerge from 'zoopharmacognosy', particularly when studying the great apes (Irwin, 2000). These animals have a huge capacity for social learning, and chimpanzees and orang-utans have been observed to apparently self-treat with bitter or unpleasant plants for a number of conditions, including parasitic infections. When active constituents have been identified, it may be possible to produce them from cultured plant tissues in the laboratory or to make equivalent compounds in the synthetic chemistry laboratory. Also of importance, The Convention on Biological Diversity, drawn up at the 1992 earth summit in Rio de Janeiro, has drawn attention to the rights of indigenous peoples and has been ratified by more than 170 nations. It was set up to protect the rights of local peoples and demands the protection of intellectual property rights and equitable sharing of any commercial benefits arising from ethnobotanical research (Prance, 2000).

With regard to discovery and development of new pharmaceutical drugs from natural products, there are, of course, many pharmaceutical companies active in this area. However, the full cost of discovering and developing new drugs is usually substantial, often running into hundreds of millions of dollars, which in turn tends to focus research on areas where the market is more lucrative (such as veterinary anthelmintics or heart and cancer drugs, rather than tropical diseases where there is an enormous need, but where profit margins are typically significantly less or non-existent). Nevertheless, one effective approach, pioneered by the World Health Organization, has been to establish collaborations with industry whereby research on 'non-commercial' or 'orphan drugs' can piggy-back research programmes on more commercially viable drugs; for example, new compounds active against veterinary helminths are provided by some companies for evaluation in WHO-funded projects working on drug discovery for human onchocerciasis. Recognizing the importance of natural products for the treatment of tropical diseases, the World Health Organization recently convened a Scientific Working Group (WHO, 2000) concerned with traditional medicine and pharmaceutical medicine perspectives on natural products for the treatment of tropical diseases. This meeting will undoubtedly lead to new initatives in natural product medicine, with the World Health Organization playing the key role in co-ordinating research and funding in collaboration with independent scientists, industry and other specialist groups such as the Research Initiative on Traditional Antimalarial Methods (RITAM) (Willcox and Bodeker, 2000).

An important initial step will be to scientifically evaluate many more traditional medicines and other natural products in preclinical antiparasite efficacy screens and mammalian toxicity screens, funded by the World Health Organization, in order to establish whether there is potential for a pharmaceutical product. From this point, promising compounds will enter the standard pharmaceutical development stage if adequate collaboration and sufficient funding is in place. However, the local usage of 'untested' traditional medicines will no doubt continue, and there is an urgent need to distinguish between the efficacious and safe products and the ineffective and/or unsafe products, particularly since many remedies are being more widely promoted in developing countries. This will require the development of new regulatory frameworks to set and monitor basic standards. In industrialized countries, these frameworks are well developed for pharmaceutical medicine products and continue to be reviewed for herbal medicine products (Keller, 2000). In developing countries, where people may have to depend on these products for debilitating or potentially fatal diseases, regulatory control may be woefully inadequate or even non-existent.

8. APPENDIX

Table 1 Medicinal plants with activity against amoebae.

Species (Family)	Origin[a]	Part (route[b])	Active ingredients	Indication	References
Acacia arabica (Leguminosae)	India	Bark (na)	Methanol extract	*Entamoeba histolytica, in vitro*	Bhakuni *et al.*, 1969
Aegele marmelos (Rutaceae)	NC	NC	Marmelostin	*E. histolytica, in vitro*	see Phillipson & O'Neill, 1987
Ainsliaea pteropoda (Compositae)	India	Whole (na)	Methanol extract	*E. histolytica, in vitro*	Dhar *et al.*, 1968
Alangium salvifolium (Alangiacea)	India	Leaf (na)	Methanol extract	*E. histolytica, in vitro*	Dhar *et al.*, 1968
Albizia lebbeck (Leguminosae)	India	Pod (na)	Methanol extract	*E. histolytica, in vitro*	Dhar *et al.*, 1968
Alhagi pseudalhagi (Leguminosae)	India	Whole (na)	Methanol extract	*E. histolytica, in vitro*	Dhar *et al.*, 1968
Allium sativum (Liliaceae)	NC	Clove (na)	Allicin	*E. histolytica, in vitro*	Mirelman *et al.*, 1987
Anemone pulsatilla (Ranunculaceae)	NC	NC (na)	Anemonin	*E. histolytica, in vitro*	see Phillipson & O'Neill, 1987
Annona muricata (Annonaceae)	Mexico	Bark (na)	Isoquinoline alkaloids	*E. histolytica, in vitro*	Heinrich *et al.*, 1992
Artemisia annua (Compositae)	China	Leaves (na)	Sesquiterpine lactone, artemisinin	*Naegleria fowleri, in vitro*	Cooke *et al.*, 1987
Asparagus filicinus (Liliaceae)	India	Whole (na)	Methanol extract	*E. histolytica, in vitro*	Dhar *et al.*, 1968

Table 1 continued

Species (Family)	Origin[a]	Part (route[b])	Active ingredients	Indication	References
Atropa belladona (Solanaceae)	India	Whole (na)	Methanol extract	*E. histolytica, in vitro*	Dhar *et al.*, 1968
Barringtonia acutangula (Lecythidaceae)	India	Stem (na)	Methanol extract	*E. histolytica, in vitro*	Dhar *et al.*, 1968
Berberis aristata (Berberidaceae)	NC	NC (na)	Alkaloid, berberine	*E. histolytica, in vitro*	Kaneda *et al.*, 1991
Brucea javanica	Thailand	Fruit (na)	Quassinoids	*E. histolytica, in vitro*	Wright *et al.*, 1988
B. antidysenterica (Simaroubaceae)	Ethiopia	NC (na)	Bruceantin, ailanthinone, yadansioside F, bruceine A,B,C,D, holacanthone, glaucarubinone	*E. histolytica, in vitro*	Gillin *et al.*, 1982
Calendula officinalis (Compositae)	India	Whole (na)	Methanol extract	*E. histolytica, in vitro*	Dhar *et al.*, 1968
Carum roxburghianum (Umbelliferae)	India	Fruit (na)	Methanol extract	*E. histolytica, in vitro*	Dhar *et al.*, 1968
Castela texana (Simaroubaceae)	Mexico	Aerial (na)	Quassinoids	*E. histolytica, in vitro*	Heinrich *et al.*, 1992
Cedrela toona (Meliaceae)	India	Leaf (na)	Methanol extract	*E. histolytica, in vitro*	Dhar *et al.*, 1968
Celosia argentea (Amaranthaceae)	India	Whole (na)	Methanol extract	*E. histolytica, in vitro*	Bhakuni *et al.*, 1969
Centella asiatica (Umbelliferae)	India	Whole (na)	Methanol extract	*E. histolytica, in vitro*	Dhar *et al.*, 1968

Table 1 continued

Species (Family)	Origin[a]	Part (route[b])	Active ingredients	Indication	References
Centipeda minima (Compositae)	China	Whole (na)	Brevilin A	*E. histolytica, in vitro*	Yu *et al.*, 1994
	India		Methanol extract	*E. histolytica, in vitro*	Bhakuni *et al.*, 1969
Cephaelis ipecacuanha [see *Psychotria ipecacuanha*]					
Chenopodium graveolens (Chenopodiaceae)	Mexico	Aerial (na)	Chloroethane extract	*E. histolytica, in vitro*	Heinrich *et al.*, 1992
Cinchona legeriana (Rubiaceae)	S. America	Leaf (na)	Isocorynantheol, dehyrochrolifuanine, cinchophylline, ochrolifuanine A	*E. histolytica, in vitro*	Keene *et al.*, 1986
Cissus setosa (Vitaceae)	India	Aerial (na)	Methanol extract	*E. histolytica, in vitro*	Dhar *et al.*, 1968
Clerodendrum squamatum (Labiatae)	India	Root (na)	Methanol extract	*E. histolytica, in vitro*	Dhar *et al.*, 1968
Coccinia indica (Cucurbitaceae)	India	Root (na)	Methanol extract	*E. histolytica, in vitro*	Bhakuni *et al.*, 1969
Cotinus coggygria (Anacardiaceae)	India	Aerial (na)	Methanol extract	*E. histolytica, in vitro*	Dhar *et al.*, 1968
Curcuma longa (Zingiberaceae)	India	Rhizome (na)	Methanol extract	*E. histolytica, in vitro*	Dhar *et al.*, 1968
Dichroa febrifuga (Hydrangeaceae)	China	Whole (po)	Febrifugine, isofebrifugine	*E. histolytica,* clinical trial	Xiao & Fu, 1986
Diospyros peregrina (Ebenaceae)	India	Bark (na)	Methanol extract	*E. histolytica, in vitro*	Dhar *et al.*, 1968

Table 1 continued

Species (Family)	Origin[a]	Part (route[b])	Active ingredients	Indication	References
Drimia indica (Liliaceae)	India	Bulb (na)	Methanol extract	*E. histolytica, in vitro*	Dhar *et al.*, 1968
Euphorbia hirta	Ivory Coast	Whole (po)	Alcohol extract	*E. histolytica*, clinical trial	Martin *et al.*, 1964
	India			*E. histolytica, in vitro*	Dhar *et al.*, 1968
E. tirucalli (Euphorbiaceae)	India	Aerial (na)	Alcohol extract	*E. histolytica, in vitro*	Dhar *et al.*, 1968
Ficus racemosa *F. religiosa* (Moraceae)	India	Bark (na)	Methanol extract	*E. histolytica, in vitro*	Dhar *et al.*, 1968
Garcinia mangostiana (Guttiferae)	NC	NC (na)	Mangostin	*E. histolytica, in vitro*	see Phillipson & O'Neill, 1987
Gossypium hirsutum (Malvaceae)	NC	Cotton seed oil (na)	Gossypol	*E. histolytica, in vitro*	Gonzalez-Garza & Said-Fernandez, 1988
Gouania polygama (Rhamnaceae)	Mexico	Leaf (na)	Ethanol extract	*E. histolytica, in vitro*	Heinrich *et al.*, 1992
Grangea maderaspatana (Compositae)	India	Whole (na)	Methanol extract	*E. histolytica, in vitro*	Bhakuni *et al.*, 1969
Hesperethusa crenulata [see *Naringi crenulata*]					
Holarrhena antidysenterica (Apocynaceae)	India	Fruit (na)	Methanol extract	*E. histolytica, in vitro*	Dhar *et al.*, 1968
Hordeum vulgare (Gramineae)	India	Seed (na)	Methanol extract	*E. histolytica, in vitro*	Dhar *et al.*, 1968

Table 1 continued

Species (Family)	Origin[a]	Part (route[b])	Active ingredients	Indication	References
Hydrolea zeylanica (Hydrophyllaceae)	India	Whole (na)	Methanol extract	*E. histolytica, in vitro*	Dhar *et al.*, 1968
Ipomoea coccinea (Convolvulaceae)	India	Aerial (na)	Methanol extract	*E. histolytica, in vitro*	Dhar *et al.*, 1968
Kirganelia reticulata (Euphorbiaceae)	India	Aerial (na)	Methanol extract	*E. histolytica, in vitro*	Dhar *et al.*, 1968
Leucas lavandulaefolia (Labiatae)	India	Whole (na)	Methanol extract	*E. histolytica, in vitro*	Bhakuni *et al.*, 1969
Melaleuca leucadendra (Myrtaceae)	India	Aerial (na)	Methanol extract	*E. histolytica, in vitro*	Bhakuni *et al.*, 1969
Murraya koenigii (Rutaceae)	India	Aerial, root (na)	Methanol extract	*E. histolytica, in vitro*	Bhakuni *et al.*, 1969
Myrica nagi (Myricaceae)	India	Stem (na)	Methanol extract	*E. histolytica, in vitro*	Dhar *et al.*, 1968
Naringi crenulata (Rutaceae)	India	Stem (na)	Methanol extract	*E. histolytica, in vitro*	Bhakuni *et al.*, 1969
Nigella sativa (Ranunculaceae)	India	Seed (na)	Methanol extract	*E. histolytica, in vitro*	Dhar *et al.*, 1968
Nyctanthes arbor-tristis (Oleaceae)	India	Leaf (po)	Ethanol extract	*E. histolytica*, rat	Chitravanshi *et al.*, 1992
Papaver somniferum (Papaveraceae)	India	Seed (na)	Methanol extract	*E. histolytica, in vitro*	Dhar *et al.*, 1968
Parthenium hysterphorus (Compositae)	India/ USA	Aerial parts (na)	Sesquiterpine lactone, parthenin	*E. histolytica, in vitro* *E. histolytica*, hamsters	Sharma & Bhutani, 1987

Table 1 continued

Species (Family)	Origin[a]	Part (route[b])	Active ingredients	Indication	References
Pavonia odorata (Malvaceae)	India	Whole (na)	Methanol extract	*E. histolytica, in vitro*	Dhar *et al.*, 1968
Pinus longifolia (Pinaceae)	India	Stem (na)	Methanol extract	*E. histolytica, in vitro*	Dhar *et al.*, 1968
Polygonatum verticillatum (Liliaceae)	India	Whole (na)	Methanol extract	*E. histolytica, in vitro*	Bhakuni *et al.*, 1969
Psychotria ipecacuanha (Rubiaceae)	S. America	Root (po)	Emetine	*E. histolytica*, established drug	Datta *et al.*, 1974 Greenwood, 1992 Keene *et al.*, 1986
Pulsatilla chiensis (Ranunculaceae)	China	NC (na)	Crude extract	*E. histolytica, in vitro*	Lan *et al.*, 1996
Quamoclit coccinea [see *Ipomoea coccinea*]					
Quassia amara *Qua. simarouba* (Simaroubaceae)	Panama NC	Stem (na) NC (po)	Quassinoids, Glaucarubicin, ailanthinone, yadansioside F, bruceine A,B,C,D, holacanthone, glaucarubinone	*E. histolytica, in vitro* and clinical trial	Wright *et al.*, 1988 Van Assendelft *et al.*, 1956
Quercus oleoides (Fagaceae)	Mexico	Bark (na)	Ethanol extract	*E. histolytica, in vitro*	Heinrich *et al.*, 1992
Ricinus communis (Euphorbiaceae)	India	Root, stem (na)	Methanol extract	*E. histolytica, in vitro*	Dhar *et al.*, 1968

Table 1 *continued*

Species (Family)	Origin[a]	Part (route[b])	Active ingredients	Indication	References
Salvia lanata (Labitae)	India	Whole (na)	Methanol extract	*E. histolytica, in vitro*	Dhar *et al.*, 1968
Sarcocca trinervis (Buxaceae)	India	Whole (na)	Methanol extract	*E. histolytica, in vitro*	Bhakuni *et al.*, 1969
Scindapsus officinalis (Araceae)	India	Fruit (na)	Methanol extract	*E. histolytica, in vitro*	Dhar *et al.*, 1968
Scutia myrtina (Rhamnaceae)	India	Aerial (na)	Methanol extract	*E. histolytica, in vitro*	Dhar *et al.*, 1968
Sida cordifolia (Malvaceae)	India	Whole (na)	Methanol extract	*E. histolytica, in vitro*	Dhar *et al.*, 1968
Simarouba amara and *Sim. glauca* [see *Quassia amara* and *Qua. simarouba*]					
Solanum seaforthianum (Solanaceae)	India	Whole (na)	Methanol extract	*E. histolytica, in vitro*	Bhakuni *et al.*, 1969
Strychnos usambarensis (Loganiaceae)	Rwanda Tanzania	Root, leaf (na)	Usambarensine, usambarine	*E. histolytica, in vitro*	Wright *et al.*, 1991
Symplocos paniculata (Symplocaceae)	India	Leaf (na)	Methanol extract	*E. histolytica, in vitro*	Dhar *et al.*, 1968
Urginia indica [see *Drimia indica*]					

Table 1 continued

Species (Family)	Origin[a]	Part (route[b])	Active ingredients	Indication	References
Vernonia amygdalina (Compositae)	Tanzania	Whole (na)	Sesquiterpine lactone, steroid glucoside, isovernoniol, vernonioside A1, A2, A4 and B1	*E. histolytica, in vitro*	Ohigashi *et al*., 1994
Withania somnifera (Solanaceae)	India	Whole (na)	Methanol extract	*E. histolytica, in vitro*	Dhar *et al*., 1968
Ziziphus rotundifolia (Rhamnaceae)	India	Fruit (na)	Methanol extract	*E. histolytica, in vitro*	Bhakuni *et al*., 1969
Zizyphus rotundifolia [see *Ziziphus rotundifolia*]					

[a] Origin of the plant or product described in the citation. May not be the only origin.
[b] Route of administration: po, *per os* (oral); na, not applicable.
NC, not cited.

Table 2 Medicinal plants with activity against ciliates.

Species (Family)	Origin[a]	Part (route[b])	Active ingredients	Indication	References
Embelia ribes (Apocynaceae)	India	Fruit (po)	Crude preparation (used with *Holarrhena antidysenterica* seeds)	*Balantidium coli*, calves	Suhruda *et al.*, 1991
Holarrhena antidysenterica (Apocynaceae)	India	Seed (po)	Crude preparation (used with *Embelia ribes* fruit)	*B. coli*, calves	Suhruda *et al.*, 1991

[a] Origin of the plant or product described in the citation. May not be the only origin.
[b] Route of administration: po, *per os* (oral).

Table 3 Medicinal plants with activity against *Giardia*.

Species (Family)	Origin[a]	Part (route[b])	Active ingredients	Indication	References
Albizia coriaria (Fabaceae)	E. Africa	Root, bark (na)	Methanol extract	*Giardia lamblia, in vitro*	Johns *et al.*, 1995
Allium sativum (Liliaceae)	Egypt	Clove extract (po)	Crude extract	*G. lamblia*, clinical trial	Soffar & Mokhtar, 1991
Anisocycla cymosa (Menispermaceae)	Zaire	Root (na)	Cocsoline, dehydrotelobine, dehydroapateline	*G. lamblia, in vitro*	Kanyinda *et al.*, 1992
Berberis aristata (Berberidaceae)	NC	NC (na)	Alkaloid, berberine	*G. lamblia, in vitro*	Kaneda *et al.*, 1991
Butea monosperma (Leguminosae)	India	Whole (po)	Mixed with *Piper longum*	*G. lamblia*, clinical trial	Agarwal *et al.*, 1997
Cassia siamea (Fabaceae)	E. Africa	Leaf (na)	Methanol extract	*G. lamblia, in vitro*	Johns *et al.*, 1995
Centipeda minima (Compositae)	China	Whole (na)	Brevilin A	*G. lamblia, in vitro*	Yu *et al.*, 1994
Coleus kilimandscharica (Lamiaceae)	E. Africa	Leaf (na)	Methanol extract	*G. lamblia, in vitro*	Johns *et al.*, 1995
Commiphora africana (Burseraceae)	E. Africa	Root, bark (na)	Methanol extract	*G. lamblia, in vitro*	Johns *et al.*, 1995
Dichroa febrifuga (Hydrangeaceae)	China	Whole plant (po)	Febrifugine, isofebrifugine	*G. lamblia, in vitro*	Review Wright & Phillipson, 1990
Harrisonia abyssinica (Simaroubaceae)	E. Africa	Root, bark (na)	Methanolic extract	*G. lamblia, in vitro*	Johns *et al.*, 1995
Lannea schweinfurthii (Anacardiaceae)	E. Africa	Root, bark (na)	Methanolic extract	*G. lamblia, in vitro*	Johns *et al.*, 1995

Table 3 continued

Species (Family)	Origin[a]	Part (route[b])	Active ingredients	Indication	References
Microglossa pyrifolia (Asteraceae)	E. Africa	Root, bark (na)	Methanolic extract	*G. lamblia, in vitro*	Johns *et al.*, 1995
Ozoroa insignis (Anacardiaceae)	E. Africa	Root, bark (na)	Methanolic extract	*G. lamblia, in vitro*	Johns *et al.*, 1995
Piper longum (Piperaceae)	India	Whole (po)	Mixed with *Butea monosperma*	*G. lamblia*, clinical trial	Agarwal *et al.*, 1997
Psiadia arabica (Compositae)	E. Africa	Root (na)	Methanolic extract	*G. lamblia, in vitro*	Johns *et al.*, 1995
Rhus natalensis (Anacardiaceae)	E. Africa	Root, bark (na)	Methanolic extract	*G. lamblia, in vitro*	Johns *et al.*, 1995
Sonchus schweinfurthii (Asteraceae)	E. Africa	Leaf (na)	Methanolic extract	*G. lamblia, in vitro*	Johns *et al.*, 1995
Solanum incanum	E. Africa	Root, bark (na)	Methanolic extract	*G. lamblia, in vitro*	Johns *et al.*, 1995
S. nigrum (Solanaceae)	E. Africa	Leaf (na)	Methanolic extract	*G. lamblia, in vitro*	Johns *et al.*, 1995
Toddalia asiatica (Rutaceae)	E. Africa	Root, bark (na)	Methanolic extract	*G. lamblia, in vitro*	Johns *et al.*, 1995
Vernonia sp. (Asteraceae)	E. Africa	Root, bark (na)	Methanolic extract	*G. lamblia, in vitro*	Johns *et al.*, 1995
Ximenia caffra (Olacaceae)	E. Africa	Root, bark (na)	Methanolic extract	*G. lamblia, in vitro*	Johns *et al.*, 1995

[a] Origin of the plant or product described in the citation. May not be the only origin.
[b] Route of administration: po, *per os* (oral); na, not applicable.
NC, not cited.

Table 4 Medicinal plants with activity against *Leishmania*.

Species (Family)	Origin[a]	Part (route[b])	Active ingredients	Indication	References
Abrus precatorius (Leguminosae)	NC	Seed (na)	Plant proteins, arbrin	*L. infantum*, inhibits ribosome translocation	Cenini *et al.*, 1988
Abuta pahni	Bolivia	Stem (na)	Ethanolic extract, alkaloidal extract	*Leishmania* sp., *in vitro*	Fournet *et al.*, 1994
A. rutescens (Menispermaceae)					
Ampelocera edentula (Ulmaceae)	Bolivia	Stem, root (top)	Hydroxytetralone	*L. amazonensis*, mice	Fournet *et al.*, 1994
Anomospermum bolivianum (Menispermaceae)	Bolivia	Bark, stem (na)	Alkaloidal extract	*Leishmania* sp., *in vitro*	Fournet *et al.*, 1994
Berberis aristata	NC	NC (ip) (im)	Alkaloid, berberine	*L. donovani*, hamsters *L. donovani*, hamsters *L. braziliensis*, hamsters	Ghosh *et al.*, 1985 Vennerstrom *et al.*, 1990
B. boliviana *B. laurina* (Berberidaceae)	Bolivia	Bark (na)	Ethanolic extract	*Leishmania* sp., *in vitro*	Fournet *et al.*, 1994
Bocconia integrifolia	Bolivia	Leaf, latex, bark (top)	Benzophenathridine, alkaloids	*L. amazonensis, in vitro*	Fournet *et al.*, 1994
B. pearcei (Papaveraceae)					
Cardiopetalum calophyllum (Annonaceae)	Bolivia	Leaf, stem (na)	Alkaloidal extract	*Leishmania* sp., *in vitro*	Fournet *et al.*, 1994

Table 4 *continued*

Species (Family)	Origin[a]	Part (route[b])	Active ingredients	Indication	References
Cola attiensis (Sterculiaceae)	Nigeria	Seed (na)	Aromatic polysulphur compounds	*L. chagasi, in vitro*	Iwu *et al.*, 1992 Iwu *et al.*, 1994
Desmodium gangeticum (Fabaceae)	Nigeria	Leaf (na)	Alkylamines	*L. chagasi, in vitro*	Iwu *et al.*, 1992 Iwu *et al.*, 1994
Dianthus caryophyllus (Caryophyllaceae)	NC	Leaf (na)	Plant proteins, dianthin 30 and 32	*L. infantum*, inhibits ribosome translocation	Cenini *et al.*, 1988
Diospyros montana (Ebenaceae)	India	Bark (na)	Naphthoquinone, diospyrin	*L. donovani, in vitro*	Hazra *et al.*, 1987
Dorstenia multiradiata (Moraceae)	Nigeria	Leaf (na)	Anthocyanidins	*L. chagasi, in vitro*	Iwu *et al.*, 1992 Iwu *et al.*, 1994
Dracaena mannii (Agavaceae)	Nigeria		Saponins		Iwu *et al.*, 1992 Iwu *et al.*, 1994
Galipea longiflora (Rutaceae)	Bolivia	Stem, root (top)	Hydroxytetralone	*L. amazonensis*, mice	Fournet *et al.*, 1994
Gongronerna latifolia (Asclepiadaceae)	Nigeria	Leaf (na)	Lignans	*L. chagasi, in vitro*	Iwu *et al.*, 1992 Iwu *et al.*, 1994
Hedera helix (Araliaceae)	NC	Leaf (na)	Saponin	*L. tropica, in vitro* *L. infantum, in vitro*	Majester-Savornin *et al.*, 1991
Jacaranda copaia (Bignoniaceae)	Guyana	Leaf (sc)	Quinoids, jacaranone, ursolic acid	*L. amazonensis, in vitro* and mice	Sauvain *et al.*, 1993
Mandevilla antennaceae (Apocynaceae)	Bolivia	Leaf, stem (na)	Ethanolic extract	*Leishmania* sp., *in vitro*	Fournet *et al.*, 1994
Munnozia fournetti	Bolivia	Leaf, stem (na)	Ethanolic extract	*Leishmania* sp., *in vitro*	Fournet *et al.*, 1994

Table 4 continued

Species (Family)	Origin[a]	Part (route[b])	Active ingredients	Indication	References
M. maronii (Asteraceae)	Bolivia	Leaf (sc)	Sesquiterpine lactone, dehydrozaluzanin C	*L. amazonensis*, mice *Leishmania* sp., *in vitro*	Fournet *et al.*, 1993
Myrsine pellucida (Myrsinaceae)	Bolivia	Bark (na)	Triterpine saponins	*L. braziliensis, in vitro*	Lavaud *et al.*, 1994
Nyctanthes arbor-tristis (Oleaceae)	India	Seed (na) (ip)	Iridoid glucosides, hydroxyloganin, arbortristosides A, B, C	*L. donovani, in vitro* and hamsters	Tandon *et al.*, 1991
Oxandra espintana (Annonaceae)	Bolivia	Bark (na)	Espintanol	*Leishmania* sp., *in vitro*	Hocquemiller *et al.*, 1991
Peganum harmala (Zygophyllaceae)	Egypt	Seed (na)	Harmaline	*Leishmania* sp., *in vitro*	Ross *et al.*, 1980 Evans & Croft, 1987
Pera benensis (Euphorbiaceae)	NC	Stem (na), root	Napthoquinone, plumbagin		Fournet *et al.*, 1992
Phytolacca americana (Phytolaccaceae)	NC	Root (na), seed	Pokeweed antiviral protein	*L. infantum*, inhibits ribosome translocation	Cenini *et al.*, 1988
Picralima nitida (Apocynaceae)	Nigeria	Leaf (na)	Indole alkaloids	*L. chagasi*, *in vitro*	Iwu *et al.*, 1992 Iwu *et al.*, 1994
Picrorhiza kurrora (Scrophulariaceae)	India Sri Lanka	Root (po)	Iridoid glycosides	*L. donovani*, hamsters immunostimulant	Puri *et al.*, 1992
Piper rushbyi (Piperaceae)	Bolivia	Whole (na)	Ethylacetate extract	*Leishmania* sp., *in vitro*	Fournet *et al.*, 1994
Plumbago zeylanica (Plumbaginaceae)	NC	NC (na) (sc)	Naphthoquinolone, plumbagin	*L. donovani*, *in vitro* *L. amazonensis*, mice	Croft *et al.*, 1985

Table 4 continued

Species (Family)	Origin[a]	Part (route[b])	Active ingredients	Indication	References
Polyalthia macropoda (Annonaceae)	Malaysia	Bark (na)	Lambdanic diterpine	*L. donovani, in vitro*	Richomme *et al*., 1991
Ricinus communis (Euphorbiaceae)	NC	Root (na)	Plant proteins	*L. infantum*, inhibits ribosome translocation	Cenini *et al*., 1988
Saponaria officinalis (Caryophyllaceae)	NC	Seed (na)	Plant proteins, saponin 6 and 9	*L. infantum*, inhibits ribosome translocation	Cenini *et al*., 1988
Solanum actaeabotrys (Solanaceae)	Bolivia	Leaf (na)	Ethanolic extract	*Leishmania* sp., *in vitro*	Fournet *et al*., 1994
Stevia yaconensis (Asteraceae)	Bolivia	Whole (na)	Ethylacetate extract	*Leishmania* sp., *in vitro*	Fournet *et al*., 1994
Vernonia squamulosa	Bolivia	Stem (na)	Ethylacetate extract	*Leishmania* sp., *in vitro*	Fournet *et al*., 1994
V. amygdalina (Compositae)	Tanzania	Whole (na)	Sesquiterpine lactone, vernodalin, vernodalol	*L. infantum, in vitro*	Ohigashi *et al*., 1994

[a] Origin of the plant or product described in the citation. May not be the only origin.
[b] Route of administration: sc, subcutaneous inoculation; po, *per os* (oral); top, topical; im, intramuscular; ip, intraperitoneal; na, not applicable. NC, not cited.

Table 5 Medicinal plants with activity against *Trichomonas*.

Species (Family)	Origin[a]	Part (route[b])	Active ingredients	Indication	References
Berbis aristata (Berberidaceae)	NC	NC (na)	Alkaloid, berberine	*Trichomonas vaginalis*, *in vitro*	Kaneda *et al*., 1991
Brucea javanica (Simaroubaceae)	China	NC (NC)		*Tri. vaginalis*, clinical trial	Xiao & Fu, 1986
Macleaya cordata (Papaveraceae)	China	NC (NC)		*Tri. vaginalis*, clinical trial	Xiao & Fu, 1986
Pulsatilla chinensis (Ranunculaceae)	China	Flower (NC)		*Tri. vaginalis*, clinical trial	Xiao & Fu, 1986

[a] Origin of the plant or product described in the citation. May not be the only origin.
[b] Route of administration: na, not applicable.
NC, not cited.

Table 6 Medicinal plants with activity against *Trypanosoma*.

Species (Family)	Origin[a]	Part (route[b])	Active ingredients	Indication	References
Abrus precatorius (Leguminosae)	NC	Seed (na)	Plant proteins, arbrin	*T. rhodesiense*, inhibits ribosome translocation	Cenini *et al.*, 1988
Abuta pahni	Bolivia	Stem (na)	Ethanolic extract	*T. cruzi, in vitro*	Fournet *et al.*, 1994
A. rutescens (Menispermaceae)	Bolivia	Stem (na)	Alkaloidal extract	*T. cruzi, in vitro*	Fournet *et al.*, 1994
Acalypha guatemalensis (Euphorbiaceae)	Guatemala	Leaf (po)	Ethanol extract	*T. cruzi*, in mice	Caceres *et al.*, 1998
Albizia gummifera (Leguminosae)	E. Africa	NC (na)	Lipophilic extract	*T. rhodesiense, in vitro*	Freiburghaus *et al.*, 1996
Allium sativum (Liliaceae)	Nigeria	Cloves (na)	Diallyl disulfide	*T. brucei, in vitro* *T. brucei,* mice	Nok *et al.*, 1996
Alstonia boonei (Apocynaceae)	Nigeria	Bark (ip)	Aqueous extract	*T. brucei,* mice	Asuzu & Anaga, 1991
Ampelocera edentula (Ulmaceae)	Bolivia	Stem, root (top)	Hydroxytetralone	*T. cruzi, in vitro*	Fournet *et al.*, 1994
Annona senegalensis (Annonaceae)	NC	NC (na)		*T. rhodesiense, in vitro*	Freiburghaus *et al.*, 1996
Anomospermum bolivianum (Menispermaceae)	Bolivia	Bark, stem (na)	Alkaloidal extract	*T. cruzi, in vitro*	Fournet *et al.*, 1994
Aspidosperma nigricans	Brazil	NC (ip/iv)	Alkaloid, olivacine	Inactive in mice	Leon *et al.*, 1978
A. olivaceum (Apocynaceae)	Brazil	NC (na)		*T. cruzi, in vitro*	Cruz *et al.*, 1975
Berberis boliviana *B. laurina*	Bolivia	Bark (na)	Ethanol extract	*T. cruzi, in vitro*	Fournet *et al.*, 1994

Table 6 continued

Species (Family)	Origin[a]	Part (route[b])	Active ingredients	Indication	References
B. aristata (Berberidaceae)	E. Africa	Leaf (na)	Alkaloid, berberine	*T. rhodesiense, in vitro*	Freiburghaus *et al.*, 1996
Bocconia integrifolia *B. pearcei* (Papaveraceae)	Bolivia	Leaf, latex, bark (top)	Benzophenathridine alkaloids	*T. cruzi, in vitro*	Fournet *et al.*, 1994
Bussea occidentalis (Leguminosae)	E. Africa	NC (na)	Lipophilic extract	*T. rhodesiense, in vitro*	Freiburghaus *et al.*, 1996
Byrsonima crassifolia (Malpighiaceae)	Guatemala	Leaf (po)	Ethanol extract	*T. cruzi, in vitro* *T. cruzi*, mice	Berger *et al.*, 1998
Cardiopetalum calophyllum (Annonaceae)	Bolivia	Leaf, stem (na)	Alkaloidal extract	*T. cruzi, in vitro*	Fournet *et al.*, 1994
Catharanthus roseus [see *Vinca major*]					
Cephaelis ipecacuanha [see *Psychotria ipecachuanha*]					
Cinchona officinalis (Rubiaceae)	S. America	Bark (na)	Quinine	*T. cruzi, in vitro*	Cavin *et al.*, 1987
Dianthus caryophyllus (Caryophyllaceae)	NC	Leaf (na)	Plant proteins, dianthin 30 and 32	*T. rhodesiense*, inhibits ribosome translocation	Cenini *et al.*, 1988
Ehretia amoena (Boraginaceae)	E. Africa	NC (na)	Lipophilic extract	*T. rhodesiense, in vitro*	Freiburghaus *et al.*, 1996
Entada abyssinica (Leguminosae)	E. Africa	NC (na)	Lipophilic extract	*T. rhodesiense, in vitro*	Freiburghaus *et al.*, 1996

Table 6 *continued*

Species (Family)	Origin[a]	Part (route[b])	Active ingredients	Indication	References
Galipea longiflora (Rutaceae)	Bolivia	Stem, root (top)	Hydroxytetralone	*T. cruzi, in vitro*	Fournet *et al*., 1994
Gliricidia sepium (Leguminosae)	Guatemala	Leaf (na)	Ethanol extract	*T. cruzi, in vitro*	Berger *et al*., 1998 Caceres *et al*., 1998
Gossypium hirsutum (Malvaceae)	NC	Cotton seed oil (na)	Gossypol	*T. cruzi, in vitro*	Montamat *et al*., 1982 Turrens, 1986
Lycium chinense (Solanaceae)	China	Root (na)	Polyamine derivative kukoamine	Inhibitor of trypanothione reductase	Ponasik *et al*., 1995
Munnozia fournetti	Bolivia	Leaf, stem (na)	Ethanol extract	*T. cruzi, in vitro*	Fournet *et al*., 1994
M. maronii (Compositae)	Bolivia	Leaf (na)	Sesquiterpine lactone, dehydrozaluzanin C	*T. cruzi, in vitro*	Fournet *et al*., 1993
Neurolaena lobata (Compositae)	Guatemala	Leaf (po)	Ethanol extract	*T. cruzi, in vitro* *T. cruzi*, mice	Berger *et al*., 1998 Caceres *et al*., 1998
Oxandra espintana (Annonaceae)	Bolivia	Bark (na)	Espintanol	*T. cruzi, in vitro*	Hocquemiller *et al*., 1991
Pera benensis (Euphorbiaceae)	Bolivia	Bark, root (na)	Plumbagin	*T. cruzi, in vitro*	Fournet *et al*., 1992
Petiveria alliaceae (Phytolaccaceae)	Guatemala	Leaf (na)	Ethanol extract, dichloromethane extract	*T. cruzi, in vitro*	Berger *et al*., 1998 Caceres *et al*., 1998
Physalis angulata (Solanaceae)	NC	NC (na)		*T. rhodesiense, in vitro*	Freiburghaus *et al*., 1996
Phytolacca americana (Phytolaccaceae)	NC	Root (na), seed, root	Pokeweed antiviral protein	*T. rhodesiense*, inhibits ribosome translocation	Cenini *et al*., 1988

Table 6 continued

Species (Family)	Origin[a]	Part (route[b])	Active ingredients	Indication	References
Picralima nitida (Apocynaceae)	W. Africa	Bark (po)	Aqueous extract	*T. brucei*, rats	Wosu & Ibe, 1989
Piper rushbyi (Piperaceae)	Bolivia	Whole (na)	Ethylacetate extract	*T. cruzi, in vitro*	Fournet *et al.*, 1994
Psychotria ipecacuanha (Rubiaceae)	S. America	Bark (na)	Emetine	*T. cruzi, in vitro*	Cavin *et al.*, 1987
Saponaria officinalis (Caryophyllaceae)	NC	Seed (na)	Plant proteins, saponin 6 and 9	*T. rhodesiense*, inhibits ribosome translocation	Cenini *et al.*, 1988
Securinega virosa (Euphorbiaceae)	E. Africa	NC (na)	Lipophilic extract	*T. rhodesiense, in vitro*	Freiburghaus *et al.*, 1996
Solanum actaeabotrys	Bolivia	Leaf (na)	Ethanolic extract	*T. cruzi, in vitro*	Fournet *et al.*, 1994
S. americanum (Solanaceae)	Venezuela	Fresh fruit (na)	Glycoalkaloids, chaconine, solamargine	*T. cruzi, in vitro*	Chataing *et al.*, 1998
Stevia yaconensis (Compositae)	Bolivia	Whole (na)	Ethylacetate extract	*T. cruzi, in vitro*	Fournet *et al.*, 1994
Tridax procumbens (Compositae)	Guatemala	Leaf (na)	Ethanol extract, dichloromethane extract	*T. cruzi, in vitro*	Berger *et al.*, 1998 Caceres *et al.*, 1998
Vernonia squamulosa	Bolivia	Stem	Ethylacetate extract	*T. cruzi, in vitro*	Fournet *et al.*, 1994
V. subuligera (Compositae)	E. Africa	NC (na)	Lipophilic extract	*T. rhodesiense, in vitro*	Freiburghaus *et al.*, 1996
Vinca major (Apocynaceae)	Madagascar	NC (na)	Vinblastine	*T. cruzi, in vitro*	Cavin *et al.*, 1987

[a] Origin of the plant or product described in the citation. May not be the only origin.
[b] Route of administration: po, *per os* (oral); iv, intravenous; ip, intraperitoneal; na, not applicable; top, topical.
NC, not cited.

Table 7 Medicinal plants with activity against *Plasmodium*.

Species (Family)	Origin[a]	Part (route[b])	Active ingredients	Indication	References
Abutilon grandiflorum (Malvaceae)	Tanzania	Root (na) (po)	Ethylacetate extract	*P. falciparum, in vitro*	Gessler *et al.*, 1994 Gessler *et al.*, 1995
Acacia clavigera (Leguminosae)	Tanzania	Bark (na)	Petroleum ether extract	*P. falciparum, in vitro*	Weenen *et al.*, 1990
Acampe pachyglossa (Orchidaceae)	Tanzania	Leaf (po)	Ethylacetate extract	*P. falciparum, in vitro*	Gessler *et al.*, 1994
Acanthospermum australe (Compositae)	Brazil	NC (po) (na)	Crude extract	*P. berghei*, mice *P. falciparum, in vitro*	Carvalho *et al.*, 1991
Achillea millefolium (Compositae)	NC	NC (na)	α Peroxyachifolid	*P. falciparum, in vitro*	Rucker *et al.*, 1991
Achyranthes aspera (Amaranthaceae)	Tanzania	Root (na)	Ethylacetate extract	*P. falciparum, in vitro*	Gessler *et al.*, 1994
Adansonia digitata (Bombaceae)	Tanzania	Bark (na)	Ethylacetate extract	*P. falciparum, in vitro*	Gessler *et al.*, 1994
Aegle marmelos (Rutaceae)	India	Seed (po)	Ethanol extract	*P. berghei, in vitro* *P. berghei, Mastomys*	Misra *et al.*, 1991
Aerva lanata (Amaranthaceae)	Tanzania	Root (na)	Ethylacetate extract	*P. falciparum, in vitro*	Gessler *et al.*, 1994
Ailanthus imberbiflora	NC	Bark (sc)	Chloroform extract	*P. gallinaceum*, chicks	Spencer *et al.*, 1947
Ail. altissima			Chloroform extract	*P. falciparum, in vitro*	O'Neill *et al.*, 1985
Ail. excelsa (Simaroubaceae)	Sudan	Leaf (na)	Methanol extract	*P. falciparum, in vitro*	El Tahir *et al.*, 1999
Albizia anthelmintica (Leguminosae)	Tanzania	Bark (na)	Methanol extract	*P. falciparum, in vitro*	Weenen *et al.*, 1990

Table 7 continued

Species (Family)	Origin[a]	Part (route[b])	Active ingredients	Indication	References
Alnus incana (Betulaceae)	Poland	Stipes, fruit (na)	Ethylacetate extract	*P. falciparum, in vitro*	Grzybek *et al.*, 1997
Alstonia coriaceae and sp. (Apocynaceae)	NC	Bark (na)	Corialstonine, corialstonidine, echitamine	*P. falciparum, in vitro*	Wright *et al.*, 1993b
Amaryllis belladonna (Amaryllidaceae)	NC	Bulbs (po)	Aqueous extract	*P. gallinaceum*, chicks	Spencer *et al.*, 1947
Ampelocissus africana (Vitaceae)	Tanzania	Bark (na)	Ethylacetate extract	*P. falciparum, in vitro*	Gessler *et al.*, 1994
Ancistrocladus abbreviatus	Ivory Coast	Root, bark (na)	Ancistrobrevine	*P. falciparum, in vitro*	Francois *et al.*, 1995
Anc. barteri		Root (po)	Ancistrocladine	*P. berghei*, mice	Francois *et al.*, 1994
Anc. heyneanus		Root, bark (na)	Ancistrobarterine A	*P. falciparum, in vitro*	Francois *et al.*, 1997b
Anc. robertsoniorum		Leaf, bark (po)	Betulinic acid	*P. berghei*, mice	Francois *et al.*, 1997b
Anc. tectorius (Ancistrocladaceae)		Leaf (po)		*P. berghei*, mice	Francois *et al.*, 1997b
Andrographis paniculata (Acanthaceae)	Malaysia	Whole plant (na)	Chloroform extract	*P. falciparum, in vitro*	Rahman *et al.*, 1999
Anisocycla cymosa (Menispermaceae)	Zaire	Root (na)	Cocsoline	*P. falciparum, in vitro*	Francois *et al.*, 1992
Annickia chlorantha (Anonaceae)	Nigeria	Bark (po)	Berberine alkaloids, saponins	*P. yoelii*, mice	Agbaje & Onabanjo, 1991
Annona muricata (Annonaceae)	Togo	Leaf (na)	Ethanol extract	*P. falciparum, in vitro*	Gbeassor *et al.*, 1990

Table 7 continued

Species (Family)	Origin[a]	Part (route[b])	Active ingredients	Indication	References
Ansellia africana (Orchidaceae)	Tanzania	Bark (na)	Ethylacetate extract	*P. falciparum, in vitro*	Gessler *et al.*, 1994
Anthemis nobilis (Compositae)	NC	NC (na)	Hydroperoxy-isonobilin	*P. falciparum, in vitro*	Rucker *et al.*, 1991
Aristolochia dululu (Aristolochiaceae)	NC	Root (po)	Aqueous extract	*P. gallinaceum*, chicks	Spencer *et al.*, 1947
Artabotrys uncinatus	China	NC (po)	Sesquiterpine lactone	*P. falciparum*, clinical trial	Jaquet *et al.*, 1994
Arta. hexapetalus (Annonaceae)	NC	Root (po)	Synthetic derivative, arteflene, yingzhaosu A,B,C,D	*P. falciparum*, clinical trial	Salako *et al.*, 1994
Artemisia annua and *Artemisis appiaceae*	China	Leaf (po/im)	Sesquiterpine lactone, peroxides, artemisinin	*P. falciparum*, clinical trial	Qinghaosu group, 1979 Li *et al.*, 1994
Art. absinthium	India	Leaf (na)	Ethanol/aqueous extract	*P. berghei*, mice	Zafar *et al.*, 1990
	NC	Aerial (na)	Homoditerpene peroxides	*P. falciparum, in vitro*	Rucker *et al.*, 1992 Rucker *et al.*, 1991
Art. afra	Tanzania	Root (na)	Methanol extract	*P. falciparum, in vitro*	Weenen *et al.*, 1990
Art. japonica	India	Aerial (na)	Petroleum ether extract	*P. falciparum, in vitro*	Valecha *et al.*, 1994
Art. maritima	India	Aerial (na)	Ethanol extract, arteinculton	*P. falciparum, in vitro* *P. falciparum, in vitro*	Valecha *et al.*, 1994 Rucker *et al.*, 1991
Art. nilegarica	India	Root (na)	Ethanol extract	*P. falciparum, in vitro*	Valecha *et al.*, 1994
Art. parviflora	India	Aerial (na)	Ethanol extract	*P. falciparum, in vitro*	Badam *et al.*, 1988

Table 7 continued

Species (Family)	Origin[a]	Part (route[b])	Active ingredients	Indication	References
Art. scoparia (Compositae)	India	Aerial (na)	Ethanol extract	*P. falciparum, in vitro*	Misra *et al.*, 1991
Aspidosperma oblongum (Apocynaceae)	Brazil	NC (na)	Ethanol extract	*P. falciparum, in vitro*	Cabral *et al.*, 1993
Atalantia monophyla (Rutaceae)	India	Aerial (na)	Limonoids, triterpene, atalantin, ataphyllinine	*P. falciparum, in vitro*	Badam *et al.*, 1988 Fujioka *et al.*, 1989
Azadirachta indica (Meliaceae)	India	Leaf, bark (na)	Limonoids, gedunin	*P. falciparum, in vitro*	Dhar *et al.*, 1998 Bray *et al.*, 1990
Azanza garckeana [see *Thespia garckeana*]					
Balanites tormentosa	NC	Root (sc)	Chloroform extract	*P. gallinaceum*, chicks	Spencer *et al.*, 1947
Bal. aegyptiaca (Zygophyllaceae)	Tanzania	Bark (na)	Dichloromethane extract	*P. falciparum, in vitro*	Weenen *et al.*, 1990
Bauhinia thonningii (Leguminosae)	Tanzania	Leaf (na)	Methanol extract	*P. falciparum, in vitro*	Weenen *et al.*, 1990
Beilschmiedia madang (Lauraceae)	Indonesia	Wood (na)	Dehatrine	*P. falciparum, in vitro*	Kitagawa *et al.*, 1993
Bidens pilosa (Compositae)	Brazil	Whole plant (na)	Flavonoids, aliphatic acetylenes	*P. falciparum, in vitro*	Brandao *et al.*, 1997
Bombax rhodognaphalon (Bombacaceae)	Tanzania	Root (na)	Petroleum ether	*P. falciparum, in vitro*	Gessler *et al.*, 1994

Table 7 continued

Species (Family)	Origin[a]	Part (route[b])	Active ingredients	Indication	References
Bougainvillea spectabilis (Nyctaginaceae)		Leaf (na) (po)	Ethanol extract	*P. berghei, in vitro* inactive *Mastomys*	Misra *et al.*, 1991
Bridelia cathartica (Euphorbiaceae)	Mozambique	Root, stem (na) (po)	Ethanol extract	*P. falciparum, in vitro* *P. falciparum*, clinical trial	Jurg *et al.*, 1991
Brucea javanica (Simaroubaceae)	Indonesia	Fruit (na)	Quassinoid, bruceantin, dihydro-bruceajavanin A, bruceantinol,	*P. falciparum, in vitro*	Kitagawa *et al.*, 1994 O'Neill *et al.*, 1985
			bruceajavanin A, bruceine A		Guru *et al.*, 1983
	China		Bruceine D,E		Lin *et al.*, 1982
Caesalpinia bonducella (Leguminosae)	Tanzania	Whole (na)	Methanol extract	*P. falciparum, in vitro*	Weenen *et al.*, 1990
Canella winterana (Canellaceae)	NC	Stem, root (po/sc)	Aqueous extract	*P. gallinaceum*, chicks	Spencer *et al.*, 1947
Canthium phyllanthoideum (Rubiaceae)	NC	Bark (na)	Aqueous extract	*P. falciparum, in vitro*	Gakunju *et al.*, 1995
Cassia abbreviata	Malawi	Root (na)	Ethylacetate extract	*P. falciparum, in vitro*	Connelly *et al.*, 1996
Cas. occidentalis		Leaf (na)	Aqueous extract	*P. falciparum, in vitro*	Gasquet *et al.*, 1993
	Tanzania				Weenen *et al.*, 1990
Cas. siamea (Leguminosae)	Togo	Leaf (na)	Aqueous extract	*P. falciparum, in vitro*	Gbeassor *et al.*, 1989
Castela spinosa	NC	Root (sc)	Chloroform extract	*P. gallinaceum*, chicks	Spencer *et al.*, 1947

Table 7 continued

Species (Family)	Origin[a]	Part (route[b])	Active ingredients	Indication	References
Cast. tweedi	NC	Root, stem (po/sc)	Chloroform	*P. gallinaceum*, chicks	Spencer *et al.*, 1947
Cast. tortusa (Simaroubaceae)	NC	Root, leaf, stem (po/sc)	Aqueous extracts	*P. gallinaceum*, chicks	Spencer *et al.*, 1947
Catha edulis (Celastraceae)	Tanzania	Aerial (na)	Methanol extract	*P. falciparum, in vitro*	Weenen *et al.*, 1990
Catharanthus roseus (Apocynaceae)	Madagascar	NC (na)	Vinblastine	*P. falciparum, in vitro*	Usanga *et al.*, 1986
Celastrus paniculatus (Celastraceae)	Thailand	Root, stem (na)	Quinonoid triterpene, pristimerin	*P. falciparum, in vitro*	Pavanand *et al.*, 1989b
Centipeda minima (Compositae)	China	Whole (na)	Brevilin A	*P. falciparum, in vitro*	Yu *et al.*, 1994
Chenopodium ambrosioides (Chenopodiaceae)	India	Aerial (po)	Ethanol extract	*P. berghei, Mastomys*, inactive *in vitro*	Misra *et al.*, 1991
Cichorium intybus (Compositae)	India	Seed (na) (po)	Ethanol extract	*P. berghei, in vitro* *P. berghei, Mastomys*	Misra *et al.*, 1991
Cinchona succirubra *Cin. calisaya* (*ledgeriana*)	S. America	Bark (po/im/iv)	Alkaloids Quinine, quinidine	Established drug	Rev. Greenwood, 1992 Rev. Dobson, 1998
Cin. corolla and others (Rubiaceae)	NC	Bark (na)	Cinchonine, cinchonidine	*P. falciparum, in vitro*	Druilhe *et al.*, 1988
Cinnamomum tamala (Lauraceae)	India	Leaf (po)	Ethanol extract	*P. berghei, in vitro* *P. berghei, Mastomys*	Misra *et al.*, 1991

Table 7 continued

Species (Family)	Origin[a]	Part (route[b])	Active ingredients	Indication	References
Cissampelos mucronata (Menispermaceae)	Tanzania	Root (na) (po)	Ethylacetate extract	*P. berghei, in vitro* *P. falciparum*, mice	Gessler *et al.*, 1994 Gessler *et al.*, 1995
Citrus grandis (Rutaceae)	Taiwan	Root, bark (na) (ip)	Acridine alkaloids	*P. yoelii, in vitro* *P. yoelii*, mice	Fujioka *et al.*, 1989
Clausena anisata (Rutaceae)	Tanzania	Bark (na)	Methanol extract	*P. falciparum, in vitro*	Weenen *et al.*, 1990
Cleome gynandra (Capparidaceae)	Tanzania	Root (na)	Ethylacetate extract	*P. falciparum, in vitro*	Weenen *et al.*, 1990
Clerodendrum myricoides (Labiatae)	Tanzania	Root (na)	Ethylacetate extract	*P. falciparum, in vitro*	Gessler *et al.*, 1994
Clutia robusta (Euphorbiaceae)	Tanzania	Root (na)	Methanol extract	*P. falciparum, in vitro*	Weenen *et al.*, 1990
Cochlospermum angolense	Angola	Root (na)	Methanol extract	*P. falciparum, in vitro*	Presber *et al.*, 1992
Coc. tinctorium (Cochlospermaceae)	Burkina Faso	Tubercules (na)	Aqueous extract	*P. falciparum, in vitro*	Benoit *et al.*, 1995
Combretum micranthum	Ivory Coast	Stem, leaf (na)	Aqueous extract	*P. falciparum, in vitro*	Benoit *et al.*, 1996
Com. psilophyllum (Combretaceae)		Root (na)	Ethylacetate extract	*P. falciparum, in vitro*	Gessler *et al.*, 1994
Conyza pyrrhopappa (Compositae)	Tanzania	Leaf (na)	Dichloromethane extract	*P. falciparum, in vitro*	Weenen *et al.*, 1990
Cooperia pedunculata [see *Zephyranthes pedunculata*]					

Table 7 continued

Species (Family)	Origin[a]	Part (route[b])	Active ingredients	Indication	References
Coptis teeta (Ranunculaceae)	India	Rhizome (na)	Aqueous extract, berberine alkaloids	*P. falciparum, in vitro,* inactive *P. berghei*, mice	Sharma *et al*., 1993
Coutarea latifolia (Rubiaceae)	S. America	Bark (na)	Ethylacetate extract	*P. falciparum, in vitro*	Noster & Kraus, 1990
Crassocephalum bojeri (Compositae)	Tanzania	Aerial (na)	Dichloromethane extract	*P. falciparum, in vitro*	Weenen *et al*., 1990
Crinum amabile	Thailand	Bulb(na)	Crinamine, augustine	*P. falciparum, in vitro*	Likhitwitayawuid *et al*., 1993
Cri. americanum	NC	Bulb (po)	Aqueous extract	*P. gallinaceum*, chicks	Spencer *et al*., 1947
Cri. portifolium	Tanzania	Whole (na)	Methanol extract	*P. falciparum, in vitro*	Weenen *et al*., 1990
Cri. stuhlmanni	Tanzania	Whole (na)	Methanol extract	*P. falciparum, in vitro*	Weenen *et al*., 1990
Cri. papillosum (Amaryllidaceae)	Tanzania	Whole (na)	Methanol extract	*P. falciparum, in vitro*	Weenen *et al*., 1990
Crossopterix febrifuga (Rubiaceae)	Tanzania	Bark (na)	Methanol extract	*P. falciparum, in vitro*	Weenen *et al*., 1990
Croton guatemalensis (Euphorbiaceae)	Guatemala	NC (na)	Methanol extract	*P. berghei*, mice	Franssen *et al*., 1997
Cryptolepis sanguinolenta (Asclepiadaceae)	Ghana	Root (na)	Cryptolepine	*P. falciparum, in vitro*	Tackie *et al*., 1993
		(ip)	Isocryptolepine	*P. berghei* and *P. vinckei petteri,* mice	Grellier *et al*., 1996
				Inactive *P. berghei*, mice	Kirby *et al*., 1995
Cucumis aculeatus (Cucurbitaceae)	Kenya	Whole (na)	Aqueous extract	*P. falciparum, in vitro*	Gakunju *et al*., 1995
Cucurbita maxima (Cucurbitaceae)	Brazil	Seed (po)	Ethanol extract	*P. berghei*, mice	Amorim *et al*., 1991

Table 7 continued

Species (Family)	Origin[a]	Part (route[b])	Active ingredients	Indication	References
Cussonia zimmermanni (Araliaceae)	Tanzania Tanzania	Root (na) Root (na)	Petroleum ether extract	*P. falciparum, in vitro* *P. berghei, in vitro*	Gessler *et al.*, 1994 Weenen *et al.*, 1990
Cyclea barbata (Menispermaceae)	Thailand	Root (na)	Bisbenzyl-isoquinolines, tetrandrine, limacine, thalrugosine, homoaromoline, cycleapeltine		Lin *et al.*, 1993
Cymbopogon citratus (Gramineae)	Nigeria	Rhizome (po/ip)	Aqueous extract	*P. yoelli*, mice	Onabanjo *et al.*, 1993
Cyperus rotundus	Tanzania	Tuber (na)	Sesquiterpine endoperosides, peroxycalamenene	*P. falciparum, in vitro*	Weenen *et al.*, 1990 ThebtarAnonth *et al.*, 1995
Cyp. scariosus (Cyperaceae)	India	Aerial (na)	Ethanol extract	*P. berghei, in vitro*	Misra *et al.*, 1991
Dialium guineense (Leguminosae)	Togo	Leaf, twig (na)	Aqueous extract	*P. falciparum, in vitro*	Gbeassor *et al.*, 1989
Dichapetalum guineense (Dichapetalaceae)	Togo	Aerial (na)	Aqueous extract	*P. falciparum, in vitro*	Gbeassor *et al.*, 1989
Dichroa febrifuga (Hydrangeaceae)	China	Whole plant (po)	Febrifugine, isofebrifugine	Clinical trial *P. gallinaceum*, chicks	Xiao & Fu, 1986 Spencer *et al.*, 1947
Diosma pilosa (Rutaceae)	Sudan	NC (na)	Quercetin, trimethoxycoumarin	*P. falciparum, in vitro*	Khalid *et al.*, 1986
Diospyros zembensis (Ebenaceae)	NC	Leaf (na)	Ethylacetate extract	*P. falciparum, in vitro*	Gessler *et al.*, 1994

Table 7 continued

Species (Family)	Origin[a]	Part (route[b])	Active ingredients	Indication	References
Dissotis brazzae (Melastomataceae)	Kenya	Stem (na), leaf	Methanol extract, aqueous extract	*P. falciparum, in vitro*	Omulokoli *et al.*, 1997
Dombeya shupangae (Sterculiaceae)	Tanzania	Root (na)	Ethylacetate extract	*P. falciparum, in vitro*	Gessler *et al.*, 1994
Enantia chlorantha [see *Annickia chlorantha*]					
Enicostema hyssopifolium (Gentianaceae)	India	Root (na) (po)	Ethanol extract	*P. berghei, in vitro* *P. berghei, Mastomys*	Misra *et al.*, 1991
Entandrophragma bussei (Meliaceae)	Tanzania	Bark (na)	Dichloromethane extract	*P. falciparum, in vitro*	Weenen *et al.*, 1990
Eryngium foetidum (Umbelliferae)	NC	Whole plant (po)	Aqueous extract	*P. gallinaceum*, chicks	Spencer *et al.*, 1947
Erythrina sacleuxii (Leguminosae)	Tanzania	Root (na)	Ethylacetate extract	*P. falciparum, in vitro*	Gessler *et al.*, 1994
Esenbeckia febrifuga (Rutaceae)	Brazil	NC (na)	Crude extract	*P. falciparum, in vitro* *P. berghei*, mice	Carvalho *et al.*, 1991
Etlingera eliator (Zingiberaceae)	NC	Stalk (na)	Aqueous and ethanol extract	*P. falciparum, in vitro*	Leaman *et al.*, 1995
Eucalyptus globus *Euc. robusta* (Myrtaceae)	India China	Aerial (na) NC (na)	Ethanol extract Robustanol A	*P. falciparum, in vitro* *P. berghei*, mice	Badam *et al.*, 1988 Cheng & Snyder, 1988
Euodia fatraina (Rutaceae)	Madagascar	Stem (na)	Ethanol extract	*P. falciparum, in vitro* *P. berghei*, mice	Ratsimamanga-Urverg *et al.*, 1991
Eupatorium rutescens	Brazil	Aerial (na)	Zingiberine	*P. falciparum, in vitro*	Rucker *et al.*, 1996

Table 7 continued

Species (Family)	Origin[a]	Part (route[b])	Active ingredients	Indication	References
Eup. squalidium (Compositae)	Brazil	NC (na)	Endoperoxide	*P. falciparum, in vitro* *P. berghei*, mice	Carvalho *et al.*, 1991
Euphorbia thymifolia (Euphorbiaceae)	India	Aerial (na) (po)	Ethanol extract	*P. berghei, in vitro* *P. berghei, Mastomys*	Misra *et al.*, 1991
Eurycoma longifolia (Simaroubaceae)	Indonesia	Root (na)	Alkaloid, methoxycarboline-propionic acid	*P. falciparum, in vitro*	Kardono *et al.*, 1991
	Malaysia	Root (na)	Quassinoid, eurycoumanol, eurycomanone, dihydro-eurycoumanol, eurycoumanol-glucopyranoside	*P. falciparum, in vitro*	Ang *et al.*, 1995
Evodia fatraina [see *Euodia fatraina*]					
Exostema caribaeum (Rubiaceae)	S. America	Bark (na)	Phenylcoumarin	*P. falciparum, in vitro*	Noster & Kraus, 1990
Ficus polita (Moraceae)	NC	Leaf (na)	Ethanol extract	*P. falciparum, in vitro*	Gbeassor *et al.*, 1990
Galipea longiflora (Rutaceae)	Bolivia	Bark (po)	Parthenin	*P. vinckei petteri*, mice	Gantier *et al.*, 1996
Garcinia gummigulta (Guttiferae)	NC	NC (na)	Crude extract	*P. falciparum, in vitro*	Valsaraj *et al.*, 1995
Gentiana sp. (Gentianaceae)	NC	Whole (sc)	Chloroform extract	*P. gallinaceum*, chicks	Spencer *et al.*, 1947

Table 7 continued

Species (Family)	Origin[a]	Part (route[b])	Active ingredients	Indication	References
Glycosmis sp. (Rutaceae)	NC	Root, bark (na) (ip)	Acridine alkaloids	*P. yoelii, in vitro* *P. yoelii*, mice	Fujioka *et al.*, 1989
Gossypium hirsutum (Malvaceae)	NC	Cotton seed oil (na)	Gossypol	*P. falciparum, in vitro*	Royer *et al.*, 1986
Grewia egglingii	Tanzania	Bark (na)	Petroleum ether extract	*P. falciparum, in vitro*	Weenen *et al.*, 1990
Gre. forbesii (Tiliaceae)	Tanzania	Leaf (na)	Methanol extract	*P. falciparum, in vitro*	Weenen *et al.*, 1990
Gynandropsis gynandra (Capparidaceae)	Tanzania	Root (na)	Ethylacetate extract	*P. falciparum, in vitro*	Weenen *et al.*, 1990
Haplophyllum tuberculatum (Rutaceae)	Sudan	NC (na)	Justicidin A	*P. falciparum, in vitro*	Khalid *et al.*, 1986
Harrisonia abyssinica (Rutaceae)	Sudan	Leaf (na)	Methanolic extract	*P. falciparum, in vitro*	El Tahir *et al.*, 1999
Harungana madagascariensis (Guttiferae)	Tanzania	Root (na)	Ethylacetate extract	*P. falciparum, in vitro*	Gessler *et al.*, 1994
Hedychium spicatum (Zingiberaceae)	India	Root (na) (po)	Ethanol extract	*P. berghei, in vitro* inactive *P. berghei, Mastomys*	Misra *et al.*, 1991
Heinsia crinita (Umbelliferae)	Tanzania	Root (na)	Ethylacetate extract	*P. falciparum, in vitro*	Gessler *et al.*, 1994
Hernandia voyronii (Hernandiaceae)	Madagascar	Bark (na)	Ethanol extract	*P. falciparum, in vitro*	Ratsimamanga-Urverg *et al.*, 1994

Table 7 continued

Species (Family)	Origin[a]	Part (route[b])	Active ingredients	Indication	References
Heterothalamus psiadioides (Compositae)	NC	NC (na)	Peroxides	*P. falciparum, in vitro*	Rucker *et al.*, 1991
Hippeastrum puniceum (Amaryllidaceae)	NC	Bulb (po)	Aqueous extract	*P. gallinaceum*, chicks	Spencer *et al.*, 1947
Hoslundia opposita (Labiatae)	Tanzania	Root (na)	Abletane esters, benzoylhosloppone and others	*P. falciparum, in vitro*	Weenen *et al.*, 1990 Achenbach *et al.*, 1992
Hymenocallis caribaea (Amaryllidaceae)	NC	Bulb (po)	Aqueous extract	*P. gallinaceum*, chicks	Spencer *et al.*, 1947
Hypericum calycinum (Guttiferae)	Switzerland	Aerial (na)	Phoroglucinol derivatives	*P. falciparum, in vitro*	Decosterd *et al.*, 1991
Jatropha gossypiifolia (Euphorbiaceae)	Togo	Leaf (na)	Aqueous extract	*P. falciparum, in vitro*	Gbeassor *et al.*, 1989
Jurinea macrocephala (Compositae)	India	Root (na) (po)	Ethanol extract	*P. berghei, in vitro* *P. berghei, Mastomys*	Misra *et al.*, 1991
Keetia zanzibarica (Rubiaceae)	Tanzania	Root (na)	Petroleum ether extract	*P. falciparum, in vitro*	Gessler *et al.*, 1994
Khaya senegalensis (Meliaceae)	Sudan	Seed, leaf (na)	Chloroform extract, terpenoids, limonoids	*P. falciparum, in vitro*	El Tahir *et al.*, 1999
Lagenaria sphaerica (Cucurbitaceae)	Tanzania	Leaf (na)	Ethylacetate extract	*P. falciparum, in vitro*	Gessler *et al.*, 1994
Lannea edulis (Anacardiaceae)	Tanzania	Root (na)	Ethylacetate extract	*P. falciparum, in vitro*	Gessler *et al.*, 1994

Table 7 continued

Species (Family)	Origin[a]	Part (route[b])	Active ingredients	Indication	References
Lansium domesticum (Meliaceae)	Indonesia	Bark (na)	Ethanol extract	*P. falciparum, in vitro*	Leaman *et al.*, 1995
Lantana camara (Verbenaceae)	Tanzania	Root (na)	Crude extract	*P. falciparum, in vitro*	Weenen *et al.*, 1990
Leonotis mollissima (Labiatae)	Tanzania	Leaf (na)	Ethylacetate extract	*P. falciparum, in vitro*	Gessler *et al.*, 1994
Lippia cheralieri		Leaf (na)	Aqueous extract	*P. falciparum, in vitro*	Gasquet *et al.*, 1993
Lip. multiflora (Verbenaceae)	Ivory Coast	Leaf (na)	Aqueous extract	*P. falciparum, in vitro*	Benoit *et al.*, 1996
Lisianthus speciosus (Gentianaceae)	Brazil	NC (na)	Crude extract	*P. falciparum, in vitro* *P. berghei*, mice	Carvalho *et al.*, 1991
Luffa aegyptiaca (Cucurbitaceae)	Togo	Leaf (na)	Ethanol extract	*P. falciparum, in vitro*	Gbeassor *et al.*, 1990
Mammea longifolia (Guttiferae)	India	NC (na)	Crude extract	*P. falciparum, in vitro*	Valsaraj *et al.*, 1995
Mannia africana (Simaroubaceae)	NC	Root (po)	Chloroform extract	*P. gallinaceum*, chicks	Spencer *et al.*, 1947
Margaritaria discoidea (Euphorbiaceae)	Tanzania	Bark (na)	Dichloromethane extract	*P. falciparum, in vitro*	Weenen *et al.*, 1990
Maytenus arbutifolia	Kenya	Root (na)	Nitidine alkaloid	*P. falciparum, in vitro*	Gakunju *et al.*, 1995
May. senegalensis (Celastraceae)	Sudan	Root, bark, leaf (na)	Limonoids/terpenoids	*P. falciparum, in vitro*	El Tahir *et al.*, 1999
	Tanzania	(po)	Ethanol extract	*P. berghei*, mice	Gessler *et* al., 1995
Melia azedarach (Meliaceae)	Sudan	NC (na)	Gedunin	*P. falciparum, in vitro*	Khalid *et al.*, 1986

Table 7 continued

Species (Family)	Origin[a]	Part (route[b])	Active ingredients	Indication	References
Mikania cordata (Compositae)	NC	Leaf (na)	Ethylacetate extract	*P. falciparum, in vitro*	Weenen *et al.*, 1990
Momordica charantia	Togo	Leaf (na)	Ethanol extract	*P. falciparum, in vitro*	Gbeassor *et al.*, 1990
Mom. dioica (Cucurbitaceae)	India	Whole (na) (po)	Ethanol extract	*P. berghei, in vitro* and *Mastomys*	Misra *et al.*, 1991
Morinda lucida (Rubiaceae)	W. Africa	Leaf (po)	Petroleum ether extract	*P. falciparum*, mice	Makinde *et al.*, 1993
Moringa pterygosperma (Moringaceae)	NC	Leaf, twig (na)	Ethanol extract	*P. falciparum, in vitro*	Gbeassor *et al.*, 1989
Nardostachys chinensis (Valerianaceae)	NC	NC (na)	Nardosinon	*P. falciparum, in vitro*	Rucker *et al.*, 1991
Nauclea latifolia (Rubiaceae)	Ivory Coast	Stem, root (na)	Crude extract	*P. falciparum, in vitro*	Benoit-Vical *et al.*, 1998
Neurolaena lobata (Compositae)	Guatemala	Leaf (po)	Methanol extract, sesquiterpine lactone, neurolenin A,B,C,D, lobatin A,B	*P. berghei*, mice *P. falciparum, in vitro*	Franssen *et al.*, 1997 Francois *et al.*, 1996b
Newbouldia laevis (Bignoniaceae)	Togo	Leaf (na)	Ethanol extract	*P. falciparum, in vitro*	Gbeassor *et al.*, 1989
Nyctanthes arbor-tristis (Oleaceae)	India India	Leaf (po) Aerial (na)	Ethanol extract Ethanol extract	*P. berghei*, *Mastomys* *P. falciparum, in vitro*	Misra *et al.*, 1991 Badam *et al.*, 1988
Ocotea usambarensis (Lauraceae)	NC	Root (na)	Aqueous extract	*P. falciparum, in vitro*	Weenen *et al.*, 1990
Odyendea zimmermannii [see *Quassia zimmermannii*]					

Table 7 continued

Species (Family)	Origin[a]	Part (route[b])	Active ingredients	Indication	References
Oricia renieri (Rutaceae)	Sudan	NC (na)	Arborinine, lupeol	*P. falciparum, in vitro*	Khalid *et al.*, 1986
Ozoroa insignis (Anacardiaceae)	Tanzania	Root (na)	Dichloromethane extract	*P. falciparum, in vitro*	Weenen *et al.*, 1990
Parinari excelsasabin (Chrysobalanaceae)	Tanzania	Bark (na)	Dichloromethane extract	*P. falciparum, in vitro*	Weenen *et al.*, 1990
Parkia filicoidea (Leguminosae)	Tanzania	Root (na)	Ethylacetate extract	*P. falciparum, in vitro*	Gessler *et al.*, 1994
Parthenium hysterophorus (Compositae)	NC	NC (na)	Sesquiterpine lactone, parthenin	*P. falciparum, in vitro*	Phillipson & Wright, 1991
Paullinia pinnata (Sapindaceae)	Angola	Whole (na)	Aqueous extract	*P. falciparum, in vitro*	Presber *et al.*, 1992
Pavetta crassipes (Rubiaceae)	Togo	Aerial (na)	Aqueous extract	*P. falciparum, in vitro*	Gbeassor *et al.*, 1989
Peucedanum ostruthium (Umbelliferae)	Sudan	NC (na)	Ostruthin, osthol	*P. falciparum, in vitro*	Khalid *et al.*, 1986
Phyllanthus reticulatus (Euphorbiaceae)	Kenya	Leaf (na)	Aqueous extract	*P. falciparum, in vitro*	Omulokoli *et al.*, 1997
Physalis minima (Solanaceae)	India	Aerial (na) (po)	Ethanol extract	*P. berghei, in vitro* inactive in *Mastomys*	Misra *et al.*, 1991
Picralima nitida (Apocynaceae)	W. Africa	Rind, seed, bark (na)	Indolealkaloids, akuammine	*P. falciparum, in vitro*	Kapadia *et al.*, 1993 Iwu & Klayman, 1992 Francois *et al.*, 1996a
Picrasma javanica (Simaroubaceae)	Thailand	Bark (na)	Methylvinylcarboline	*P. falciparum, in vitro*	Pavanand *et al.*, 1988

Table 7 continued

Species (Family)	Origin[a]	Part (route[b])	Active ingredients	Indication	References
Picrolemma pseudocoffea	French Guyana	Root (na) (sc)	Sergeolide	*P. falciparum, in vitro* *P. berghei*, mice	Fandeur *et al.*, 1985
Pic. sprucei (Simaroubaceae)	NC	Root (sc) (na)	Aqueous extract, chloroform extract	*P. gallinaceum*, chicks	Spencer *et al.*, 1947
Piliostigma thonningii [see *Bauhinia thonningii*]					
Piper hispidum	C. America	Leaf (na)	Dihydrochalcone, asebogenin	*P. falciparum, in vitro*	Jenett-Siems *et al.*, 1999
Pip. sarmentosum	Malaysia	Leaf (na)	Chloroform extract	*P. falciparum, in vitro*	Rahman *et al.*, 1999
Pip. umbellata (Piperaceae)	Brazil	Leaf (na)	Ethanol extract	*P. berghei*, mice	Amorim *et al.*, 1991
Pisum sativum (Leguminosae)	Nigeria	Leaf (na)	Methanol extract	*P. falciparum, in vitro*	Abatan & Makinde, 1986
Pithecellobium acemosum (Leguminosae)	NC	NC (na)	Ethanol extract	*P. falciparum, in vitro*	Cabral *et al.*, 1993
Plantago major (Plantaginaceae)	Tanzania	Whole (na)	Dichloromethane extract	*P. falciparum, in vitro*	Weenen *et al.*, 1990
Pogonopus tubulosus (Rubiaceae)	S. America	Bark (na)	Tubulosine, psychotrine, cephaeline	*P. falciparum, in vitro*	Sauvain *et al.*, 1996
Pothomorphe umbellata [see *Piper umbellata*]					
Prunus persica (Rosaceae)	India	Seed (na)	Ethanol extract	*P. berghei, Mastomys*	Misra *et al.*, 1991
Pseudocedrela kotosifyi (Meliaceae)	Sudan	Leaf (na)	Methanolic extract, terpenoids, limonoids	*P. falciparum, in vitro*	El Tahir *et al.*, 1999

Table 7 continued

Species (Family)	Origin[a]	Part (route[b])	Active ingredients	Indication	References
Psidium guajava (Myrtaceae)	Tanzania	Leaf (na)	Petroleum ether extract	*P. falciparum, in vitro*	Weenen *et al.*, 1990
	NC	Leaf (na)	Ethylacetate extract	*P. falciparum, in vitro*	Gessler *et al.*, 1994
Quassia sp. (Simaroubaceae)					
	NC	Root (po)	Aqueous extract	*P. gallinaceum*, chicks	Spencer *et al.*, 1947
	NC	Kernel, bark, root (po/sc)	Aqueous extract, chloroform extract	*P. gallinaceum*, chicks	Spencer *et al.*, 1947
	French Guyana	Bark (na)	Cedronin	*P. falciparum, in vitro* *P. vinkei petteri*, mice	Moretti *et al.*, 1994
	NC	Bark (na)	Gutolactone	*P. falciparum, in vitro*	Cabral *et al.*, 1993
	NC	Wood, bark, stem (po/sc)	Quassinoids, sergeolide, glaucarubinone, bruceantin	*P. gallinaceum*, chicks *P. berghei*, mice	Spencer *et al.*, 1947 Trager & Polonsky, 1981
	Guatemala		Soularubinone, glaucarubinone, simalikalactone D	*P. falciparum, in vitro*	Franssen *et al.*, 1997 O'Neill *et al.*, 1986 Wright *et al.*, 1993a
Rauwolfia mombasiana (Apocynaceae)	Tanzania	Root (na)	Methanol extract	*P. falciparum, in vitro*	Weenen *et al.*, 1990
Remijia peruviana (Rubiaceae)	NC	Bark (po)	Aqueous extract	*P. gallinaceum*, chicks	Spencer *et al.*, 1947
Rhamnus staddo (Rhamnaceae)	Tanzania	Root (na)	Aqueous extract	*P. falciparum, in vitro*	Weenen *et al.*, 1990

Table 7 continued

Species (Family)	Origin[a]	Part (route[b])	Active ingredients	Indication	References
Rosa rugosa (Rosaceae)	NC	NC (na)	Rugosal A	*P. falciparum, in vitro*	Rucker *et al.*, 1991
Salacia madagascariensis (Celastraceae)	Tanzania	Root (na)	Petroleum ether extract	*P. falciparum, in vitro*	Gessler *et al.*, 1994
Sansevieria guineensis (Dracaenaceae)	Guatemala	NC (po)	Methanol extract	*P. berghei*, mice	Franssen *et al.*, 1997
Scadoxus multiflorus (Amaryllidaceae)	Tanzania	Whole (na)	Methanol extract	*P. falciparum, in vitro*	Weenen *et al.*, 1990
Schultesia lisianthoides (Gentianaceae)	NC	Whole plant (po)	Aqueous extract	*P. gallinaceum*, chicks	Spencer *et al.*, 1947
Sclerocarya caffra (Anancardiaceae)	Tanzania	Bark (na)	Methanol extract	*P. falciparum, in vitro*	Weenen *et al.*, 1990
Senecio selloi (Compositae)	Brazil	Aerial (na)	Zingiberine endoperoxides	*P. falciparum, in vitro*	Rucker *et al.*, 1996
Senna petersiana (Leguminosae)	Malawi	Leaf (na)	Methanol extract	*P. falciparum, in vitro*	Connelly *et al.*, 1996
Severinia sp. (Rutaceae)	NC	Root, bark (na) (ip)	Acridine alkaloids	*P. yoelii, in vitro* *P. yoelii*, mice	Fujioka *et al.*, 1989
Sida rambifolia (Malvaceae)	India	Root (na) (po)	Ethanol extract	*P. berghei, in vitro* inactive in *Mastomys*	Misra *et al.*, 1991
Simaba sp.					
Sim. cedron					
Sim. cuneata *Sim. insigni*					
Sim. multiflora *Sim. trichilioides*					

Table 7 continued

Species (Family)	Origin[a]	Part (route[b])	Active ingredients	Indication	References
Sim. guianensis [see *Quassia* sp.] (Simaroubaceae)					
Simarouba sp.					
Sima. glauca,					
Sima. berteroana					
Sima. tulae					
Sima. amara [see *Quassia* sp.] (Simaroubaceae)					
Siparuna andina	C. America	Leaf (na)	Petroleum ether	*P. falciparum, in vitro*	Jenett-Siems *et al.*, 1999
Sip. pauciflora	C. America	Leaf (na)	Aqueous methanol	*P. falciparum, in vitro*	Jenett-Siems *et al.*, 1999
Sip. tonduziana (Monimiaceae)	C. America	Leaf (na)	Extracts	*P. falciparum, in vitro*	Jenett-Siems *et al.*, 1999
Solanum nigrum (Solanaceae)	India	Aerial (na) (po)	Ethanol extract	*P. berghei, in vitro* inactive in *Mastomys*	Misra *et al.*, 1991
Sorindeia madagascariensis (Anacardiaceae)	Tanzania	Root (na)	Petroleum ether extract	*P. falciparum, in vitro*	Weenen *et al.*, 1990
Spathodea campanulata (Bignoniaceae)	Nigeria	Bark (na)	Hexane extract	*P. falciparum, in vitro*	Makinde *et al.*, 1987
Spilanthes oleraceae (Chenopodiceae)	NC	Flower (na)	Aqueous extract	*P. falciparum, in vitro*	Gasquet *et al.*, 1993
Spirostachys africana (Euphorbiaceae)	Mozambique	Root (na)	Ethanol extract Aqueous extract	*P. falciparum, in vitro* *P. falciparum*, clinical trial	Jurg *et al.*, 1991

Table 7 continued

Species (Family)	Origin[a]	Part (route[b])	Active ingredients	Indication	References
Streblus asper (Moraceae)	India	Bark (na)	Aqueous extract	*P. berghei*, mice	Das & Beuria, 1991
Strychnos usambarensis (Strychnaceae)	Rwanda Tanzania	Root, leaf (na)	Strychnopentamine, dihydro-usambarensine	*P. falciparum, in vitro,* inactive *P. berghei*, mice	Wright *et al.*, 1991
Suregada zanzibariensis (Euphorbiaceae)	Kenya	Leaf (na)	Aqueous extract	*P. falciparum, in vitro*	Omulokoli *et al.*, 1997
Tachia guianensis (Gentianaceae)	Brazil	NC (na)	Crude extract	*P. falciparum, in vitro,* *P. berghei*, mice	Carvalho *et al.*, 1991
Tamarindus indica (Leguminosae)	Tanzania	Fruit (na) Leaf (na)	Methanol extract Ethylacetate extract	*P. falciparum, in vitro* *P. falciparum, in vitro*	Weenen *et al.*, 1990 Gessler *et al.*, 1994
Terminalia spinosa (Combretaceae)	Kenya	Bark (na)	Aqueous extract	*P. falciparum, in vitro*	Omulokoli *et al.*, 1997
Thespia garckeana (Malvaceae)	Malawi	Leaf (na)	Napthoquinones	*P. falciparum, in vitro*	Connelly *et al.*, 1996
Tiliacora triandra (Menispermaceae)	Thailand	Root (na)	Bisbenzyl-isoquinolines, tiliacorine, tiliacorinine, nor-tiliacorinine A and others	*P. falciparum, in vitro*	Pavanand *et al.*, 1989a
Tinospora cordifolia	India	Whole (na)	Ethanol extract	*P. berghei, in vitro*	Misra *et al.*, 1991
Tin. crispa (Menispermaceae)	Malaysia	Stem (na)	Methanol extract	*P. falciparum, in vitro,* *P. berghei*, mice	Rahman *et al.*, 1999
Toddalia asiatica (Rutaceae)	Kenya	Root, bark (na)	Nitidine	*P. falciparum, in vitro*	Gakunju *et al.*, 1995
Trichilia emetica (Meliaceae)	Sudan	Leaf, bark (na)	Methanol extract, terpenoids, limonoids	*P. falciparum, in vitro*	El Tahir *et al.*, 1999

Table 7 continued

Species (Family)	Origin[a]	Part (route[b])	Active ingredients	Indication	References
Triclisia patens (Menispermaceae)	Sierra Leone	Whole plant (na)	Bisbenzylisoquinoline, pycnamine, aromoline, phaeanthine	*P. falciparum, in vitro*	Phillipson & Wright, 1991 Partridge *et al.*, 1988 Ekong *et al.*, 1991
Tridax procumbens (Compositae)	Tanzania	Whole (na)	Dichloromethane extract	*P. falciparum, in vitro*	Weenen *et al.*, 1990
Triphyophyllum peltatum (Dioncophyllaceae)	Ivory Coast	Root, bark (po/iv)	Naphthyl-isoquinolines Dioncopeltine A, dioncophylline C	*P. berghei*, mice *P. falciparum, in vitro*	Bringmann *et al.*, 1987 Francois *et al.*, 1997a,b Bringmann *et al.*, 1998 Francois *et al.*, 1996c Francois *et al.*, 1994
Uapaca nitida (Euphorbiaceae)	Tanzania	Root, bark, leaf (na)	Ethanol extract	*P. falciparum, in vitro*	Kirby *et al.*, 1993
Urtica dioica (Urticaceae)	Poland	Rhizome (na)	Ethylacetate extract	*P. falciparum, in vitro*	Grzybek *et al.*, 1997
Uvaria lucida and *Uvaria* sp. (Annonaceae)	Tanzania	Stem/root (na)	Farnesylindole, uvaretin, diuvaretin	*P. falciparum, in vitro*	Nkunya *et al.*, 1991
Vangueria infausta (Rubiaceae)	Tanzania	Root (na) Bark	Methanol extract Dichloromethane extract	*P. falciparum, in vitro*	Weenen *et al.*, 1990
Vepris lanceolata (Rutaceae)	NC	Root, leaf (na)	Ethanol extract	*P. falciparum, in vitro*	Gessler *et al.*, 1994
Vernonia amygdalina	Tanzania	Leaf (na)	Dichloromethane Sesquiterpine lactone, vernodalin, vernodalol	*P. falciparum, in vitro* *P. falciparum, in vitro*	Weenen *et al.*, 1990 Ohigashi *et al.*, 1994

Table 7 continued

Species (Family)	Origin[a]	Part (route[b])	Active ingredients	Indication	References
Ver. brasiliana	Brazil	NC (na)	Crude extract	*P. falciparum, in vitro* *P. berghei*, mice	Carvalho *et al.*, 1991
Ver. colorata (Compositae)	Tanzania	Bark (na)	Methanol extract	*P. falciparum, in vitro*	Weenen *et al.*, 1990
Viburnum opulus (Caprifoliaceae)	Poland	Stipes (na)	Ethylacetate extract	*P. falciparum, in vitro*	Grzybek *et al.*, 1997
Vismia orientala (Guttiferae)	Tanzania	Leaf (na)	Methanol extract	*P. falciparum, in vitro*	Weenen *et al.*, 1990
Xanthium strumarium (Compositae)	India	Aerial (na)	Sesqueterpine lactones	*P. falciparum, in vitro*	Badam *et al.*, 1988
Ximenia americana	Ivory Coast	Stem, leaf (na)	Aqueous extract	*P. falciparum, in vitro*	Benoit *et al.*, 1996
Xim. cafra (Olacaceae)		Leaf (na)	Methanol extract	*P. falciparum, in vitro*	Weenen *et al.*, 1990
Xylopia frutescens (Annonaceae)	C. America	Stem (na)	Aqueous methanol and petroleum ether extracts	*P. falciparum, in vitro*	Jenett-Siems *et al.*, 1999
Zanthoxylum chalybeum	Tanzania	NC (na) (po)		*P. falciparum, in vitro* *P. berghei*, mice	Gessler *et al.*, 1994
Zan. gilleti	Tanzania	Bark (na)	Methanol extract	*P. falciparum, in vitro*	Weenen *et al.*, 1990
Zan. xylubeum (Rutaceae)	Tanzania	Bark (na)	Methanol extract	*P. falciparum, in vitro*	Weenen *et al.*, 1990
Zephyranthes pedunculata (Amaryllidaceae)	NC	Bulb (po/sc)	Aqueous extract, chloroform extract	*P. gallinaceum*, chicks	Spencer *et al.*, 1947

[a] Origin of the plant or product described in the citation. May not be the only origin.
[b] Route of administration: sc, subcutaneous inoculation; po, *per os* (oral); ip, intraperitoneal; im, intramuscular; na, not applicable.
NC, not cited; rev, review.

Table 8 Medicinal plants with antisporozoal activity.

Species (Family)	Origin[a]	Part (route[b])	Active ingredients	Indication	References
Artemisia annua (Compositae)	China	Leaf (na)	Artemesinin	*Toxoplasma gondii, in vitro*	Sarciron *et al.*, 2000
		(po)		*Tox. gondii*, mice	
	China	Leaf (na)	Derivatives	*Tox. gondii, in vitro*	Ou-Yang *et al.*, 1990

[a] Origin of the plant or product described in the citation. May not be the only origin.
[b] Route of administration: po, *per os* (oral); na, not applicable.

Table 9 Medicinal plants with activity against *Pneumocystis carinii.*

Species (Family)	Origin[a]	Part (route[b])	Active ingredients	Indication	References
Citrus sp. (Rutaceae)	NC	Root, bark (na)	Acridine alkaloids, atalaphillinine, glycobismine	*Pneumocystis carinii, in vitro*	Queener *et al.*, 1991
Ginkgo biloba (Ginkgoaceae)	NC	Leaves (na)	Sesquiterpene, bilobalide	*Pne. carinii, in vitro*	Atzori *et al.*, 1993
		(ip)		*Pne. carinii*, rats	
Glycosmis sp. (Rutaceae)	NC	Root, bark (na)	Acridine alkaloids, atalaphillinine, glycobismine	*Pne. carinii, in vitro*	Queener *et al.*, 1991
Severinia sp. (Rutaceae)	NC	Root, bark (na)	Acridine alkaloids, atalaphillinine, glycobismine	*Pne. carinii, in vitro*	Queener *et al.*, 1991

[a] Origin of the plant or product described in the citation. May not be the only origin.
[b] Route of administration: ip, intraperitoneal; na, not applicable.
NC, not cited.

Table 10 Medicinal plants with activity against cestodes.

Species (Family)	Origin[a]	Part (route[b])	Active ingredients	Indication	References
Agrimonia pilosa (Rosaceae)	China	Root, sprout, buds (na)	Agrimophol	*Taenia solium, in vitro*, clinical trial	Xiao & Fu, 1986
Albizia anthelmintica (Leguminosae)	Ethiopia	Bark (po)	Crude preparation with honey	*Tae. saginata*, clinical trial	Desta, 1995
Allium sativum (Alliaceae)	Egypt	Clove extract (po)		*Hymenolepis nana*, clinical trial	Soffar & Mokhtar, 1991
Aningeria adolfifriedericii [see *Pouteria adolfifriedericii*]					
Asparagus aethiopicus (Liliaceae)	Ethiopia	Root (po)	Crude preparation with honey	*Tae. saginata*, clinical trial	Desta, 1995
Berchemia discolor (Rhamnaceae)	Ethiopia	Leaf (po)	Crude preparation with honey	*Tae. saginata*, clinical trial	Desta, 1995
Commiphora resinflua (Burseraceae)	Ethiopia	Resin (po)	Crude preparation with honey	*Tae. saginata*, clinical trial	Desta, 1995
Cucurbita moschata	China	Seeds (NC)	Cucurbitine	*Tae. solium*, clinical trial	Xiao & Fu, 1986
C. pepo (Cucurbitaceae)	Ethiopia	Seed (po)	Crude preparation with honey	*Tae. saginata*, clinical trial	Desta, 1995
Cussonia sp. (Araliaceae)	Ethiopia	Bark (po)	Crude preparation with honey	*Tae. saginata*, clinical trial	Desta, 1995
Cynodon dactylon (Gramineae)	Ethiopia	Whole (po)	Crude preparation with honey	*Tae. saginata*, clinical trial	Desta, 1995
Diospyros mollis (Ebenaceae)	S.E. Asia	Fruit (po)	Dinaphthyl derivative, diospyrol	*H. nana*, mice	Sen *et al.*, 1974

Table 10 continued

Species (Family)	Origin[a]	Part (route[b])	Active ingredients	Indication	References
Dodonaea viscosa (Sapindaceae)	Ethiopia	Root (po)	Crude preparation with honey	*Tae. saginata*, clinical trial	Desta, 1995
Echinops gigantean *Echinops* sp. (Compositae)	Ethiopia	Root (po)	Crude preparation with honey	*Tae. saginata*, clinical trial	Desta, 1995
Embelia schimperi (Myrsinaceae)	Ethiopia Tanzania/ Kenya	Fruit (po) Fruit (po)	Crude preparation Embelin	*Tae. saginata*, clinical trial *H. diminuta*, rats and *in vitro*	Desta, 1995 Bogh *et al.*, 1996
Flemingia vestita (Leguminosae)	India	Root tuber peel (na)	Isoflavone, genistein	Paralyses *Echinobothrida railletina, in vitro*	Tandon *et al.*, 1997
Galium sp. (Rubiaceae)	Ethiopia	Leaf (po)	Crude preparation with honey	*Tae. saginata*, clinical trial	Desta, 1995
Glinus lotoides (Molluginaceae)	Ethiopia	Fruit (po)	Crude preparation with honey	*Tae. saginata*, clinical trial	Desta, 1995
Grewia ferruginea (Tiliaceae)	Ethiopia	Bark (po)	Crude preparation with honey	*Tae. saginata*, clinical trial	Desta, 1995
Guizotia scabra (Compositae)	Ethiopia	Root (po)	Crude preparation with honey	*Tae. saginata*, clinical trial	Desta, 1995
Hagenia abyssinica (Rosaceae)	Ethiopia	Flower (po)	Crude preparation with honey	*Tae. saginata*, clinical trial	Desta, 1995
Helichrysum schimperi (Compositae)	Ethiopia	Root (po)	Crude preparation with honey	*Tae. saginata*, clinical trial	Desta, 1995
Jasminum abyssinicum (Oleaceae)	Ethiopia	Root (po)	Crude preparation with honey	*Tae. saginata*, clinical trial	Desta, 1995

Table 10 continued

Species (Family)	Origin[a]	Part (route[b])	Active ingredients	Indication	References
Kalanchoe quartiniana (Crassulaceae)	Ethiopia	Root (po)	Crude preparation with honey	*Tae. saginata*, clinical trial	Desta, 1995
Maesa lanceolata (Myrsinaceae)	Ethiopia	Flower (po)	Crude preparation with honey	*Tae. saginata*, clinical trial	Desta, 1995
Mallotus philippinensis (Euphorbiaceae)	Pakistan	Fruit (po)	Powdered fruit	Mixed cestodes, goats	Akhtar & Ahmad, 1992
Myrsine africana (Myrsinaceae)	Ethiopia	Flower (po)	Crude preparation with honey	*Tae. saginata*, clinical trial	Desta, 1995
Nigella sativa (Ranunculaceae)	Pakistan	Seed (po)	Powdered seeds	*Tae. saginata*, clinical trial	Akhtar & Riffat, 1991
Plantago lanceolata (Plantaginaceae)	Ethiopia	Whole (po)	Crude preparation with honey	*Tae. saginata*, clinical trial	Desta, 1995
Pouteria adolfifriedericii (Sapotaceae)	Ethiopia	Fruit (po)	Crude preparation with honey	*Tae. saginata*, clinical trial	Desta, 1995
Prunus persica (Rosaceae)	Ethiopia	Leaf (po)	Crude preparation with honey	*Tae. saginata*, clinical trial	Desta, 1995
Punica granatum (Punicaceae)	India Ethiopia	Rind, root (na) Root (po)	Isopelletierine Crude preparation	*Tae. solium*, *in vitro* *Tae. saginata*, clinical trial	Hukkeri *et al.*, 1993 Desta, 1995
Rhamnus staddo (Rhamnaceae)	Ethiopia	Leaf (po)	Crude preparation with honey	*Tae. saginata*, clinical trial	Desta, 1995
Ricinus communis (Euphorbiaceae)	Ethiopia	Root (po)	Crude preparation with honey	*Tae. saginata*, clinical trial	Desta, 1995

Table 10 continued

Species (Family)	Origin[a]	Part (route[b])	Active ingredients	Indication	References
Securidaca longipedunculata (Polygalaceae)	Ethiopia	Root (po)	Crude preparation with honey	*Tae. saginata*, clinical trial	Desta, 1995
Smilax goetzeana (Smilacaceae)	Ethiopia	Root (po)	Crude preparation with honey	*Tae. saginata*, clinical trial	Desta, 1995
Solanum marginatum (Solanaceae)	Ethiopia	Root (po)	Crude preparation with honey	*Tae. saginata*, clinical trial	Desta, 1995
Syzygium guinensis (Myrtaceae)	Ethiopia	Root (po)	Crude preparation with honey	*Tae. saginata*, clinical trial	Desta, 1995
Thymus serrulatus (Labiatae)	Ethiopia	Leaf (po)	Crude preparation with honey	*Tae. saginata*, clinical trial	Desta, 1995
Zanthoxylum alatum (Rutaceae)	India	Stem (na)	Ether extract	*H. nana, in vitro,* *H. nana*, rats	Singh *et al.*, 1982

[a] Origin of the plant or product described in the citation. May not be the only origin.
[b] Route of administration: po, *per os* (oral); na, not applicable.
NC, not cited.

Table 11 Medicinal plants with activity against trematodes.

Species (Family)	Origin[a]	Part (route[b])	Active ingredients	Indication	References
Abrus precatorius (Leguminosae)	Zimbabwe	NC (po)	Crude extract	*Schistosoma haematobium*, hamsters	Nyazema *et al.*, 1994
Agrimonia pilosa (Rosaceae)	China	Root, sprout, buds (na)	Agrimophol	*S. japonicum, in vitro* *S. japonicum*, mice	Xiao & Fu, 1986 Xiao *et al.*, 1995
Artemisia annua (Compositae)	China	Leaves (NC)	Qinghaosu	*Clonorchis sinensis*, rats *S. japonicum*, mice	see Xiao & Fu, 1986 You *et al.*, 1992
Cucurbita moschata (Cucurbitaceae)	China	Seeds (NC)	Cucurbitine	*S. japonicum* cercariae, mice	see Xiao & Fu, 1986
Deverra triradiata (Umbelliferae)	Egypt	NC (na)	Ethanol extract	*S. mansoni* cercariae, *in vitro*	Shabana *et al.*, 1988
Euodia rutaecarpa (Rutaceae)	China	Fruit (na)	Quinolone alkaloid, atanine	*S. mansoni* miracida and cercariae, *in vitro*	Perrett & Whitfield, 1995b
Evodia rutaecarpa [see *Euodia rutaecarpa*]					
Flemingia vestita (Leguminosae)	India	Root tuber peel (na)	Isoflavone, genistein	*Paramphistomum* sp., *in vitro, Fasciolopsis buski, in vitro, Artyfechinostomum sufrartyfex, in vitro*	Tandon *et al.*, 1997 Roy & Tandon, 1996
Hemerocallis thunbergii (Hemerocallidaceae)	China	NC	Hemerocallin	*S. japonicum*, mice	Chen *et al.*, 1962
Lysimachia clethroides (Primulaceae)	Korea	Root (na)	Ethanol extract	*Clo. sinensis, in vitro*	Soh *et al.*, 1980
Millettia thoningi (Leguminosae)	Ghana	Seed (na)	Isoflavonoids, alpinumisoflavone	*S. mansoni* miracida and cercariae, *in vitro*	Perrett & Whitfield, 1995a

Table 11 continued

Species (Family)	Origin[a]	Part (route[b])	Active ingredients	Indication	References
Ozoroa insignis (Anacardiaceae)	Zimbabwe	NC (po)	Crude extract	*S. haematobium*, hamsters	Nyazema *et al.*, 1994
Panicum turgidum (Gramineae)	Egypt	NC (na)	Ethanol extract	*S. mansoni* cercariae, *in vitro*	Shabana *et al.*, 1988
Pituranthos tortuosus triradiata [see *Deverra triradiata*]					
Pterocarpus angolensis (Leguminosae)	Zimbabwe	NC (po)	Crude extract	*S. haematobium*, hamsters	Nyazema *et al.*, 1994
Vernonia amygdalina (Compositae)	Tanzania	Whole (na)	Sesquitepine lactone, vernodalin, vernodalol, steroid glucoside, vernonioside B1, vernoniol B1	*S. japonicum, in vitro*	Ohigashi *et al.*, 1994
Zanthoxylum alatum (Rutaceae)	India	Stem (na)	Ether extract	*F. buski, in vitro, F. buski*, mice	Singh *et al.*, 1982
Zingiber officinale (Zingiberaceae)	Nigeria	Rhizome (na)	Gingerol	*S. mansoni* miracida, *in vitro* and in *Biomphalaria glabrata*	Adewunmi *et al.*, 1990

[a] Origin of the plant or product described in the citation. May not be the only origin.
[b] Route of administration: po, *per os* (oral); na, not applicable.
NC, not cited.

Table 12 Medicinal plants with activity against gastrointestinal nematodes.

Species (Family)	Origin[a]	Part (route[b])	Active ingredients	Indication	References
Acorus calamus	India	Rhizome (na)	Crude extract	*Ascaris lumbricoides, in vitro*	Raj, 1974
Aco. gramineus (Acoraceae)	S.E. Asia	Rhizome (na)	Phenylpropanoid	*Ostertagia circumcincta, in vitro*	Perrett & Whitfield, 1995c
			Alpha asarone	*Nippostrongylus brasiliensis, in vitro*	
			Beta asarone	*Trichostrongylus colubriformis, in vitro*	
Agati gratifolia [see *Sesbania gratifolia*]					
Alpinia galanga (Zingiberaceae)	India	Rhizome (na)	Alcohol extract	*A. lumbricoides, in vitro*	Raj, 1975
Amomum aromaticum (Zingiberaceae)	India	Rhizome, root (na) (po)	Methanol extract	*Ascaridia galli, in vitro* *Asc. galli,* chicks	Dhar *et al.*, 1968
Andrographis paniculata (Acanthaceae)	India	Rhizome (na)	Alcohol extract	*A. lumbricoides, in vitro*	Raj, 1975
Anthocephalus indicus [see *Breonia indicus*]					
Artemisia herba-alba	Iraq/Egypt, S.W. Asia	Stem, leaf (po)	Aqueous extract	*Enterobius vermicularis,* clinical trial	Al-Waili, 1988
Art. maritima (Compositae)	China	NC (NC)	Santonin given with cathartic	*A. lumbricoides,* clinical trial	Xiao & Fu, 1986
Artocarpus altilis (Moraceae)	Jamaica	Leaf (na)	Aqueous methanol extract	*Strongyloides stercoralis* larvae, *in vitro*	Robinson *et al.*, 1990

Table 12 continued

Species (Family)	Origin[a]	Part (route[b])	Active ingredients	Indication	References
Breonia indicus (Rubiaceae)	India	Bark (na) (po)	Methanol extract	*Asc. galli, in vitro* *Asc. galli,* chicks	Dhar *et al.*, 1968
Butea frondosa (Leguminosae)	India	Seed (na)	Palasonin	*A. lumbricoides, in vitro*	Raj & Kurup, 1968
Calamintha unbrosa [see *Clindopodium unbrosa*]					
Carica papaya (Caricaceae)	Asia	Seed, leaf (na) (po)	Benzylisothiocyanate, carpasemine	*A. lumbricoides, in vitro* *Asc. galli, in vitro* *A. lumbricoides* and *Trichuris trichiura,* clinical trial	Dar *et al.*, 1965 Kumar *et al.*, 1991 Pohowalla & Singh, 1959
Carum copticum (Umbelliferae)	India	Seed (na)	Aqueous extract	*A. lumbricoides, in vitro*	Raj, 1974
Cinnamomum zeylanicum (Lauraceae)	India	Bark (na)	Alcoholic extract	*A. lumbricoides, in vitro*	Raj, 1975
Citrus decumana (Rutaceae)	India	Rind (na)	Alcoholic extract	*A. lumbricoides, in vitro*	Raj, 1975
Clindopodium unbrosa (Labiatae)	India	Whole (na) (po)	Methanol extract	*Asc. galli, in vitro* *Asc. galli,* chicks	Dhar *et al.*, 1968
Cuscuta americana (Convolvulaceae)	Jamaica	Leaf (na)	Aqueous methanol extract	*Str. stercoralis* larvae, *in vitro*	Robinson *et al.*, 1990
Dalbergia latifolia (Leguminosae)	India	Bark (na) (po)	Methanol extract	*Asc. galli, in vitro* *Asc. galli,* chicks	Dhar *et al.*, 1968

Table 12 *continued*

Species (Family)	Origin[a]	Part (route[b])	Active ingredients	Indication	References
Datura metel (Solanaceae)	India	Whole (na) (po)	Methanol extract	*Asc. galli, in vitro* *Asc. galli*, chicks	Dhar *et al.*, 1968
Desmodium triflorum (Leguminosae)	India	Rind (na)	Alcoholic extract	*A. lumbricoides, in vitro*	Raj, 1975
Euodia rutaecarpa (Rutaceae)	China	Fruit (na)	Quinolone alkaloid, atanine	*Ostertagia circumcincta* larvae, *in vitro*	Perrett & Whitfield, 1995b
Evodia rutaecarpa [see *Euodia rutaecarpa*]					
Ficus insipidia and *F. carica*	C. and S. America	Latex (po)	Ficin	*Syphacia obvelata*, in mice	de Amorin *et al.*, 1999
F. religiosa (Moraceae)	India	Bark (na) (po)	Methanol extract	*Asc. galli, in vitro* *Asc. galli*, chicks	Dhar *et al.*, 1968
Flemingia vestita (Leguminosae)	India	Root (na)	Ethanol extract	*A. suum, in vitro*	Yadav *et al.*, 1992
Helleborus niger (Ranunculaceae)	India	Stem (na)	Aqueous extract	*A. lumbricoides, in vitro*	Raj, 1974
Hunteria umbellata (Apocynaceae)	Nigeria	Bark (na)	Ethanol extract	*A. lumbricoides, in vitro*	Onuaguluchi, 1964
Hydnocarpus wightiana (Flacourtiaceae)	India	Seed (na)	Alcoholic extract	*A. lumbricoides, in vitro*	Raj, 1975
Kaempferia galanga (Zingiberaceae)	India	Rhizome (na)	Alcoholic extract	*A. lumbricoides, in vitro*	Raj, 1975
Lippia nodiflora (Verbenaceae)	India	Rhizome (na)	Alcoholic extract	*A. lumbricoides, in vitro*	Raj, 1975

Table 12 continued

Species (Family)	Origin[a]	Part (route[b])	Active ingredients	Indication	References
Mangifera indica (Anacardiaceae)	India	Kernel (na)	Aqueous extract	*A. lumbricoides, in vitro*	Raj, 1974
Melia toosendan (Meliaceae)	China	Bark (NC)	Chuanliansu	*A. lumbricoides*, clinical trials	Xiao & Fu, 1986
Mimosa pudica (Leguminosae)	Jamaica	Leaf (na)	Aqueous methanol extract	*Str. stercoralis* larvae, *in vitro*	Robinson *et al.*, 1990
Morinda citrifolia (Rubiaceae)	India	Leaf (na)	Alcohol extract	*A. lumbricoides, in vitro*	Raj, 1975
Pollia serzogonian (Commelinaceae)	India	Rhizome (na)	Alcohol extract	*A. lumbricoides, in vitro*	Raj, 1975
Polyadoa umbellata [see *Hunteria umbellata*]					
Punica granatum (Punicaceae)	India	Rind (na)	Alcohol extract Aqueous extract	*A. lumbricoides, in vitro* *Asc. galli, in vitro*	Raj, 1975 Hukkeri *et al.*, 1993
Quercus lanceaefolia (Fagaceae)	India	Bark (na)	Methanol extract	*Asc. galli, in vitro,* *Asc. galli,* chicks	Dhar *et al.*, 1968
Quisqualis indica (Combretaceae)	China	Seed (NC)	Quisqualic acid	*A. lumbricoides*, clinical trials	Xiao & Fu, 1986
Salvia serotina (Labiatae)	Jamaica	Leaf (na)	Aqueous methanol extract	*Str. stercoralis* larvae, *in vitro*	Robinson *et al.*, 1990
Saussurea lappa (Compositae)	Pakistan	Root (po)	Powdered root	*A. lumbricoides*, clinical trial	Akhtar & Riffat, 1991
Scutia myrtina (Rhamnaceae)	India	Aerial (na)	Methanol extract	*Asc. galli, in vitro,* *Asc. galli,* chicks	Dhar *et al.*, 1968

Table 12 continued

Species (Family)	Origin[a]	Part (route[b])	Active ingredients	Indication	References
Sesbania gratifolia (Leguminosae)	India	Seed (na)	Aqueous extract	*A. lumbricoides, in vitro*	Raj, 1974
Symplocos paniculata (Symplocaceae)	India	Leaf (na) (po)	Methanol extract	*Asc. galli, in vitro,* *Asc. galli,* chicks	Dhar *et al.*, 1968
Tephrosia purpurea (Leguminosae)	India	Rhizome (na)	Alcoholic extract	*A. lumbricoides, in vitro*	Raj, 1975
Zanthoxylum liebmanniaum (Rutaceae)	Mexico	Bark (po) (na)	Crude extract Alpha-sanshool	*A. suum*, sheep *A. suum, in vitro*	Navarette & Hong, 1996
Zingiber zerumbeth	India	Rhizome (na)	Alcoholic extract	*A. lumbricoides, in vitro*	Raj, 1975
Zin. officinale (Zingiberaceae)	India	Rhizome (na)	Aqueous extract	*A. lumbricoides, in vitro*	Raj, 1974

[a] Origin of the plant or product described in the citation. May not be the only origin.
[b] Route of administration: po, *per os* (oral); na, not applicable.
NC, not cited.

Table 13 Medicinal plants with activity against tissue-dwelling nematodes.

Species (Family)	Origin[a]	Part (route[b])	Active ingredients	Indication	References
Andrographis paniculata (Acanthaceae)	India	Dried leaf (na)	Aqueous extract	*Dipetalonema reconditum* microfilariae, *in vitro* and dogs	Dutta & Sukul, 1982
Areca catechu (Palmae)	S.E. Asia	Nuts (na)	Fatty acids	*Toxocara canis, in vitro*	Kiuchi *et al.*, 1987
Argyreia speciosa (Convolvulaceae)	India	Whole plant (na)	Ethanol extract	*Setaria cervi, in vitro*	Parveen *et al.*, 1989a Parveen *et al.*, 1992
Carapa procera (Meliaceae)	Cameroon	Dried fruit (na)	Methanol extract	*Onchocerca volvulus, in vitro*	Titanji *et al.*, 1987 Titanji *et al.*, 1989
Cardiospermum halicacabum (Sapindaceae)	Thailand	Aerial (na)	Aqueous extract Ethanol extract	*Brugia pahangi* adult worms, *in vitro* *Bru. pahangi* microfilariae, *in vitro*	Khunkitti *et al.*, 2000
Cassia aubrevellei (Leguminosae)	Liberia	Root, bark (po)	Aqueous and alchoholic extract	*Onchocerca volvulus, in vitro* and clinical trial	Kilian *et al.*, 1989 Kilian, 1987
Cinnamomum culilawan (Lauraceae)	New Guinea	Bark (top)	Crude extract	Filarial lymphangitis (rubeifacient)	McMillan, 1968
Enicostema litorale (Gentianaceae)	India	Whole (ip)	Aqueous extract	*Conispiculum guindiensis*, lizard	Kulangara & Subramaniam, 1960
Erythrophleum ivorense (Leguminosae)	Cameroon	Stem (na)	Methanol, hexane, ethylacetate extract	*O. volvulus, in vitro*	Titanji *et al.*, 1987
Hilleria latifolia (Phytolaccaceae)	Cameroon	Dried aerial parts (na)	Methanol extract	*O. volvulus, in vitro*	Titanji *et al.*, 1987
Morus sp. (Moraceae)	China	Leaf (po)	Aqueous extract	Filarial lymphangitis, clinical trial	Wang *et al.*, 1989

Table 13 continued

Species (Family)	Origin[a]	Part (route[b])	Active ingredients	Indication	References
Pachyelasma tessmanii (Leguminosae)	Cameroon	Fruit (na)	Methanol extract	*O. volvulus, in vitro*	Titanji *et al.*, 1987
Pachypodanthium staudii (Annonaceae)	Cameroon	Bark (na)	Hexane extract	*O. volvulus, in vitro*	Titanji *et al.*, 1987 Titanji *et al.*, 1989
			Oliverine		Comley *et al.*, 1990
Raphia faninifera (Palmae)	Cameroon	Fruit, root (na)	Hexane extract	*O. volvulus, in vitro*	Titanji *et al.*, 1987
Streblus asper (Moraceae)	India	Bark (na)	Strebloside, asperoside	*Litomosoides carinii, Sigmodon, Acanthocheilonema viteae* and *Brugia malayi, Mastomys*	Chatterjee *et al.*, 1992
		Bark (po)	Ethanol extract	*Setaria cervi, in vitro*	Parveen *et al.*, 1989a,b Parveen *et al.*, 1992
Zingiber officinale (Zingiberaceae)	India	Fresh rhizome (top)	Alcoholic extract	*Dirofilaria immitis* microfilariae, *in vitro* and dogs	Datta & Sukul, 1987

[a] Origin of the plant or product described in the citation. May not be the only origin.
[b] Route of administration: po, *per os* (oral); top, topical; ip, intraperitoneal; na, not applicable.
NC, not cited.

Table 14 Medicinal plants reported to cause the physical extrusion of tissue-dwelling nematodes.

Species (Family)	Origin[a]	Part (route[b])	Active ingredients	Indication	References
Carica papaya (Caricaceae)	India	Leaves (top) with opium and salt	Crude preparation	Guinea worm extraction, clinical trial	Sanghui, 1989
Combretum mucronatum (Combretaceae)	Ghana	Root (po)	Crude preparation	Guinea worm extraction, clinical trial	Ampofo, 1977
Elaeophorbia drupifera (Euphorbiaceae)	Ghana	Leaf (po) (used with *Hilleria latifolia*)	Crude preparation	Guinea worm extraction, clinical trial	Ampofo, 1977
Hilleria latifolia (Phytolaccaceae)	Ghana	Leaf (po) (used with *Elaeophorbia drupifera*)	Crude preparation	Guinea worm extraction, clinical trial	Ampofo, 1977

[a] Origin of the plant or product described in the citation. May not be the only origin.
[b] Route of administration: po, *per os* (oral); top, topical.

Table 15 Other natural products with antiprotozoal activity.

Product	Source	Indication	References
Magainin MSI-103	Analogue of peptide from *Xenopus laevis*	*Acanthamoeba polyphaga, in vitro*	Schuster & Jacobs, 1992
Magainin MSI-94	Analogue of peptide from *X. laevis*	*A. polyphaga, in vitro*	Schuster & Jacobs, 1992
Cecropin A	Insect protein from *Hyalophora cecropia*	*Leishmania aethiopica, in vitro*	Kimbrell, 1991
SB-37	Synthetic cecropin b-type peptide	*T. cruzi, in vitro*	Jaynes *et al.*, 1988
Shiva-1	Synthetic cecropin b-type peptide	*T. cruzi, in vitro*	Jaynes *et al.*, 1988
DC-1	Synthetic cecropin b-type peptide	*T. cruzi, in vitro*	Barr *et al.*, 1995
DC-2	Synthetic cecropin b-type peptide	*T. cruzi,* in mice	Barr *et al.*, 1995
DC-2R	Synthetic cecropin b-type peptide	*T. cruzi,* in mice	Barr *et al.*, 1995
Netropsin	Isolated from *Streptomyces netropsis* and *Str. chromogenus*	*T. congolense, T. brucei* and *T. equiperdum*	See Lombardi & Crisanti, 1997
SB-37	Synthetic cecropin b-type peptide	*P. falciparum, in vitro*	Jaynes *et al.*, 1988
Shiva-1	Synthetic cecropin b-type peptide	*P. falciparum, in vitro*	Jaynes *et al.*, 1988
Synthetic magainin 2	Peptide from *Xenopus laevis* skin	*Plasmodium* oocyte development in *Anopheles*	Gwadz *et al.*, 1989
Synthetic cecropin B	Peptide from *Hyalophora cecropia*	*Plasmodium* oocyte development in *Anopheles*	Gwadz *et al.*, 1989
Distamycin	Pyrrole-amidine oligopeptide from *Streptomyces distallicus*	*P. falciparum, in vitro*	Lombardi & Crisanti, 1997
Netropsin	From *Streptomyces netropsis* and *Str. chromomgenus*	*P. falciparum*	Ginsburg *et al.*, 1993
Hectate 1	Synthetic melittin-type peptide	*Cryptosporidium parvum, in vitro*	Arrowood *et al.*, 1991
Shiva-1	Synthetic cecropin-type peptide	*C. parvum, in vitro*	Arrowood *et al.*, 1991
SB-37	Synthetic cecropin-type peptide	*C. parvum, in vitro*	Arrowood *et al.*, 1991
Magainin 1	*Xenopus laevis*	*Bonamia astreae*	Morvan *et al.*, 1994

Table 16 Other natural products with anthelmintic activity.

Product	Source	Indication	References
Ivermectin[a]	Avermectins from *Streptomyces avermitilis*	*Str. stercoralis* and *A. lumbricoides,* clinical trial	Marti *et al.*, 1996
		Visceral larvae migrans, clinical trial	Maruyama *et al.*, 1996
	Avermectins from *Streptomyces avermitilis*	*O. volvulus* and *Loa loa* microfilariae, clinical trial	Richard-Lenoble *et al.*, 1988; WHO, 1995
		Wuchereria bancrofti, clinical trial	Nguyen *et al.*, 1996
		Bru. malayi, clinical trial	Mak *et al.*, 1993
Moxidectin[a]	Milbemycins from *Streptomyces cyanogriseus*	Mixed gastrointestinal nematodes, lambs (*Haemonchus*, *Ostertagia*, *Cooperia*, *Trichostrongylus*, *Oesophagostomum*, *Chabertia*, *Strongyloides*)	Bauer & Conraths, 1994
	Milbemycins from *Streptomyces cyanogriseus*	*O. volvulus* and *O. lienalis* microfilariae, *in vitro* and mice	Tagboto & Townson, 1996
		Bru. malayi and *Bru. pahangi*, *Mastomys*	Schares *et al.*, 1994
Synthetic cecropin A	Peptides for *Hyalophora cecropia*	*Bru. pahangi* microfilariae, *in vitro*	Chalk *et al.*, 1995
Synthetic cecropin B	Peptides for *Hyalophora cecropia*	*Bru. pahangi* microfilariae, *Aedes aegypti* and *in vitro*	Chalk *et al.*, 1995

[a] These products belong to a group of compounds known as macrocyclic lactones, of which ivermectin is classified as an avermectin and moxidectin as a milbemycin. There have been many similar compounds described, some of which occur naturally and some of which are semisynthetic.

ACKNOWLEDGEMENTS

This investigation was supported in part by the UNDP/World Bank/WHO Special Programme for Research and Training in Tropical Diseases (TDR).

REFERENCES

Abatan, M.O. and Makinde, M.J. (1986). Screening of *Azadirachta indica* and *Pisium sativum* for possible antimalarial activities. *Journal of Ethnopharmacology* **17**, 85–93.

Achenbach, H., Waibel, R., Nkunya, M.H.H. and Weenen, H. (1992). Antimalarial compounds from *Hoslundia opposita. Phytochemistry* **40**, 3781–3784.

Adewunmi, C.O., Babajide, O.O. and Furu, P. (1990). Molluscicidal and antischistosomal activities of *Zingiber officinale*. *Planta Medica* **56**, 374–376.

Agarwal, A.K., Triparthi, D.M., Sahai, R., Gupta, N., Saxena, R.P., Puri, A., Singh, M., Misra, R.N., Dubey, C.B. and Saxena, K.C. (1997). Management of giardiasis by a herbal drug 'Pippali Rasayana': a clinical study. *Journal of Ethnopharmacology* **56**, 233–236.

Agbaje, E.O. and Onabanjo, A.O. (1991). The effects of extracts of *Enantia chlorantha* in malaria. *Annals of Tropical Medicine and Parasitology* **85**, 585–590.

Akhtar, M.S. and Ahmad, I. (1992). Comparative efficacy of *Mallotus philipinensis* fruit (Kamala) or Nilzan R drug against gastrointestinal cestodes of Beetal goats. *Small Ruminant Research* **8**, 121–128.

Akhtar, M.S. and Riffat, S. (1991). Field trials of *Saussurea lappa* roots against nematodes and *Nigella sativa* seeds against cestodes in children. *Journal of the Pakistan Medical Association* **41**, 185–187.

Albonico, M., Crompton, D.W.T. and Savioli, L. (1998). Control strategies for human intestinal nematode infections. In *Advances in Parasitology* (J.R. Baker, R. Muller and D. Rollinson, eds), pp. 278–341. London: Academic Press.

Al-Khayat, A.H.A., Kirby, G.C., Warhurst, D.C. and Phillipson, J.D. (1991). The *in vitro* antimalarial effects of combinations of some protein synthesis inhibitors. *Transactions of the Royal Society of Tropical Medicine and Hygiene* **85**, 310.

Al-Waili, N.S. (1988). *Artemisia herba-alba* extract for treating *Enterobius vermicularis* infection. *Transactions of the Royal Society of Tropical Medicine and Hygiene* **82**, 217–218.

Amorim, C.Z., Marques, A.D. and Cordeiro, R.S.B. (1991). Screening of the antimalarial activity of plants of the Cucurbitaceae family. *Memorias do Instituto Oswaldo Cruz* **86**(S2), 177–180.

Amorin, A., Barba, H.R., Carauta, J.P.P., Lopes, D., Kaplan, M.A.C. (1999). Anthelmintic activity of the latex of *Ficus* species. *Journal of Ethnopharmacology* **64**, 255–258.

Ampofo, O. (1977). Plants that heal. *World Health* November 26–30.

Ang, H.H., Chan, K.L. and Mak, J.W. (1995). Effect of 7-day daily replacement of culture medium containing *Eurycoma longifolia* Jack constituents on the Malaysian *Plasmodium falciparum* isolates. *Journal of Ethnopharmacology* **49**, 171–175.

Anonymous (1994). Pharmaceuticals from plants: great potential, few funds. *The Lancet* **343**, 1513–1514.

Arrowood, M.J., Jaynes, J.M. and Healey M.C. (1991). *In vitro* activity of lytic peptides against the sporozoites of *Cryptosporidium parvum. Antimicrobial Agents and Chemotherapy* **35**, 224–227.

Asuzu, I.U. and Anaga, A.O. (1991). Pharmacological screening of the aqueous extract of *Alstonia boonei* bark. *Fitoterapia* **62**, 411–414.

Atzori, C., Bruno, A., Chichino, G., Bombardelli, E., Scaglia, M. and Ghione, M. (1993). Activity of bilboalide, a sesquiterpene from *Ginkgo biloba*, on *Pneumocystis carinii*. *Antimicrobial Agents and Chemotherapy* **37**, 1492–1496.

Ayensu, F.S. (1978). *Medicinal Plants of West Africa*. Algonac, Michigan: Reference Publications Inc. 330pp.

Badam, L., Deolankar, R.P., Rojatkar, S.R., Nagsampgi, B.A. and Wagh, U.V. (1988). *In vitro* antimalarial activity of medicinal plants of India. *Indian Journal of Medical Research* **87**, 379–383.

Bandi, C., McCall, J.W., Genchi, C., Corona, S., Venco, L. and Sacchi, L. (1999). Effects of tetracycline on the filarial worms *Brugia pahangi* and *Dirofilaria immitis* and their bacterial endosymbionts *Wolbachia*. *International Journal for Parasitology*, **29**, 357–364.

Barr, S.C., Rose, D. and Jaynes, J.M. (1995). Activity of lytic peptides against intracellular *Trypanosoma cruzi* amastigotes *in vitro* and parasitaemias in mice. *Journal of Parasitology* **81**, 974–978.

Bauer, C. and Conraths, F.J. (1994). Comparative efficacy of moxidectin and mebendazole against gastrointestinal nematodes in experimentally infected lambs. *Veterinary Record* **135**, 136–138.

Bechinger, B. (1997). Structure and functions of channel-forming peptides: magainins, cecropins, melittin and alamethicin. *Journal of Membrane Biology* **156**, 197–211.

Benoit, F., Valentin, A., Pelissier, Y., Marion, C., Dakuyo, Z., Mallie, M. and Bastide, J.M. (1995). Antimalarial activity *in vitro* of *Cochlosperum tinctorium* tubercule extracts. *Transactions of the Royal Society of Tropical Medicine and Hygiene* **89**, 217–218.

Benoit, F., Valentin, A., Pelissier, Y., Diafouka, F., Marion, C., Kone-Bamba, D., Kone, M., Mallie, M., Yapo, A. and Bastide, J.M. (1996). *In vitro* antimalarial activity of vegetal extracts used in West African traditional medicine. *American Journal of Tropical Medicine and Hygiene* **54**, 67–71.

Benoit-Vical, F., Valentin, A., Cournac, V., Pelissier, Y., Mallie, M. and Bastide, J.M. (1998). *In vitro* antiplasmodial activity of stem and root extracts of *Nauclea latifolia* S.M. (Rubiaceae). *Journal of Ethnopharmacology*. **61**, 173–178.

Berger, I., Barrientos, A.C., Caceres, A., Hernandez, M., Rastrelli, L., Passreiter, C.M. and Kubelka, W. (1998). Plants used in Guatemala for the treament of protozoal infections. *Journal of Ethnopharmacology* **62**, 107–115.

Bhakuni, D.S., Dhar, M.L., Dhar, M.M., Dhawan, B.N. and Mehrotra, B.N. (1969). Screening of Indian plants for biological activity: Part 11. *Indian Journal of Experimental Biology* **7**, 250–262.

Bianco, A.E., Nwachukwu, M.A., Townson, S., Doenhoff, M.J. and Muller, R.L. (1986). Evaluation of drugs against *Onchocerca* microfilariae in an inbred mouse model. *Tropical Medicine and Parasitology* **37**, 39–45.

Bodeker, G. and Willcox, M. (2000). New research initiative of plant-based antimalarials. *The Lancet* **355**, 761.

Bogh, H., Andreassen, J. and Lemmich, J. (1996). Anthelmintic usage of extracts of *Embelia schimperi* from Tanzania. *Journal of Ethnopharmacology* **50**, 35–42.

Boyce, N. (2000). Drugs on tap from morning dew. *New Scientist* **2266**, 22.

Brandao, M.G., Krettli, A.U., Soares, L.S., Nery, C.G. and Marinuzzi, H.C. (1997). Antimalarial activity of extracts and fractions from *Bidens pilosa* and other *Bidens* species (Asteraceae) correlated with the presence of acetylene and flavinoid compounds. *Journal of Ethnopharmacology* **57**, 131–138.

Bray, D.H., Connolly, J.D., O'Neill, M.J., Phillipson, J.D. and Warhurst, D.C. (1990). Plants as sources of antimalarial compounds, 7. Activity of some species of Meliaceae plants and their constituent limonoids. *Phytotherapy Research* **4**, 29–35.

Bringmann, G., Saeb, W., Ake Assi, L., Francois, G., Narayanan, A.S.S., Peters, K. and Peters, E.M. (1987). Betulinic acid: isolation from *Triphyophyllum peltatum* and *Anicistrocladus heyneanus*, antimalarial activity and crystal structure of the benzyl ester. *Planta Medica* **63**, 255–257.

Bringmann, G., Francois, G., Ake Assi, L. and Schlauer, J. (1998). The alkaloids of *Triphyophyllum peltatum* (Dioncophyllaceae). *Chimia* **52**, 18–28.

Buckner, F.S., Wilson, A.J., White, T.C. and Van Voorhis, W.C. (1998). Introduction of resistance to azole drugs in *Trypanosoma cruzi*. *Antimicrobial Agents and Chemotherapy* **42**, 3245–3250.

Cabral, J.A., McChesney, D.J. and Milhous, W.K. (1993). A new antimalarial quassinoid from *Simaba guianensis*. *Journal of Natural Products* **56**, 1954–1961.

Caceres, A., Lopez, B., Gonzalez, S., Berger, I., Tada, I. and Maki, J. (1998). Plants used in Guatemala for the treatment of protozoal infections. 1. Screening of activity to bacteria, fungi and American trypanosomes of 13 native plants. *Journal of Ethnopharmacology* **62**, 195–202.

Carvalho, L.H., Brandao, M.G., Santos-Filho, D., Lopes, J.L. and Krettli, A.U. (1991). Antimalarial activity of crude extracts from Brazilian plants studied *in vivo* in *Plasmodium berghi*-infected mice and *in vitro* against *Plasmodium falciparum* in culture. *Brazilian Journal of Medical and Biological Research* **24**, 1113–1123.

Cavin, J.C., Krassner, S.M. and Rodriguez, E. (1987). Plant-derived alkaloids against *Trypanosoma cruzi*. *Journal of Ethnopharmacology* **19**, 89–94.

Cenini, P., Bolognesi, A. and Stirpe, F. (1988). Ribosome inactivating proteins from plants inhibit ribosome activity of *Trypanosoma* and *Leishmania*. *Journal of Protozoology* **35**, 384–387.

Chalk, R., Townson, H. and Ham, P.J. (1995). *Brugia pahangi*: The effects of cecropins on microfilariae *in vitro* and in *Aedes aegypti*. *Experimental Parasitology* **80**, 401–406.

Chang, H.M. and Nut, P.P.H. (1986). *Pharmacology and Application of Chinese Materia Medica* (2 volumes). Singapore: World Scientific.

Chataing, B., Concepcion, J.L., Lobaton, R. and Usubillaga, A. (1998). Inhibition of *Trypanosoma cruzi* growth *in vitro* by *Solanum* alkaloids: a comparison with ketoconazole. *Planta Medica* **64**, 31–36.

Chatterjee, R.K., Fatma, N., Murthy, P.K., Sinha, P., Kulshrestha, D.K. and Dhawan, B.N. (1992). Macrofilaricidal activity of the stembark of *Streblus asper* and its major active constituents. *Drug Development Research* **26**, 67–78.

Chawira, N. and Warhurst, D.C. (1987). The effect of artemisinin combined with standard antimalarials against chloroquine-sensitive and chloroquine-resistant strains of *Plasmodium falciparum in vitro*. *Journal of Tropical Medicine and Hygiene* **90**, 1–8.

Chawira, N., Warhurst, D.C., Robinson, B.L. and Peters, W. (1987). The effect of combinations of qinghaosu (artemisinin) with standard antimalarial drugs in the suppressive treatment of malaria in mice. *Transactions of the Royal Society of Tropical Medicine and Hygiene* **81**, 554–558.

Chen, C., Zheng, X., Quian, Y., Xiao, S., Shao, B. and Huang, L. (1962). Studies on *Hemerocallis thunbergii* Baker III. Isolation and characterization of active principle against *Schistosoma japonicum*. *Acta Pharmaceutica Sinica* **9**, 579–586.

Chitravanshi, V.C., Singh, A.P., Ghoshal, S., Krishna-Prasad, B.N., Srivastava, V. and Tandon, J.S. (1992). Therapeutic action of *Nyctanthes arbor-tristis* against caecal amoebiasis of rat. *International Journal of Pharmacognosy* **30**, 71–75.

Chung, C.T.A. and Staba, E.J. (1986). Effects of age and growth regulators on growth and alkaloid production in *Cinchona ledgeriana* leaf-shoot organ cultures. *Planta Medica* **53**, 206–209.

Comley, J.W.C. (1990). New macrofilaricidal leads from plants? *Tropical Medicine and Parasitology* **41**, 1–9.

Comley, J.W.C., Titanji, V.P.K., Ayafor, J.F. and Singh, V.K. (1990). *In vitro* antifilarial activity of some medicinal plants. *Acta Leidensia* **59**, 361–363.

Connelly, M.P.E., Fabiano, E., Patel, I.H., Kinyanjui, S.M., Mberu, E.K. and Watkins, W.M. (1996). Antimalarial activity in crude extracts of Malawian medicinal plants. *Annals of Tropical Medicine and Parasitology*. **90**, 597–602.

Cooke, D.W., Lallinger, G.J. and Durack, D.T. (1987). *In vitro* sensitivity of *Naegleria fowl-eri* to qinghaosu and dihydroqinghaosu. *Journal of Parasitology* **73**, 411–413.

Croft, S.L., Evans, A.T. and Neal, R.A. (1985). The activity of plumbagin and other electron carriers against *Leishmania donovani* and *Leishmania mexicana amazonensis*. *Annals of Tropical Medicine and Parasitology* **79**, 651–653.

Cruz, F.S., Vasconcellos, M.E. and Leon, W. (1975). Inhibition and development of *Trypanosoma cruzi* by olivacine and olivacine pamoate. *Journal of Protozoology* **22**, 86A–87A.

Daly, J.W. (1998). Thirty years of discovery of arthropod alkaloids in amphibian skin. *Journal of Natural Products* **61**, 162–172.

Dalziel, J. (1937). *The Useful Plants of West Tropical Africa*. London: The Crown Agents for the Colonies. 612pp.

Dar, R.N., Garg, L.C. and Pathak, R.D. (1965). Anthelmintic activity of *Carica papaya* seeds. *Indian Journal of Pharmacy* **27**, 335.

Das, M.K. and Beuria, M.K. (1991). Antimalarial property of an extract of the plant *Streblus asper* in murine malaria. *Transactions of the Royal Society of Tropical Medicine and Hygiene* **85**, 40–41.

Datta, A. and Sukul, N.C. (1987). Antifilarial effects of *Zingiber officinale* on *Dirofilaria immitis*. *Journal of Helminthology* **61**, 268–270.

Datta, D.V., Singh, S.A.K. and Chhuttani, P.N. (1974). Treatment of amoebic liver abscess with emetine hydrochloride, niridazole and metronidazole. A controlled clinical trial. *American Journal of Tropical Medicine and Hygiene* **23**, 586–589.

de Amorin, A., Borba, H.R., Carauta, J.P.P., Lopes, D. and Kaplan, M.A.C. (1999). Anthelmintic activity of the latex of *Ficus* species. *Journal of Ethnopharmacology* **64**, 255–258.

Decosterd, L.A., Hoffmann, E., Kyburz, R., Bray, B. and Hostettmann, K. (1991). A new phloroglucinol derivative from *Hypericum calycinum* with antifungal and *in vitro* antimalarial activity. *Planta Medica* **57**, 548–551.

Derbyshire, D. (2000). Now for some clinical evidence. *The Daily Telegraph*, December 13, 2000.

Desta, B. (1995). Ethiopian traditional herbal drugs. Part 1: Studies on the toxicity and therapeutic activity of local taenicidal medications. *Journal of Ethnopharmacology* **45**, 27–33.

Dhar, M.L., Dhar, M.M., Dhawan, B.N., Mehrotra, B.N. and Ray, C. (1968). Screening of Indian plants for biological activity: Part 1. *Indian Journal of Experimental Biology* **6**, 232–247.

Dhar, R., Zhang, K., Talwar, G.P., Garg, S. and Kumar, N. (1998). Inhibition of the growth and development of asexual and sexual stages of drug sensitive and resistant strains of the human malaria parasite *Plasmodium falciparum* by Neem (*Azadirachta indica*) fractions. *Journal of Ethnopharmacology* **61**, 31–39.

Dobson, M.J. (1998). Bitter-sweet solutions for malaria: exploring natural remedies from the past. *Parasitologica* **40**, 69–81.

Druilhe, P., Brandicourt, O., Chongsuphajaisiddhi, T. and Berthe, J. (1988). Activity of a combination of three cinchona bark alkaloids against *Plasmodium falciparum in vitro*. *Antimicrobial Agents and Chemotherapy* **32**, 250–254.

Dutta, A. and Sukul, N.C. (1982). Filaricidal properties of a wild herb, *Andrographis paniculata*. *Journal of Helminthology* **56**, 81–84.

Ekong, R., Partridge, S.J., Anderson, M.M., Kirby, G.C., Warhurst, D.C., Russel, P.F. and Phillipson, J.D. (1991). *Plasmodium falciparum*: effects of phaeanthine, a naturally-occurring bisbenzylisoquinoline alkaloid, on chloroquine-resistant and -sensitive parasites *in vitro*, and its influence on chloroquine activity. *Annals of Tropical Medicine and Parasitology* **85**, 205–213.

El Tahir, A., Satti, G.M.H. and Khalid, S.A. (1999). Antiplasmodial activity of selected Sudanese medicinal plants with emphasis on *Maytenus senegalensis* (Lam.) Excell. *Journal of Ethnopharmacology* **64**, 227–233.

Evans, A.T. and Croft, S.L. (1987). Antileishmanial activity of harmaline and other tryptamine derivatives. *Phytotherapy Research* **1**, 25–27.

Faedo, M., Larsen, M. and Waller, P.J. (1997). The potential of nematophagous fungi to control the free-living stages of nematode parasites of sheep: comparison between Australian isolates of *Arthrobotrys* sp. and *Duddingtonia flagrans*. *Veterinary Parasitology* **72**, 149–155.

Fandeur, T., Moretti, C. and Polonsky, J. (1985). *In vitro* and *in vivo* assessment of the antimalarial activity of sergeolide. *Planta Medica*, **57**, 20–23.

Feldman, S.T., Speaker, M. and Cleveland, P. (1991). Effects of magainins on *Acanthamoeba castellanii*. *Reviews of Infectious Diseases* **13**(S5), 439.

Fernandez, A.S., Larsen, M., Henningsen, E., Nansen, P., Gronvold, J., Bjorn, H. and Wolstrup, J. (1999). Effect of *Duddingtonia flagrans* against *Ostertagia ostertagi* in cattle grazing at different stocking rates. *Parasitology* **119**, 105–111.

Flores Crespo, J., Herrera Rodrigues, D., Vazquez Prats, V., Flores Crespo, R., Liebano Hernandez, E. and Mendoza de Gives, P. (1999). *In vitro* predatory activity of 8 fungal isolates aginst the nematode *Panagrellus redivivus*. *Revista Latinoamericana de Microbiologica* **41**, 239–244.

Foster, S. (1994). Economic prospects for a new antimalarial drug. *Transactions of the Royal Society of Tropical Medicine and Hygiene* **88S**, 55–56.

Fournet, A., Angelo, A., Munoz, V., Roblot, F., Hocquemiller, R. and Cave, A. (1992). Biological and chemical studies of *Para benensis*, a Bolivian plant used in folk medicine as a treatment of cutaneous leishmaniasis. *Journal of Ethnopharmacology* **37**, 159–164.

Fournet, A., Munoz, V., Roblot, F., Hocquemiller, R., Cave, A. and Gantier, J. (1993). Antiprotozoal activity of dehydrozaluzanin C, a sesquiterpene lactone isolated from *Munnoiia maronii* (Asteraceae). *Phytotherapy Research* **7**, 111–115.

Fournet, A., Barrios, A.A. and Munoz, V. (1994). Leishmanicidal and trypanocidal activities of Bolivian medicinal plants. *Journal of Ethnopharmacology* **41**, 19–37.

Francois, G., Kanyinda, B., Dochez, C., Wery, M. and Vanhaelen, M. (1992). Activity of cocsoline a bisbenzylisoquinoline alkaloid from *Anisocycla cymosa* against *Plasmodium falciparum*. *Planta Medica* **58**(S1), A634–A635.

Francois, G., Bringmann, G., Phillipson, J.D., Ake Assi, L., Dochez, C., Rubenacker, M., Schneider, C., Wery, M., Warhurst, D.C. and Kirby, D.C. (1994). Activity of extracts and napthylisoquinoline alkaloids from *Ancistrocladus abbreviatus* and *A. barteri* against *Plasmodium falciparum in vitro*. *Phytochemistry* **35**, 1461–1464.

Francois, G., Bringmann, G., Dochez, C., Schneider, C., Timperman, G. and Ake Assi, L. (1995). Activities of extracts and naphthylisoquinoline alkaloids from *Triphyophyllum peltatum*, *Ancistrocladus abbreviatus* and *Ancistrocladus barteri* against *Plasmodium berghei*. *Journal of Ethnopharmacology* **46**, 115–120.

Francois, G., Ake Assi, L., Holenz, J. and Bringmann, G. (1996a). Constituents of *Picralima nitida* display pronounced inhibitory activities against asexual erythrocytic forms of *Plasmodium falciparum in vitro. Journal of Ethnopharmacology* **54**, 113–117.

Francois, G., Passreiter, C.M., Woerdenbag, H.J. and Van Looveren, M. (1996b). Antiplasmodial activities and cytotoxic effects of aqueous extracts and sesquiterpine lactones from *Neurolaena lobata. Planta Medica* **62**, 126–129.

Francois, G., Timperman, G., Holenz, J., Ake Assi, L., Geuder, T., Maes, L., Dubois, J., Hanocq, M. and Bringmann, G. (1996c). Naphthylisoquinoline alkaloids exhibit strong growth-inhibiting activities against *Plasmodium falciparum* and *P. berghei in vitro.* Structure–activity relationships of dioncophylline C. *Annals of Tropical Medicine and Parasitology* **90**, 115–123.

Francois, G., Timperman, G., Eling, W., Assi, L.A., Holenz, J. and Bringmann, G. (1997a). Naphthylisoquinoline alkaloids against malaria: evaluation of the curative potentials of dioncophylline C and dioncopeltine against *Plasmodium berghei in vivo. Antimicrobial Agents and Chemotherapy* **41**, 2533–2539.

Francois, G., Timperman, G., Haller, R.D., Bar, S., Isahakia, M.A., Robertson, S.A., Zhao, C., DeSouza, N.J., Assi, L.A., Holenz, J. and Bringmann, G. (1997b). Growth inhibition of asexual erythrocytic forms of *Plasmodium falciparum* and *P. berghei in vitro* by naphthylisoquinoline alkaloid-containing extracts of *Anicistroclaudus* and *Triphyophyllum* species. *International Journal of Pharmacology* **35**, 55–59.

Franssen, F.F., Smeijsters, L.J., Berger, I. and Medinilla-Aladana, B.E. (1997). *In vivo* and *in vitro* antiplasmodial activity of some plants traditionally used in Guatemala against malaria. *Antimicrobial Agents and Chemotherapy* **41**, 1500–1503.

Freiburghaus, F., Kaminsky, R., Nkunya, M.H.H. and Brun, R. (1996). Evaluation of African medicinal plants for their *in vitro* trypanocidal activity. *Journal of Ethnopharmacology* **55**, 1–11.

Frieburghaus, F., Ogwal, E.N., Nkuna, M.H.H., Kaminsky, R. and Brun, R. (1996). *In vitro* antitrypanosomal activity of African medicinal plants used in traditional medicine in Uganda to treat sleeping sickness. *Tropical Medicine and International Health* **1**, 765–771.

Fujioka, H., Nishiyama, Y., Furukawa, H. and Kumada, N. (1989) *In vitro* and *in vivo* activities of ataphillinine and related acridine alkaloids against malaria. *Antimicrobial Agents and Chemotherapy* **33**, 6–9.

Gakunju, D.M.N., Mberu, E.K., Dossagi, S.F., Gray, A.I., Waigh, R.D., Waterman, P.G. and Watkins, W.M. (1995). Potent antimalarial activity of alkaloid nitidine, isolated from a Kenyan herbal remedy. *Antimicrobial Agents and Chemotherapy* **39**, 2606–2609.

Gantier, J.L., Fournet, A., Munos, M.H. and Hocquemiller, R. (1996). The effect of some 2-substituted quinolones isolated from *Galipea longiflora* on *Plasmodium vinckei petteri* infected mice. *Planta Medica* **62**, 285–286.

Gasquet, M., Delmas, F., Timon-David, P., Keita, A., Guindo, M., Koita, N., Diallo, D. and Doumbo, O. (1993). Evaluation *in vitro* and *in vitro* of a traditional antimalarial, "Malarial 5". *Fitoterapia* **64**, 423–426.

Gbeassor, M., Kossou, K., Amegbo, K.A., DeSouza, C., Koumaglo, K. and Demke, A. (1989). Antimalarial effects of eight African medicinal plants. *Journal of Ethnopharmacology* **25**, 115–118.

Gbeassor, M., Kedjagni, A.Y., Koumaglo, K., DeSouza, C., Agbo, K., Aklikokou, K. and Amegbo, K.A. (1990). *In vitro* antimalarial activity of six medicinal plants. *Phytotherapy Research* **4**, 115–117.

Gessler, M.C., Nkunya, M.H.H., Mwasumbi, L.B., Heinrich, M. and Tanner, M. (1994). Screening Tanzanian medicinal plants for antimalarial activity. *Acta Tropica* **56**, 65–77.

Gessler, M.M., Tanner, M., Chollet, J., Nkunya, M.H.H. and Heinrich, M. (1995). Tanzanian medicinal plants used traditionally for the treatment of malaria: *in vivo* antimalarial and *in vitro* cytotoxic avtivities. *Phytotherapy Research* **9**, 504–508.

Ghosh, A.K., Bhattacharya F.K. and Ghosh, D.K. (1985). *Leishmania donovani*: amastigote inhibition and mode of action of berberine. *Experimental Parasitology* **60**, 404–413.

Gillin, F.D., Reiner, D.S. and Suffness, M. (1982). Bruceantin, a potent amoebicide from a plant, *Brucea antidysenterica. Antimicrobial Agents and Chemotherapy* **22**, 342–345.

Ginsburg, H., Nissani, E., Krugliak, M. and Williamson, D.H. (1993). Selective toxicity to malaria parasites by non-intercalating DNA-binding ligands. *Molecular and Biochemical Parasitology* **58**, 7–15.

Gonzalez-Garza, M.T. and Said-Fernandez, S. (1988). *Entamoeba histolytica*: potent *in vitro* antiamoebic effect of gossypol. *Experimental Parasitology* **66**, 253–255.

Gotaskie, G.E. and Andreassi, B.F. (1994). Paclitaxel: a new antimitotic chemotherapeutic agent. *Cancer Practice: a Multidisciplinary Journal of Cancer Care* **2**, 27–33.

Goto, H., Gomes, C.M., Corbett, C.E., Monteiro, H.P. and Gidlund, M. (1998). Insulin-like growth factor I is a growth-promoting factor for *Leishmania* promastigotes and amastigotes. *Proceedings of the National Academy of Sciences of the USA* **95**, 13211–13216.

Greenwood, D. (1992). The quinine connection. *Journal of Antimicrobial Chemotherapy* **30**, 417–427.

Grellier, P., Ramiaramanana, L., Millerioux, U., Deharo, E., Schrevil, J., Frappier, F., Trigalo, F., Bodo, B. and Pousset, J.L. (1996). Antimalarial activity of cryptolepine and isocryptolepine, alkaloids isolated from *Cryptolepis sanguinolenta. Phytotherapy Research* **10**, 317–321.

Grove, D.I. (1990). *A History of Human Helminthology*. CAB International, Wallingford, Oxon, UK.

Groves, M.J. and Bisset, N.G. (1991). A note on the use of topical digitalis prior to William Withering. *Journal of Ethnopharmacology* **35**, 99–103.

Grzybek, J., Wongpanich, V., Mata-Greenwood, E., Angerhofer, C.K., Pezzuto, J.M. and Cordell, G.A. (1997). Biological evaluation of selected plants from Poland. *International Journal of Pharmacology* **35**, 1–5.

Guru, P.Y., Warhurst, D.C., Harris, A. and Phillipson, J.D. (1983). Antimalarial activity of bruceantin *in vitro*. *Annals of Tropical Medicine and Parasitology* **77**, 433–435.

Gwadz, R.W., Kaslow, D., Lee, J., Maloy, W.L., Zasloff, M. and Miller, L.H. (1989). Effects of magainins and cecropins on the sporogonic development of malaria parasites in mosquitoes. *Infection and Immunity* **57**, 2628–2633.

Harvey, A.L. (1999). Deadly remedies. *Biologist* **46**, 102–104.

Hay, F.S., Niezen, J.H., Miller, C., Bateson, L. and Robertson, H. (1997). Infestation of sheep dung by nematophagous fungi and implications for the control of free-living stages of gastro-intestinal nematodes. *Veterinary Parasitology* **70**, 247–254.

Hazra, B., Saha, A.K., Ray, R., Roy, D.K., Sur, P. and Banerjee, A. (1987). Antiprotozoal activity of diospyrin towards *Leishmania donovani* promastigotes *in vitro*. *Transactions of the Royal Society of Tropical Medicine and Hygiene* **81**, 738–741.

Heinrich, M., Kuhnt, M., Wright, C.W., Rimpler, H., Phillipson, J.D., Schandelmaier, A. and Warhurst, D.C. (1992). Parasitological and microbiological evaluation of Mixe Indian medicinal plants (Mexico). *Journal of Ethnopharmacology* **36**, 81–85.

Hien, T.T. and White, N.J. (1993). Qinghaosu. *The Lancet* **341**, 603–608.

Hocquemiller, R., Cortes, D., Arango, G.J., Myint, S.H. and Cave, A. (1991). Isolement et synthese de l'espintanol nouveau monoterpine antiparasitaire. *Journal of Natural Products* **54**, 445–452.

Hoerauf, A., Nissen-Pahle, K., Schmetz, C., Henkle-Duhrsen, K., Blaxter, M.L., Buttner, D.W., Gallin, M.Y., Al-Qaoud, K.M., Lucius, R. and Fleischer, B. (1999). Tetracycline therapy targets intracellular bacteria in the filarial nematode *Litomosoides sigmodontis* and results in filarial infertility. *Journal of Clinical Investigation*, **103**, 11–18.

Hukkeri, V.I., Kalyani, G.A., Hatpaki, B.C. and Manvi, F.V. (1993). *In vitro* anthelmintic activity of aqueous extract of fruit rind of *Punica granatum*. *Fitoterapia* **64**, 69–70.

Huston, C.D. and Petri, W.A., jr (1998). Host–pathogen interaction in amoebiasis and progress in vaccine development. *European Journal of Clinical Microbiology and Infectious Diseases* **17**, 601–614.

Irwin, A. (2000). How man apes animal medicine. *The Daily Telegraph*, December 13, 2000.

Iwu, M.M. and Klayman, D.L. (1992). Evaluation of the *in vitro* antimalarial activity of *Picralima nitida* extracts. *Journal of Ethnopharmacology* **36**, 133–135.

Iwu, M.M., Jackson, J.E., Tally, J.D. and Klayman, D.L. (1992). Evaluation of plant extracts for antileishmanial activity using a mechanism-based radiorespirometric microtechnique (RAM). *Planta Medica* **58**, 436–441.

Iwu, M.M., Jackson, J.E. and Schuster, B.G. (1994). Medicinal plants in the fight against leishmaniasis. *Parasitology Today* **10**, 65–68.

Jaquet, C., Stoher, H.R., Chollet, J. and Peters, W. (1994). Antimalarial activity of the bicyclic peroside Ro42-1611 (arteflene) in experimental models. *Tropical Medicine and Parasitology* **45**, 266–271.

Jaynes, J.M., Burton, C.A., Barr, S.B., Jeffers, G.W., Julian, G.R., White, K.L., Enwright, F.M., Klei, T.R. and Laine, R.A. (1988). *In vitro* cytocidal effect of novel lytic peptides on *Plasmodium falciparum* and *Trypanosoma cruzi*. *FASEB Journal* **2**, 2878–2883.

Jenett-Siems, K., Mockenhaupt, F.P., Bienzle, U., Gupta, M.P. and Eich, E. (1999). *In vitro* antiplasmodial activity of Central American medicinal plants. *Tropical Medicine and International Health* **4**, 611–615.

Johns, T., Faubert, G.M., Kokwaro, J.O., Mahunnah, R.L.A. and Kimanani, E.B. (1995). Anti-giardial activity of gastrointestinal remedies of the Luo of East Africa. *Journal of Ethnopharmacology* **46**, 17–23.

Jurg, A., Tomas, T. and Pividal, J. (1991). Antimalarial activity of some plant remedies in use in Marracuene, southern Mozambique. *Journal of Ethnopharmacology* **33**, 79–83.

Kaneda, Y., Torii, M., Tanaka, T. and Aikawa, M. (1991). *In vitro* effects of berberine sulphate on the growth and structure of *Entamoeba histolytica*, *Giardia lamblia* and *Trichomonas vaginalis*. *Annals of Tropical Medicine and Parasitology* **85**, 417–425.

Kanyinda, B., Francois, G., Vanhaelen, M. and Wery, M. (1992). Activity of three bisbenzylisoquinoline alkaloids from *Anisocycla cymosa* against *Giardia lamblia*. *Planta Medica* **58**(S1), A635.

Kapadia, G.J., Angerhofer, C.K. and Ansa-Asamoah, R. (1993). Akuammine: an antimalarial indolemonoterpene alkaloid of *Picralima nitida* seeds. *Planta Medica* **69**, 565–566.

Kaplan, D.T., Keen, N.T. and Thomason, I.J. (1980a). Association of glyceollin with the incompatible response of soybean roots to *Meloidogyne incognita*. *Physiological Plant Pathology* **16**, 309–318.

Kaplan, D.T., Keen, N.T. and Thomason, I.J. (1980b). Studies on the mode of action of glyceollin in soybean incompatibility to the root knot nematode, *Meloidogyne incognita*. *Physiological Plant Pathology* **16**, 319–325.

Kardono, L.B.S., Angerhofer, C.K., Tsauri, S., Padmawinata, K., Pezzuto, J.M. and Kinghorn, A.D. (1991). Cytotoxic and antimalarial constituents of the roots of *Eurycoma longifolia*. *Journal of Natural Products* **54**, 1360–1367.

Kazura, J.W., Bockarie, M., Alexander, N., Perry, R., Bockarie, F., Dagoro, H., Dimber, Z., Hyun, P. and Alpers, M.P. (1997). Transmission intensity and its relationship to infection and disease due to *Wuchereria bancrofti* in Papua New Guinea. *Journal of Infectious Diseases* **176**, 242–246.

Keene, A.T., Phillipson, J.D., Warhurst, D.C., Koch, M. and Seguin, E. (1986). *In vitro* amoebicidal testing of natural products; Part 2. Alkaloids related to emetine. *Planta Medica* **53**, 201–206.

Keller, K. (2000). The registration of herbal medicine products in the European Union. In: *Traditional Medicine and Pharmaceutical Medicine Perspectives on Natural Products for the Treatment of Tropical Diseases*. Geneva: WHO/TDR Scientific Working Group. Abstract.

Khalid, S.A., Farouk, A., Geary, T.G. and Jensen, J.B. (1986). Potential antimalarial candidates from African plants: an *in vitro* approach using *Plasmodium falciparum*. *Journal of Ethnopharmacology* **15**, 201–209.

Khunkitti, W., Fujimaki, Y. and Aoki, Y. (2000). *In vitro* activity of extracts of the medicinal plant *Cardiospermum halicacabum* against *Brugia pahangi*. *Journal of Helminthology* **74**, 241–246.

Kilian, H.D. (1987). *Preliminary Data on the Effects of an Extract from* Cassia aubrevellei *in Onchocerciasis. Annual Report*, pp. 33–34. Hamburg: Liberia Research Unit of the Tropical Institute.

Kilian, H.D., Jahn, K., Buttner, D.W. and Kraus, L. (1989). *In vivo* and *in vitro* effects of extracts of *Cassia aubrevillei* in onchocerciasis. *O-NOW! Symposium on Onchocerciasis*. September 20–22, Leiden, The Netherlands.

Kimbrell, D.A. (1991). Insect antibacterial proteins: not just for insects and against bacteria. *BioEssays* **13**, 657–663.

Kirby, G.C. (1996). Medicinal plants and the control of protozoal disease, with particular reference to malaria. *Transactions of the Royal Society of Tropical Medicine and Hygiene* **90**, 605–609.

Kirby, G.C., O'Neill, M.J., Phillipson, J.D. and Warhurst, D.C. (1989). *In vitro* studies on the mode of action of quassinoids with activity against chloroquine-resistant *Plasmodium falciparum*. *Biochemical Pharmacology* **38**, 4367–4374.

Kirby, G.C., Khumalo-Ngwenya, M.B., Grawehr, A., Fison, T.W. and Warhurst, D.C. (1993). Antimalarial activity from 'Mhekara' (*Uapaca nitida* Mull-Arg.) a Tanzanian tree. *Journal of Ethnopharmacology* **40**, 47–51.

Kirby, G.C., Paine, A., Warhurst, D.C., Noamese, B.K. and Phillipson, J.D. (1995). *In vitro* and *in vivo* antimalarial activity of cryptolepine, a plant-derived indoloquinoline. *Phytotherapy Research* **9**, 359–363.

Kitagawa, I., Minagawa, K., Zhang, R., Hori, K., Doi, M., Inoue, M., Ishida, T., Kimura, M., Uji, T. and Shibuya, H. (1993). Dehatrine and antimalarial bisbenzyl- isoquinoline alkaloid from the Indonesian medicinal plant *Beischmiedia madang*, isolated as a mixture of two rotational isomers. *Chemical and Pharmaceutical Bulletin* **41**, 997–999.

Kitagawa, I., Mahmud, T., Simanjutak, P., Hori, K., Uji, T. and Shibuya, H. (1994). Indonesian medicinal plants. VIII. Chemical structures of three new triterpenoids, brucejavanin A, dihydrobrucejavanin A and brucejavanin B, and a new alkaloid glycoside, bruceacanthinoside, from the stems of *Brucea javanica* (Simaroubacaea). *Chemical and Pharmaceutical Bulletin* **42**, 1416–1421.

Kiuchi, F., Miyashita, N., Tsuda, Y., Kondo, K. and Yoshimura, H. (1987). Studies on crude drugs effective on visceral larva migrans. I. Identification of larvicidal principles in betel nuts. *Chemical and Pharmacological Bulletin* **35**, 2880–2886.

Kozek, W.J.P. and Marroquin, H.F. (1977). Intracytoplasmic bacteria in *Onchocerca volvulus*. *American Journal of Tropical Medicine and Hygiene* **26**, 663–678.

Kulangara, A.C. and Subramaniam, R. (1960). Preliminary studies on the effects of certain compounds on the filarial worm of the lizard including an estimate of the toxicity of sodium fluoride. *Indian Journal of Medical Research* **48**, 698–704.

Kumar, D., Mishra, S.K. and Triparthi, H.C. (1991). Mechanism of anthelmintic action of benzylisothicyanate. *Fitoterpia* **62**, 403–410.

Lan, J., Yuan, J., Shao, Z.J., Zhong, D.H., Wang, P.X. and Qi, X.C. (1996). Experimental study of five species of Chinese traditional drugs against *Entamoeba histolytica. Chinese Journal of Parasitic Diseases Control* **9**, 43–46.

Larsen, M., Faedo, M., Waller, P.J. and Hennessy, D.R. (1998). The potential of nematophagous fungi to control the free-living stages of nematode parasites of sheep: studies with *Duddingtonia flagrans. Veterinary Parasitology* **76**, 121–128.

Laughlin, J.C. (1994). Agricultural production of artemisinin – a review. *Transactions of the Royal Society of Tropical Medicine and Hygiene* **88**(S1), 21–22.

Lavaud, C., Massiot, G., Barrera, J.B., Moretti, C., Men-Olivier, L. and Le Men-Olivier, L. (1994). Triterpine saponins from *Myrsine pellucida. Phytochemistry* **37**, 1671–1677.

Leaman, D.J., Arnason, J.T., Yusuf, R., Sangat-Roemantyo, H., Soedjito, H., Angerhofer, C.K. and Pezzuto, J.M. (1995). Malaria remedies of the Kenyah of Apo Kayan, east Kalimantan, Indonesia Borneo: A quantitative assessment of local consensus as an indicator of biological efficacy. *Journal of Ethnopharmacology* **49**, 1–16.

Leon, L., Vasconcellos, M.E., Leon, W., Cruz, F.S., Docampo, R. and De Souza, W. (1978). *Trypanosoma cruzi*: effect of olivacine macromolecules synthesis, ultrastructure and respiration of epimastigotes, *Experimental Parasitology* **45**, 151–159.

Li, G., Guo, X., Fu, L., Jian, H. and Wang, X. (1994). Clinical trials of artemisinin and its derivatives in the treatment of malaria in China. *Transactions of the Royal Society of Tropical Medicine and Parasitology* **88**(S1), 5–6.

Likhitwitayawuid, K., Angerhofer, C.K., Chai, H., Pezzuto, J.M. and Cordell, G.A. (1993). Cytotoxic and antimalarial alkaloids from the bulbs of *Crinum amabile. Journal of Natural Products* **56**, 1331–1338.

Lin, L., Zhang, J., Chen, Z. and Xu, R. (1982). Studies on chemical constituents of *Brucea javanica* (L) Merr. I. Isolation and identification of bruceaketolic acid and four other quassinoids. *Acta Chimica Sinica* **40**, 73–78.

Lin, L.Z., Sheih, H.L., Angerhofer, C.K., Pezzuto, J.M., Cordell, G.A., Xue, L., Johnson, M.E. and Ruangrungsi, N. (1993). Cytotoxic and antimalarial bisbenzylisoquinoline alkaloids from *Cyclea barbata. Journal of Natural Products* **56**, 22–29.

Lindley, D. (1987). Merck's new drug free to WHO for river blindness programme. *Nature*, **329**, 752.

Lombardi, P. and Crisanti, A. (1997). Antimalarial activities of synthetic analogues of distamycin. *Pharmacology and Therapeutics* **76**, 125–133.

Mabberley, D.J. (1997). *The Plant-Book, a Portable Dictionary of the Vascular Plants*, 2nd edn. Cambridge: Cambridge University Press.

Majester-Savornin, B., Elias, R., Diaz-Lanza, A.M., Balansard, G., Gasquet, M. and Delmas, F. (1991). Saponins of the ivy plant, *Hedra helix* and their leishmanicidal activity. *Planta Medica* **57**, 260–262.

Mak, J.W., Navaratnam, V., Grewel, J.S., Mansor, S.M. and Ambu, S. (1993). Treatment of subperiodic *Brugia malayi* infection with a single dose of ivermectin. *American Journal of Tropical Medicine and Hygiene* **48**, 591–596.

Makinde, J.M., Amusan, O.O.G. and Adesogan, E.K. (1987). The antimalarial activity of *Spathodea campanulata* stem bark extract on *Plasmodium berghei berghei* in mice. *Planta Medica* **54**, 122–124.

Makinde, J.M., Awe, S.O. and Salako, L.A. (1993). Seasonal variation in the antimalarial activity of *Morinda lucida* on *Plasmodium berghei berghei* in mice. *Fitoterapia* **65**, 124–130.

Marti, H., Haji, H.J., Savioli, L., Chwaya, H.M., Mgeni, A.F., Ameir, J.S. and Hatz, C. (1996). A comparative trial of a single dose of ivermectin versus three days of albendazole for the treatment of *Strongyloides stercoralis* and other soil transmitted helminth infections in children. *American Journal of Tropical Medicine and Hygiene* **55**, 477–481.

Martin, M., Ridet, J., Chartol, A., Biot, J., Porte, L. and Bezon, A. (1964). Action therapeutique de l'extrait d'*Euphorbia hirta* dans l'amibiase intestinale. A propos de 150 observations. *Medicine Tropicale* **24**, 250–261.

Maruyama, H., Nawa, Y., Noda, S., Mimori, T., Choi, W. and Choi, W.Y. (1996). An outbreak of visceral larvae migrans due to *Ascaris suum* in Kyushu, Japan. *Lancet* **347**, 1766–1767.

McCall, J.W., Jun, J.J. and Bandi, C. (1999). *Wolbachia* and the antifilarial properties of tetracycline. An untold story. *Italian Journal of Zoology* **66**, 7–10.

McLaren, D.J., Worms, M.J., Laurence, B.R. and Simpson, M.G. (1975). Microorganisms in filarial larvae (Nematoda). *Transactions of the Royal Society of Tropical Medicine and Hygiene* **69**, 509–514.

McMillan, B. (1968). Lawang bark as a rubefacient in the treatment of filarial lymphangitis in New Guinea. *Medical Journal of Australia* **13**, 63–64.

Meshnick, S.R., Jefford, C.W., Posner, G.H., Avery, M.A. and Peters, W. (1996). Second-generation antimalarial endoperoxides. *Parasitology Today* **60**, 301–315.

Michael, E., Bundy, D.A.P. and Grenfell, B.T. (1996). Re-assessing the global prevalence and distribution of lymphatic filariasis. *Parasitology* **112**, 409–428.

Mirelman, D., Monheit, D. and Varon, S. (1987). Inhibition of growth of *Entamoeba histolytica* by allicin, the active principle of garlic extract *Allium sativum*. *Journal of Infectious Diseases* **156**, 243–244.

Misra, P., Pal, N.L., Guru, P.Y., Katiyar, J.C. and Tandon, J.S. (1991). Antimalarial activity of traditional plants against erythrocytic stages of *Plasmodium berghei*. *International Journal of Pharmacognosy* **1**, 19–23.

Montamat, E.E., Burgos, C., Gerez de Burgos, N.M., Rovai, L.E. and Blanco, A. (1982). Inhibitory action of gossypol on enzymes and growth of *Trypanosoma cruzi*. *Science* **218**, 288–289.

Morales-Ramirez, P., Madrigal-Bujaidar, E., Mercader-Martinez, J., Cassini, M., Gonzalez, G., Chamorro-Cevallos, G. and Salazar-Jacobo, M. (1992). Sister-chromatid exchange induction produced by ab *in vivo* and *in vitro* exposure to alpha-asarone. *Mutation Research* **279**, 269–273.

Morelli, I., Bonari, E., Pagni, A.M., Tomei, P.E. and Menichini, F. (1983). *Selected Medicinal Plants*. Rome: FAO.

Moretti, C., Deharo, E., Sauvain, M., Jardel, C., Timon David, P. and Gasquet, M. (1994). Antimalarial activity of cedronin. *Journal of Ethnopharmacology* **43**, 57–61.

Morvan, A., Bachere, E., DaSilva, P.P., Pimenta, P. and Mialhe, E. (1994). *In vitro* activity of the antimicrobial peptide magainin 1 against *Bonamia ostraea* the intrahaemocytic parasite of the oyster *Ostreae edulis*. *Molecular Marine Biology and Biotechnology* **3**, 327–333.

Navarrete, A. and Hong, E. (1996). Anthelmintic properties of alpha-sanshool from *Zanthoxylum liebmannianum*. *Planta Medica* **62**, 250–251.

Nguyen, N.L., Moulia-Pelat, J.P. and Cartel, J.L. (1996). Control of bancroftian filariasis in an endemic area of Polynesia by ivermectin 400 micrograms/kg. *Transactions of the Royal Society of Tropical Medicine and Hygiene* **90**, 689–691.

Nkunya, M.H.H., Weenen, H., Bray, D.H., Mgani, Q.A. and Mwasumbi, L.B. (1991). Antimalarial activity of Tanzanian plants and their active constituents: the genus *Uvaria*. *Planta Medica* **57**, 341–346.

Noble, R.L. (1990). The discovery of the vinca alkaloids – chemotherapeutic agents against cancer. *Biochemistry and Cell Biology* **68**, 1344–1351.

Nok, A.J., Williams, S. and Onyenekwe, P.C. (1996). *Allium sativum* induced death of African trypanosomes. *Parasitology Research* **82**, 634–637.

Noster, S. and Kraus, L.J. (1990). *In vitro* antimalarial activity of *Coutarea latifolia* and *Exostema caribaeum* extracts on *Plasmodium falciparum*. *Planta Medica* **56**, 63–65.

Nyazema, N.Z., Ndamba, J., Anderson, C., Makaza, N. and Kaondera, K.C. (1994). The doctrine of signatures or similitudes: a comparison of the efficacy of praziquantel and traditional herbal remedies used for treatment of urinary schistosomiasis in Zimbabwe. *International Journal of Pharmacognosy* **32**, 142–148.

Ohigashi, H., Huffman, M.A., Izutsu, D., Koshimizu, K., Kawanaka, M., Sugiyama, H., Kirby, G.C., Warhurst, D.C., Allen, D., Wright, C.W., Phillipson, J.D., Timon-David, P., Delmas, F., Elias, R. and Balansard, G. (1994). Toward the chemical ecology of medicinal plant use in chimpanzees: the case of *Vernonia amygdalina*, a plant used by wild chimpanzees possibly for parasite-related diseases. *Journal of Chemical Ecology* **20**, 541–553.

Oliver-Bever, B.E.P. (1986). Anti-infective activity of higher plants. In *Medicinal Plants in Tropical West Africa* (B.E.P. Oliver-Bever, ed.), pp. 123–190. Cambridge: Cambridge University Press.

Omulokoli, E., Khan, B. and Chhabra, S.C. (1997). Antiplasmodial activity of four Kenyan medicinal plants. *Journal of Ethnopharmacology* **56**, 133–137.

Onabanjo, A.O., Agbaje, E.O. and Odusote, O.O. (1993). Effect of aqueous extracts of Cymbopogon citrates in malaria. *Journal of Protozoology Research* **3**, 40–45.

O'Neill, M.J. (1986). Phytoalexins: antiparasitics of higher plants. *Parasitology Today* **2**, 358–359.

O'Neill, M.J., Bray, D., Boardman. P., Phillipson, J.D. and Warhurst, W.D. (1985). Plants as sources of antimalarial drugs. Part I. *In vitro* test method for the evaluation of crude extracts from plants. *Planta Medica* **61**, 394–398.

O'Neill, M.J., Bray, D., Boardman. P., Phillipson, J.D., Warhurst, W.D., Peters, W. and Suffness, M. (1986). Plants as sources of antimalarial drugs: *in vitro* antimalarial activity of some quassinoids. *Antimicrobial Agents and Chemotherapy* **30**, 101–104.

Onuaguluchi, G. (1964). Anti-ascaris activity of certain extracts from the bark of *Polyadoa umbellata* (Dalziel) (Erin-Yoruba). *West African Medical Journal* **13**, 162–165.

Ou-Yang, K.E., Krug, E.C., Marr, J.J. and Berens, R.L. (1990). Inhibition of growth of *Toxoplasma gondii* by qinghaosu and derivatives. *Antimalarial Agents and Chemotherapy* **34**, 1961–1965.

Partridge, S.J., Russel, P.F., Kirby, G.C., Bray, D.H., Warhurst, D.C., Phillipson, J.D., O'Neill, M.J. and Schiff, P.L. (1988). *In vitro* antiplasmodial activity of *Triclisia patens* and some of its constituent alkaloids. *Journal of Pharmacy and Pharmacology* **40**, 53.

Parveen, N., Singhal, K.C., Khan, N.U., Parveen, N. and Raychaudhuri, S.P. (1992). Screening of some plant extracts for their potential antifilarial activity using *Setaria cervi* as test organism. *Recent Advances in Medicinal, Aromatic and Spice Crops* **2**, 505–510.

Parveen, N., Singhal, K.C. and Khan, N.U. (1989a). Screening of some plant extracts for their potential antifilarial activity using *Setaria cervi* as test organism. *International Conference on Recent Advances in Medicinal Aromatic and Spice Crops.* New Delhi, India, 28–31 January.

Parveen, N., Singhal, K.C., Khan, N.U. and Singhal, P. (1989b). Potential antifilarial activity of *Streblus asper* against *Setaria cervi* (Nematoda: Filaroidea). *Indian Journal of Pharmacology* **21**, 16–21.

Pavanand, K., Yongvanitchit, K., Webster, H.K., Dechatiwongse, T., Nutakul, W., Jewvachdamrongkul, Y. and Bansiddhi, J. (1988). *In vitro* antimalarial activity of a Thai medicinal plant *Picrasma javanica* l. *Phytotherapy Research* **2**, 33–36.

Pavanand, K., Webster, H.K. and Yongvanitchit, K. (1989a). Antimalarial activity of *Tiliacora triandra* diels against *Plasmodium falciparum in vitro. Phytotherapy Research* **3**, 215–217.

Pavanand, K., Webster, H.K., Yongvanitchit, K., Kun-anake, A., Dechatiwongse, T., Nutakul, W. and Bansiddhi, J. (1989b). Shizonticidal activity of *Celastrus peniculatus* Wild. against *Plasmodium falciparum in vitro. Phytotherapy Research* **3**, 136–139.

Perrett, S. and Whitfield, P.J. (1995a). Aqueous degradation of isoflavonoids in an extract of *Milletia thonningii* (Leguminosae), which is larvicidal towards schistosomes. *Phytotherapy Research* **9**, 401–404.

Perrett, S. and Whitfield, P.J. (1995b). Atanine (3-dimethyl allyl-4-methoxy-2-quinolone), an alkaloid with anthelmintic activity from the Chinese medical plant *Euvodia rutaecarpa. Planta Medica* **61**, 276–278.

Perrett, S. and Whitfield, P.J. (1995c). Anthelmintic and pesticidal activity of *Acorus gramineus* (Araceae) is associated with phenyl propanoid asarones. *Phytotherapy Research* **9**, 405–409.

Phillipson, J.D. (1994). Natural products as drugs. *Transactions of the Royal Society of Tropical Medicine and Hygiene* **88**(S1), 17–19.

Phillipson, J.D. and O'Neill, M.J. (1986). Novel antimalarial drugs from plants? *Parasitology Today* **2**, 355–358.

Phillipson, J.D. and O'Neill, M. (1987) Antimalarial and amoebicidal natural products. In *Biologically Active Natural Products* (K. Hostettman and P.S. Lea, eds), Oxford: Clarendon Press, 49–64.

Phillipson, J.D. and Wright, C.W. (1991). Medicinal plants in tropical medicine 1. Medicinal plants against protozoal diseases. *Transactions of the Royal Society of Tropical Medicine and Hygiene* **85**, 18–21.

Phillipson, J.D., Wright, C.W., Kirby, G.C. and Warhurst, D.C. (1995). Phytochemistry of some plants used in traditional medicine for the treatment of protozoal diseases. In *Phytochemistry of Plants used in Traditional Medicine* (K. Hostettman, A. Marston, M. Maillard and M. Hamburger, eds), Oxford University Press.

Pohowalla, J.N. and Singh, S.D. (1959). Worm infestations in infants and children of preschool age in Indore. *Indian Journal of Pediatrics* **26**, 459–466.

Ponasik, J.A., Strickland, C., Faerman C., Savvides, S., Karplus, P.A. and Ganem, B. (1995). Kukoamine A and other hydrophobic acylpolyamines: potent and selective inhibitors of *Crithidia fasciculate* trypanothione reductase. *Biochemical Journal* **311**, 371–375.

Prance, G.T. (2000). Ethnobotany and the future of conservation. *Biologist* **42**, 65–68.

Presber, W., Hegenscheid, B., Hernandez-Alvarez, H., Herrmann, D. and Brendel, C. (1992). Inhibition of the growth of *Plasmodium falciparum* and *Plasmodium berghei in vitro* by an extract of *Cochlospermum angolense* (Welw). *Acta Tropica* **50**, 331–338.

Puri, A., Saxena, R.P., Sumati, Guru, P.Y., Kulshreshtha D.K., Saxena, K.C. and Dhawan, B.N. (1992). Immunostimulant activity of picroliv, the iridoid glycoside fraction of *Picrorhiza kurroa*, and its protective action against *Leishmania donovani* infection in hamsters. *Planta Medica* **58**, 528–532.

Qinghaosu Antimalarial Coordinating Group. (1979). Antimalarial studies on qinghaosu. *Chinese Medical Journal* **92**, 811–816.

Queener, S.F., Fujioka, H., Nishiyama, Y., Furukawa, H., Bartlett, M.S. and Smith, J.W. (1991). *In vitro* activities of acridone alkaloids against *Pneumocystis carinii*. *Antimicrobial Agents and Chemotherapy* **35**, 377–379.

Rahman, N.N.N.A., Furuta, T., Kojima, S., Takane, K. and Mohd, M.A. (1999). Antimalarial activity of extracts of Malaysian medicinal plants. *Journal of Ethnopharmacology* **64**, 249–254.

Raj, K.R. (1974). Screening of some indigenous plants for anthelmintic action against human *Ascaris lumbricoides*. *Indian Journal of Physiology and Pharmacology* **18**, 129–131.

Raj, K.R. (1975). Screening of indigenous plants for anthelmintic action against human *Ascaris lumbricoides*. Part II. *Indian Journal of Physiology and Pharmacology* **19**, 47–49.

Raj, K.R. and Kurup, P.A. (1968). Anthelmintic activity, toxicity and other pharmacological properties of palasonin, the active principle of *Butea frondosa* seeds and its piperazine salt. *Indian Journal of Medical Research* **56**, 1818–1825.

Ratsimamanga-Urverg, S., Rasoanaivo, P., Rakoto-Ratsimamanga, A., LeBras, J., Ramiliarisoa, O., Savel, J. and Coulaud, J.P. (1991). Antimalarial activity and cytotoxicity of *Evodia fatraina* stem bark extracts. *Journal of Ethnopharmacology* **33**, 231–236.

Ratsimamanga-Urverg, S., Rasoanaivo, P., Millijaona, R., Rakotoarimanga, J., Rafatro, H., Rabijaona, B. and Rakoto-Ratsimamanga, A. (1994). *In vitro* antimalarial activity, chloroquine potentiating effect and cytotoxicity of alkaloids of *Hernandia voyronii* Jum. (Hernandiaceae). *Phytotherapy Research* **8**, 18–21.

Rich, J.R., Keen, N.T. and Thomason, I.J. (1977). Association of coumestans with the hypersensitivity of Lima bean roots to *Pratylenchus scribneri*. *Physiological Plant Pathology* **10**, 105–116.

Richard-Lenoble, D., Kombila, M., Rupp, E.A., Pappayliou, E.S., Gaxotte, P., Nguiri, C., Aziz, M.A. and Pappayliou, E.S. (1988). Ivermectin in loiasis and concomitant *O. volvulus* and *M. perstans* infections. *American Journal of Tropical Medicine and Hygiene* **39**, 480–483.

Richomme, P., Godet, M., Foussard, F., Toupet, L., Sevenet, T. and Bruneton, J. (1991). A novel leishmanicidal labdane from *Polyalthia macropoda*. *Planta Medica* **57**, 552–554.

Rivas-Alcala, R., Mackenzie, C.D., Gomez-Rojo, E., Green, B.M. and Taylor, H.R. (1984). The effects of diethylcarbamazine, mebendazole and levamisole on *Onchocerca volvulus in vivo* and *in vitro*. *Tropenmedizin und Parasitologie* **35**, 71–77.

Robinson, R.D., Williams, L.A.D., Lindo, J.F., Terry, S.I. and Mansingh, A. (1990). Inactivation of *Strongyloides stercoralis* filariform larvae *in vitro* by six Jamaican plant extracts and three commercial anthelmintics. *West Indian Medical Journal* **39**, 213–217.

Ross, S.A., Megalla, S.E., Bishay, D.W. and Awad, A.H. (1980). Studies for determining antibiotic substances in some Egyptian plants. Part II antimicrobial alkaloids from the seeds of *Perganum harmala* L. *Fitoterapia* **51**, 309–312.

Roy, B. and Tandon, V. (1996). Effect of root-tuber extract of *Flemingia vestita*, leguminous plant, on *Artyfechinostomum sufrartyfex* and *Fasciolopis buskii*. A scanning electron microscopy study. *Parasitology Research* **82**, 248–252.

Royer, R.E., Deck, L.M., Campos, N.M., Hunsaker, L.A. and Vander-Jagt, D.L. (1986). Biologically active derivatives of gossypol: synthesis and antimalarial activities of periacylated gossylic nitriles. *Journal of Medicinal Chemistry* **29**, 1799–1801.

Rucker, G., Walter, R.D., Manns, D. and Mayer, R. (1991). Antimalarial activity of some natural peroxides. *Planta Medica* **57**, 295–296.

Rucker, G., Manns, D. and Wilbert, S. (1992). Homoditerpene peroxides from *Artemisia absinthium*. *Phytochemistry* **31**, 340–342.

Rucker, G., Schenkel, E.P., Manns, D., Mayer, R., Heiden, K. and Heinzmann, B.M. (1996). Sesquiterpene peroxides from *Senecio selloi* and *Eupatorium rutescens*. *Planta Medica* **62**, 565–566.

Salako, L.A., Guiguemde, R., Mittelholzer, M.L., Haller, L., Sorensen, F. and Sturchler, D. (1994). Ro 42-1611 in the treatment of patients with mild malaria: a clinical trial in Nigeria and Bourkina Faso, *Tropical Medicine and Parasitology* **45**, 284–287.

Sanghui, P.K. (1989). Epidemiological studies on guinea worm in some newly discovered villages of Jhabua district (M.P.) and test of *Carica papaya* leaves on guinea worm infection. *Indian Journal of Medical Sciences* **43**, 123–124.

Sarciron, M.E., Saccharin, C., Petavy, A.F. and Peyron, F. (2000). Effects of artesunate, dihydroartemisinin and artesunate-dihydroartemisinin combination against *Toxoplasma gondii*. *American Journal of Tropical Medicine and Hygiene* **62**, 73–76.

Sauvain, M., Dedet, J., Kunesch, N., Poisson, J., Gantier, J., Gayral, P. and Kunesch, G. (1993). *In vitro* and *in vivo* leishmanicidal activities of natural and synthetic quinoids. *Phytotherapy Research* **7**, 167–171.

Sauvain, M., Moretti, C., Bravo, J., Callapa, J., Munoz, V., Ruiz, E., Richard, B. and Le Men-Oliver, L. (1996). Antimalarial activity of alkaloids from *Pogonopus tubulosus*. *Phytotherapy Research* **10**, 198–201.

Schares, G., Hofmann, B. and Zahner, H. (1994). Antifilarial activity of macrocyclic lactones: comparative studies with ivermectin, doramectin, Milbemycin A4 oxime, and moxidectin in *Litomosoides carinii, Acanthocheilonema viteae, Brugia malayi* and *Brugia pahangi* infections of *Mastomys coucha*. *Tropical Medicine and Parasitology* **45**, 97–106.

Schuster, F.L. and Jacobs, J.L. (1992). Effects of magainins on amoeba and cyst stages of *Acanthamoeba polyphaga*. *Antimicrobial Agents and Chemotherapy* **36**, 1263–1271.

Sen, H.G., Joshi, B.S., Parthasarathy, P.C. and Kamat, U.N. (1974). Anthelmintic efficacy of diospyrol and its derivatives. *Arzneimittel Forschung* **24**, 2000–2003.

Shabana, M.M., Aboutable, E.A., Mirhom, Y.W., Genenah, A.A. and Yousif, F. (1988). Study of wild Egyptian plants of potential medicinal activity. IV. Molluscicidal and cercaricidal activities of some selected plants. *Egyptian Journal of Bilharziasis* **10**, 11–20.

Sharma, G.L. and Bhutani, K.K. (1987). Plant based antiamoebic drugs: Part II. Amoebicidal activity of parthenin isolated from *Parthenium hysterophorus*. *Planta Medica* **54**, 120–122.

Sharma, S.K., Satyanarayana, S., Yadav, R.N.S. and Dutta, L.P. (1993). Screening of *Coptis teeta* Wall. for antimalarial effect: a preliminary report. *Indian Journal of Malariology* **30**, 179–181.

Sharp, D. (1996). Malaria range set to spread in a warmer world. *The Lancet* **347**, 1612.

Singh, S., Srivastata, M.C. and Tewari, J.P. (1982). Anthelmintic activity of *Zanthoxylum alatum*. *Indian Drugs* **19**, 348–351.

Soffar, S.A. and Mokhtar, G.M. (1991). Evaluation of the antiparasitic effects of aqueous garlic (*Allium sativum*) extract in *Hymenolepis nana* and giardiasis. *Journal of the Egyptian Society of Parasitology* **21**, 497–502.

Soh, C., Oh, H. and Kim, N. (1980). Effect of *Lysimachia clethroides in vitro* on several trematodes and nematodes. *Yonsei Reports on Tropical Medicine* **11**, 58–64.

Sowunmi, A., Salako, L.A., Laoye, O.J. and Aderounmu, A.F. (1990). Combination of quinine, quinidine and cinchonine for the treatment of acute falciparum malaria: correlation with susceptibility of *Plasmodium falciparum* to the cinchona alkaloids *in vitro*. *Transactions of the Royal Society for Tropical Medicine and Hygiene* **84**, 626–629.

Spencer, C.F., Koniuszy, F.R., Rogers, E.F., Shavel, J., jr, Easton, N.R., Kaczka, E.A., Kuehl, F.A., jr, Phillips, R.F., Walti, A. and Folkers, K. (1947). Survey of plants for antimalarial activity. *Lloydia* **10**, 145–174.

Subbaiah, T.V. and Amin, A.H. (1967). Effect of berberine sulphate on *Entamoeba histolytica*. *Nature* **215**, 527–528.

Suhruda, J., Satyanarancharyulu, N., Rao, B.V., Choudhuri, P.C. and Rajaiah, M. (1991). Studies on the efficacy of baberang (*Embelia ribes*) and kurchi (*Holarrhena antidysenterica*) in experimental balantidosis in calves. *Indian Journal of Veterinary Medicine* **11**, 1–3.

Swerdlow, J.L. (2000). Medicines in nature. *National Geographic* **4**, 98–117.

Tackie, A.N., Boye, G.L., Sharaf, M.H.M., Schiff, P.L., Crouch, R.C., Spitzer, D.T., Johnson, R.L., Dunn, J., Minick, D. and Martin, G.E. (1993). Cryptospirolepine a unique spiro-non acyclic alkaloid isolated from *Cryptolepis sanguinolenta*. *Journal of Natural Products* **56**, 653–670.

Tagboto, S.K. and Townson, S. (1996) *Onchocerca volvulus* and *O. lienalis*: the microfilaricidal activity of moxidectin compared with that of ivermectin *in vitro* and *in vivo*. *Annals of Tropical Medicine and Parasitology* **90**, 479–505.

Tandon, J.S., Srivastava, V. and Guru. P.Y. (1991). Iridoids: a new class of leishmanicidal agents from *Nyctanthes arbortristis*. *Journal of Natural Products* **54**, 1102–1104.

Tandon, V., Pal, P., Roy, B., Rao, H.P.S. and Reddy, K.S. (1997). *In vitro* anthelmintic activity of root-tuber extract of *Fleminga vestita*, an indigenous plant in Shillong, India. *Parasitology Research* **83**, 492–498.

Taylor, M.J. and Hoerauf, A. (1999). *Wolbachia* bacteria of filarial nematodes. *Parasitology Today* **15**, 437–442.

Taylor, J.M., Jones, W.I., Hogan, E.C., Gross, M.A., David, D.A. and Cook, E.L. (1967). Toxicity of oil of calamus (Jammu variety). *Toxicology and Applied Pharmacology* **10**, 405.

ThebtarAnonth, C., ThebtarAnonth, Y., Wanauppathamkul, S. and Yuthavong, Y. (1995). Antimalarial sesquiterpenes from tubers of *Cyperus rotundus*: structure of 10, 12-peroxycalamene, a sesquiterpene endoperoxide. *Phytochemistry* **40**, 125–128.

Titanji, V.P.K., Ayafor, J.F., Mulufi, J.P. and Mbacham, W.F. (1987). *In vitro* killing of *Onchocerca volvulus* (Filaroidea) adults and microfilariae by selected Cameroonian medicinal plant extracts. *Fitoterpia* **58**, 338–339.

Titanji. V.P.K., Evehe, M.S., Ayafor, J.F. and Kimbu, S.F. (1989) Novel *Onchocerca volvulus* filaricides from *Carapa procera*. *Polyalthia suavenolens* and *Pachypodanthium staudii*. *O-NOW! Symposium on onchocerciasis*. September 20–22, Leiden, The Netherlands.

Townson, S. (1988). The development of a laboratory model for onchocerciasis using *Onchocerca gutturosa*: *in vitro* culture, collagenase effects, drug studies and cryopreservation. *Tropical Medicine and Parasitology* **39**, 475–479.

Townson, S. (2000). Drug discovery for human onchocerciasis: what strategy for the evaluation of natural products? In: *Traditional Medicine and Pharmaceutical Medicine Perspectives on Natural Products for the Treatment of Tropical Diseases*. Geneva: WHO/TDR Scientific Working Group. Abstract.

Townson, S., Connelly, C., Dobinson, A. and Muller, R. (1987). Drug activity against *Onchocerca gutturosa* males *in vitro*: a model for chemotherapeutic research on onchocerciasis. *Journal of Helminthology* **61**, 271–281.

Townson, S., Hutton, D., Siemienska, J., Hollick, L., Scanlon, T., Tagboto, S.K. and Taylor, M.J. (2000). Antibiotics and *Wolbachia* in filarial nematodes: antifilarial activity of rifampicin, oxytetracycline and chloramphenicol against *Onchocerca gutturosa, Onchocerca lienalis* and *Brugia Pahangi*. *Annals of Tropical Medicine and Parasitology* **94**, 801–806.

Townson, S., Siemienska, J., Hollick, L. and Hutton, D. (1999). The activity of rifampicin, oxytetracycline and chloramphenicol against *Onchocerca lienalis* and *O. gutturosa*. *Transactions of the Royal Society of Tropical Medicine and Hygiene* **93**, 123–124.

Trager, W. and Polonsky, J. (1981). Antimalarial activity of quassinoids against chloroquine-resistant *Plasmodium falciparum in vitro. American Journal of Tropical Medicine and Hygiene* **30**, 531–537.

Trigg, P.I. and Wernsdorfer, W.H. (1999). Malaria control priorities and constraints. *Parasitologia* **41**, 329–332.

Turrens, J.F. (1986). The potential of antispermatogenic drugs against trypanosomatids. *Parasitology Today* **2**, 351–352.

Usanga, E.A., O'Brien, E. and Luzzato, L. (1986). Mitotic inhibitors arrest the growth of *Plasmodium falciparum. FEBS Letters* **209**, 23–27.

Valecha, N., Biswas, S., Badoni, V., Bhandari, K.S. and Sati, O.P. (1994). Antimalarial activity of *Artemisia japonica, Artemisia maritima* and *Artemisia nilegarica. Indian Journal of Pharmacology* **26**, 144–146.

Valsaraj, R., Pushpagandan, P., Nyaman, U., Smitt, U.V., Adsersen, A. and Gudisken, L. (1995). New antimalarial drugs from Indian medicinal plants. *International Seminar on Recent Trends in Pharmaceutical Sciences*, Ootacamund, 18–20 February.

Van Assendelft, F., Miller, J.W., Mintz, D.T., Schack, J.A., Ottolenghi, P. and Most, H. (1956). The use of glaucarubicin (a crystalline glycoside isolated from *Simarouba glauca*) in the treatment of human colonic amoebiasis. *American Journal of Tropical Medicine and Hygiene* **5**, 501–503.

Veech, J.A. (1982). Phytoalexins and their role in the resistance of plants to nematodes. *Journal of Nematology* **14**, 2–9.

Vennerstrom, J.L. and Klayman, D.L. (1988). Protoberberine alkaloids as antimalarials. *Journal of Medicinal Chemistry* **31**, 1084–1087.

Vennerstrom, J.L., Lovelace, J.K., Waits, V.B., Hanson, W.L. and Klayman, D.L. (1990). Berberine derivatives as antileishmanial drugs. *Antimicrobial Agents and Chemotherapy* **34**, 918–921.

Vincent, A.L., Portaro, J.K. and Ash, L.R. (1975). A comparison of the body wall ultrastructure of *Brugia pahangi* with that of *Brugia malayi. Journal of Parasitology* **63**, 567–570.

Vohora, S.B., Shaukat, A., Shah, S.A. and Dandiya, P.C. (1990). Central nervous system studies on an ethanol extract of *Acorus calamus* rhizomes. *Journal of Ethnopharmacology* **28**, 52–62.

Waller, P.J. and Faedo, M. (1996). The prospects for the biological control of nematode parasites of livestock. *International Journal for Parasitology* **26**, 915–925.

Waller, P.J. and Larsen, M. (1993). The role of nematophagous fungi in the biological control of nematode parasites of livestock. *International Journal for Parasitology* **23**, 539–546.

Wang, P.V., Chen, J.T., Liu, L.H., Zhen, T.M., Lu, G.Y., Zhao, X.L., Chen, C., Tang, X.Y., Fu, G.C., Sun, X.C., Xu, Z.J., Wu, X.Q. and Yang, F.J. (1989). Treatment of filarial elephantiasis by the injection of 25% extracts from mulberry leaves. *Chinese Journal of Parasitic Diseases Contro*l **2**, 264–267.

Watt, J.M. and Breyer-Brandwijk, M.C. (1962). *The Medicinal and Poisonous Plants of Southern and Eastern Africa*, 2nd edn. London: E. & S. Livingstone.

Weenen, H., Nkunya, M.H.H., Bray, D.H., Mwasumbi, L.B., Kinabo, L.S. and Kilimali, V.A.E.B. (1990). Antimalarial activity of Tanzanian medicinal plants. *Planta Medica* **56**, 368–370.

Whitfield, P.J. (1996). Medicinal plants and the control of parasites. *Transactions of the Royal Society of Tropical Medicine and Hygiene* **90**, 596–600.

WHO (1990). *WHO Model Prescribing Information*. Drugs used in parasitic diseases. Geneva: World Health Organization.

WHO (1993). Public health impact of schistosomiasis: disease and mortality. WHO Expert Committee on the Control of Schistosomiasis. *Bulletin of the World Health Organization* **71**, 657–662.
WHO (1995). Onchocerciasis and its control. Report of a WHO Expert Committee on onchocerciasis control. *World Health Organization Technical Report Series* 852. Geneva: World Health Organization.
WHO (1998). Control and surveillance of African trypanosomiasis. Report of a WHO Committee. *World Health Organization Technical Report Series* 881, I–VI, 1–114. Geneva: World Health Organization.
WHO (2000). *Traditional Medicine and Pharmaceutical Medicine Perspectives on Natural Products for the Treatment of Tropical Diseases*. WHO/TDR Scientific Working Group, Geneva: World Health Organization. Abstract.
Willcox, M.L. and Bodeker, G. (2000). Plant-based malaria control: research initiative on traditional antimalarial methods. *Parasitology Today* **16**, 220–221.
Wosu, L.O. and Ibe, C.C.(1989). Use of extracts of *Picralima nitida* bark in the treatment of experimental trypanosomiasis: a preliminary study. *Journal of Ethnopharmacology* **25**, 263–268.
Wright, C.W., O'Neill, M.J., Phillipson, J.D. and Warhurst, D.C. (1988) Use of microdilution to assess *in vitro* antiamoebic activities of *Brucea javanica* fruits, *Simarouba amara* stem, and a number of quassinoids. *Antimicrobial Agents and Chemotherapy* **32**, 1725–1729.
Wright, C.W., Bray, D.H., O'Neill, M.J., Warhurst, D.C., Phillipson, J.D., Quentin-Lecrecq, J. and Angenot, L. (1991). Antiamoebic and antiplasmodial activities of alkaloids isolated from *Strychnos usambarensis. Planta Medica* **57**, 337–340.
Wright, C.W., Anderson, M.M., Allen, D., Phillipson, J.D., Kirby, G.C., Warhurst, D.C. and Chang, H.R. (1993a). Quassinoids exhibit greater selectivity against *Plasmodium falciparum* than against *Entamoeba histolytica, Giardia intestinalis* or *Toxoplasma gondii in vitro. Journal of Eukaryotic Microbiology* **40**, 244–246.
Wright, C.W., Allen, D., Phillipson, J.D., Kirby, G.C., Warhurst, D.C., Massiot, G. and Men-Oliver, L. (1993b). *Alstonia* species: are they effective in malaria treatment? *Journal of Ethnopharmacology* **40**, 41–45.
Xiao, P. and Fu, S. (1986). Traditional antiparasitic drugs in China. *Parasitology Today* **2**, 353–358.
Xiao, S.H., You, J.O., Yang, Y.Q. and Wang, C.Z. (1995). Experimental studies on early treatment of schistosomal infections with artemether. *Southeast Asian Journal of Tropical Medicine and Public Health* **26**, 306–318.
Xu, L.Q., Yu, S.H., Jiang, Z.X., Yang, J.L., Lai, C.Q., Zhang, X.J. and Zheng, C.Q. (1995). Soil-transmitted helminthsiases: nationwide survey in China. *Bulletin of the World Health Organization* **73**, 507–513.
Yadav, A.K., Tandon, V. and Rao, H.S.P. (1992). *In vitro* anthelmintic activity of fresh tuber extract of *Fleminga vestita* against *Ascaris suum. Fitoterpia* **63**, 395–398.
You, J.O., Mei, J.Y. and Xiao, S.H. (1992). Effect of artemether against *Schistosoma japonicum. Acta Pharmacologica Sinica* **13**, 280–284.
Yu, H.W., Wright, C.W., Cai, Y., Yang, S.L., Phillipson, J.D., Kirby, G.C. and Warhurst, D.C. (1994). Antiprotozoal activities of *Centipeda minima. Phytotherapy Research* **8**, 436–438.
Zafar, M.M., Hamdard, M.E. and Hameed, A. (1990). Screening of *Artemisia absinthium* for antimalarial effects on *Plasmodium berghei* in mice: a preliminary report. *Journal of Ethnopharmacology* **4**, 223–226.

Index

Page entries in *italic* refer to tables and figures.

Contents of Volumes in This Series

Volume 40

Part 1 *Cryptosporidium parvum* and related genera

Part 2 *Enterocytozoon bieneusi* and Other Microsporidia

Part 3 *Cyclospora cayetanensis* and related species

Volume 41

Volume 42

Volume 43

Volume 44

Volume 45

Volume 46

Volume 47

Volume 48

Volume 49

Volume 50